D0522042

CT ANGIOGRAPHY
OF THE CHEST

CT ANGIOGRAPHY OF THE CHEST

MARTINE REMY-JARDIN, MD, PHD

JACQUES REMY, MD

JOHN R. MAYO, MD

NESTOR L. MÜLLER, MD, PHD

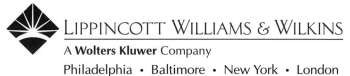

LIPPINCOTT WILLIAMS & WILKINS
A **Wolters Kluwer** Company
Philadelphia · Baltimore · New York · London
Buenos Aires · Hong Kong · Sydney · Tokyo

Acquisitions Editor: Joyce Rachel-John
Developmental Editor: Murray E. Hill
Production Editor: Rakesh Rampertab
Manufacturing Manager: Tim Reynolds
Cover Designer: Mark Lerner
Compositor: Lippincott Williams & Wilkins Desktop Division
Printer: Maple Press

© 2001 by LIPPINCOTT WILLIAMS & WILKINS
530 Walnut Street
Philadelphia, PA 19106 USA
LWW.com

Printed in the USA

Library of Congress Cataloging-in-Publication Data

CT angiography of the chest / Martine Rémy-Jardin ... [et al.].
    p. ; cm.
  Includes bibliographical references and index.
  ISBN 0-7817-2731-6
  1. Chest—Blood-vessels—Tomography. 2. Lungs—Blood-vessels—Diseases—Diagnosis.
I. Rémy-Jardin, Martine.
  [DNLM: 1. Angiography—methods. 2. Radiography, Thoracic—methods. 3
Tomography, X-Ray Computed—methods. WF 975 C9594 2001]
RC941 .C87 2001
617.5'407572—dc21   2001038342

10 9 8 7 6 5 4 3 2 1

To our children

Maxime Remy, Darrell and Danielle Mayo, and
Alison and Philip Müller

CONTENTS

CONTRIBUTING AUTHORS

John R. Mayo, MD   Associate Professor, Department of Radiology, University of British Columbia; and Head, General Radiology, Department of Radiology, Vancouver General Hospital, Vancouver, British Columbia, Canada

Nestor L. Müller, MD, PhD   Professor and Chairman, Department of Radiology, University of British Columbia; and Head, Department of Radiology, Vancouver General Hospital, Vancouver, British Columbia, Canada

Jacques Remy, MD   Professor of Radiology, Department of Radiology, University of Lille; and Co-Director, Imaging Research Laboratory, Department of Radiology, Hospital Calmette, 59037 Lille Cedex, France

Martine Remy-Jardin, MD, PhD   Professor of Radiology, Department of Radiology, University of Lille, 59037 Lille Cedex; and Head, Department of Radiology, Hospital Calmette, 59037 Lille, France

PREFACE

The advent of spiral CT scanners in the late 1980s and multislice scanners in the late 1990s has allowed depiction of pulmonary and systemic vessels during the bolus phase of contrast enhancement. This has resulted in a new application for cross-sectional imaging, CT angiography. Because of its non-invasive nature, its ease of performance and interpretation, CT angiography is rapidly replacing conventional diagnostic angiography in an increasing number of clinical settings.

This book, written by chest radiologists from Europe and North America, provides a practical overview of the state-of-the-art of CT angiography in the chest. Written for the general radiologist, pulmonologist, and residents in both specialties, this book provides a foundation for acquiring and interpreting chest CT angiograms. The first two chapters concisely summarize the basics, outlining the technical aspects of CT angiography and describing normal and variant thoracic vascular anatomy. Eight chapters describe the current clinical utility of CT angiography for acute and chronic pulmonary embolism, pulmonary hypertension, thoracic aortic disease, acquired pulmonary vascular abnormalities, congenital vascular anomalies, hemoptysis, thoracic outlet disorders, and SVC syndromes. Current recommended scanning protocols for single and multislice spiral CT scanners are conveniently summarized in an appendix. Although the book is written to provide an overview of chest CT angiography, it is augmented with an extensive review of the literature for interested readers.

The authors hope that this book will encourage the clinical use of chest CT angiography and stimulate further research.

ACKNOWLEDGMENT

We acknowledge the support and guidance provided by our editor at Lippincott Williams & Wilkins, Ms. Joyce-Rachel John. We also wish to thank Nathalie Velluet, Nelly Coquel, and Jenny Silver for their secretarial assistance.

We are grateful to our colleagues and spouses for their patience and encouragement and to our friends who contributed illustrations.

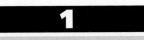

ACQUISITION, INJECTION, AND RECONSTRUCTION TECHNIQUES

INTRODUCTION

The introduction of computed tomography (CT) in the early 1970s represented a major advance for diagnostic imaging of the chest. The improved contrast sensitivity and cross-sectional perspective of CT greatly improved the detection and characterization of thoracic abnormalities. However, conventional stop-and-shoot scanners were slow, acquiring raw scan data during a 2-second x-ray tube rotation and requiring up to 4 seconds of interscan delay to move the table to the next scan location. The slow rate of scanning limited the volume within the patient that could be scanned during a single breath-hold or the bolus phase of vascular contrast enhancement. Additionally, although spatial resolution was submillimeter within the transverse plane (x-axis, y-axis), along the longitudinal plane (z-axis) it was much lower. For these reasons, CT angiography (CTA) performed on these scanners only provided adequate visual-ization of relatively large vessels oriented perpendicular to the imaging plane, such as the descending thoracic aorta. Despite these limitations, by the early 1990s it had been demonstrated that CTA was useful for the diagnosis of thoracic aortic disease because of the increased contrast resolution and the cross-sectional imaging plane (1–3). However, the general application of CTA to the thoracic vasculature was not possible with conventional CT scanners.

In the late 1980s, a new CT raw scan data acquisition technique was developed, spiral or helical CT (4). This new method of raw data acquisition used simultaneous x-ray tube rotation and table motion to obtain a continuous helical band of x-ray attenuation measurements within the patient. Slip rings delivered power to the x-ray tube and transmitted x-ray attenuation measurements from the detector array to the scanner electronics. Slip-ring gantry technology eliminated the starting and stopping motion of the x-ray tube and detector array that was required by the previous generation of stop-and-shoot scanners. This increased the rotational velocity of the gantry to one second. High-speed gantry rotation combined with continuous table motion meant that large volumes of tissue could be rapidly scanned. In the thorax, this permitted single breath-hold imaging of the entire lungs, eliminating breath-to-breath misregistration which had been a major problem with previous stop-and-shoot scanners. Studies demonstrated that spiral CT acquisition technology significantly (p less than 0.05) increased the detection of focal lung lesions such as pulmonary nodules (5,6). Rapid data acquisition allowed CTA of entire organs (e.g., pulmonary vasculature) with high-density contrast enhancement (7). Finally, as a continuous helical band of x-ray attenuation data was obtained through the scanned volume, images could be reconstructed at any location along the z-axis of the patient. In contrast to stop-and-shoot scanners, one set of spiral scan raw data could yield multiple overlapping reconstructed images without any additional radiation exposure (8,9). These overlapping reconstructions along the z-axis increased the longitudinal spatial resolution and decreased the effect of volume averaging. The combination of rapid breath-hold scanning of the thorax during the bolus phase of vascular contrast enhancement and the improved z-axis spatial resolution provided improved visualization of all noncardiac thoracic vascular structures with the first generation of single-slice spiral CT scanners. In the thorax, the most important initial vascular application of these enhanced CT imaging capabilities was the diagnosis of pulmonary embolism (7).

The initial implementation of spiral scanning used one-second x-ray tube rotation and a single row of x-ray detectors (single-slice spiral CT). The introduction of multislice spiral CT using subsecond x-ray tube rotation times, multirow detectors, higher heat capacity x-ray tubes, and more powerful computing systems has further improved spiral CTA techniques (10,11). In conjunction with cardiac gated reconstruction algorithms (12), essentially motion-free CT angiograms using isometric voxels can be obtained on current equipment. These improvements allow all thoracic cardiovascular structures to be noninvasively examined in any orientation with minimal motion artifact and isometric submillimeter spatial resolution.

In this chapter, we will describe single-slice and multislice spiral CT techniques, with special emphasis on user-programmable variables that influence the image quality of CTA. Suggested imaging protocols for a variety of clinical indications can be found in Appendix A.

SINGLE-SLICE SPIRAL CT TECHNIQUE

In conventional stop-and-shoot CT, slice collimation, reconstruction field of view, reconstruction algorithm, and x-ray tube current are the critical user-specified parameters

TABLE 1-1. USER-PROGRAMMABLE CT SCAN ACQUISITION PARAMETERS

Stop and Shoot	Spiral
▪ kVp, mA	▪ kVp, mA
▪ Scan time	▪ Scan time
▪ Field-of-view	▪ Field-of-view
▪ Reconstruction algorithm	▪ Reconstruction algorithm
▪ Slice collimation	▪ Slice collimation
▪ Table increments	▪ Pitch
	▪ Interpolation algorithm
	▪ Reconstruction interval

kVp, peak kilovoltage; mA, milliampere.

(13). Changes in these parameters affect spiral CT image quality in an identical fashion. Similarly, the trade off between image noise and patient radiation dose is the same for both conventional and spiral CT. However, spiral CT introduces new user-programmable factors of pitch, data interpolation algorithm, and reconstruction interval (Table 1-1).

In conventional stop-and-shoot CT, the collimation and table increment between slices primarily determine the longitudinal resolution. To avoid excessive radiation dose buildup, the slice collimation and the table increment are usually the same, yielding contiguous slices. In spiral CT slices, the x-ray beam collimation, interpolation algorithm, and pitch define the shape of the slice sensitivity profile (SSP), defining the potential longitudinal spatial resolution in the raw data set (14). The extent to which the available longitudinal resolution is rendered in the reconstructed images is determined by the reconstruction interval (8,9).

Collimation

Collimation in spiral CT is defined, in a similar fashion to conventional CT, as the full width of the SSP at a specified signal intensity. The rectangular shape of the SSP in stop-and-shoot CT scanners made the full width at half height a reasonable signal-intensity reference point. However, in spiral CT, the broadening of the SSP caused by convolution of the table motion on the slice profile makes the full width at half-height measurement a somewhat optimistic measure of the SSP. In response, some manufacturers have suggested using the full width at one-tenth maximum intensity to define the SSP for spiral CT (15). At this time, there is no established standard for measuring the width of the SSP.

Pitch

Pitch describes the relationship between table motion and collimation. Pitch is a unitless parameter defined as table travel per 360-degree gantry rotation divided by the collimation. For example, in a single-slice spiral scanner using a 1-second scan time, the combination of 3-mm collimation and 6-mm-per-second table feed results in a pitch of 2. Since the number of views obtained in each 360-degree x-ray tube rotation is fixed in the design of the scanner (approximately 1,000 views in most current scanners), the pitch is related to the sampling frequency along the longitudinal axis. The combination of pitch, collimation, and helical interpolation algorithm define the available longitudinal spatial resolution in a single-slice spiral CT raw scan data set. In CTA, since there is a limited time that the bolus phase of contrast enhancement is available, the combination of pitch and collimation also determines the volume that can be scanned. For example, the diagnosis of central or segmental pul-

monary embolism requires that all central, segmental, and proximal subsegmental vessels be scanned, a volume of approximately 12 cm. In practice the scan time is limited by the duration of the bolus phase of intravenous contrast (approximately 50 seconds) and the breath-hold time of the patient (approximately 25 seconds). These constraints determine the selection of collimation and pitch. Within this volume/time constraint, there are different combinations of pitch and collimation parameters that can be used. For example, in the assessment of pulmonary embolism, 5-mm collimation with a pitch 1 or 3-mm collimation with a pitch 1.7 can cover the required volume within the available time. However, the longitudinal spatial resolution is improved when the data is acquired using narrower collimation (3 mm) and increased pitch (1.7) (Figure 1-1).

The selection of narrow collimation and increased pitch has been shown to improve the detection of segmental and subsegmental vessels (16). In addition to broadening of the SSP, scans obtained at elevated pitch (e.g., 1.5 to 3.0) are also degraded by helical artifact (Figure 1-2). Helical artifact

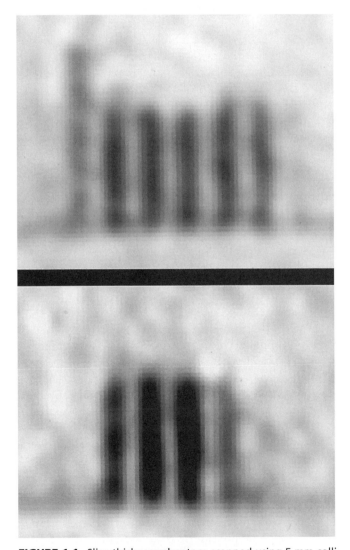

FIGURE 1-1. Slice thickness phantom scanned using 5-mm collimation pitch 1.0 (*top*) and 3-mm collimation pitch 1.7 (*bottom*). These two protocols scan the same volume of tissue in the same time. However, the larger number of vertical lines seen with 5-mm pitch 1.0 indicates that these slices are thicker than those obtained using 3-mm pitch 1.7. The narrower slice thickness using 3-mm pitch 1.7 reduces volume averaging and improves the detection of small vessels running oblique to the image plane.

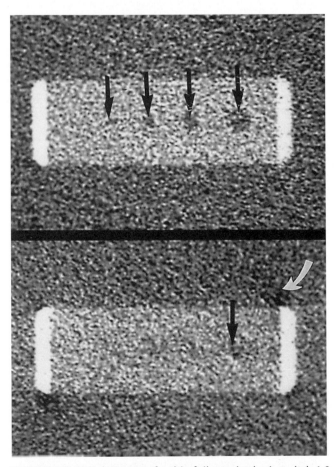

FIGURE 1-2. Spiral CT scan of a thin foil acquired using pitch 1.0 (*top*) and pitch 3.0 (*bottom*). Four holes (*arrows*) are seen using pitch 1.0 compared to one hole (*arrow*) using pitch 3.0. This illustrates the decreased contrast resolution associated with increasing pitch. There is also increased helical artifact (*curved arrow*) evident on the image acquired using pitch 3.0.

is caused by undersampling in the longitudinal plane and generates streaks and bands in the reconstructed image. This artifact will not be eliminated by increased radiation exposure. Despite the image degradation arising from helical artifact, it has been shown that the improvement in longitudinal spatial resolution associated with decreasing the collimation outweighs the effects of increasing the pitch for CTA. Therefore, most CTA studies are performed using as narrow collimation as possible and pitch values of 1.5 to 2.0.

Interpolation Algorithm

The choice of interpolation algorithm also affects single-slice spiral CTA image quality. In spiral CT the table is moving continuously while the attenuation data are acquired. Transverse slices are then created at specified locations by interpolation of the spiral data set. The relative noise and slice sensitivity profile in the reconstructed images depend on the angular interval (360 degrees or 180 degrees) of the interpolation algorithm (14). Compared to the noise in a nonspiral acquisition, there is a 17% decrease in noise with a 360-degree interpolation algorithm and a 12% increase in noise with a 180-degree interpolation algorithm. The effect on the slice sensitivity profile is opposite, with greater broadening of the slice profile with 360-degree interpolation compared with 180-degree interpolation. In single-slice spiral CTA, the dominant effect on image quality is broadening of the slice profile, which causes increased volume averaging. This can obscure obliquely oriented medium and small vessels when the 360-degree interpolation algorithm is used. Use of the 180-degree interpolation algorithm improves visualization of these segmental and subsegmental vessels. The 12% increase in image noise associated with the 180-degree interpolation algorithm can be compensated for by timing the scan acquisition to the bolus phase of intravenous contrast enhancement and, if necessary, increasing the tube current (mA). Currently, the 180-degree linear algorithm is used in most clinical scanners.

Reconstruction Parameters

The longitudinal spatial resolution of spiral CT can be improved by reconstructing the data at rotational increments of less than 360 degrees, creating images that partially overlap with each other. Calculations indicate significant improvements in longitudinal spatial resolution when up to five images are reconstructed for each tube rotation (8). The only drawback to overlapping images is the increased computer time for reconstruction and the increased number of images to review. Reconstruction times of less than one second and review of images on a Picture Archiving and Communications System (PACS) workstation minimize these problems. Therefore, most single-slice CTA studies are viewed using overlapping images.

Summary

The acquisition and reconstruction parameters used for CTA on single-slice spiral CT scanners are determined by the requirements of volume of coverage and duration of the bolus phase of intravenous contrast. In general, the volume of interest is covered during the contrast bolus using the narrowest collimation possible and a pitch of 1.5 to 2.0. The 180-degree linear interpolation algorithm is used and overlapping images are reconstructed. The resulting image set is reviewed using a workstation in paging format to facilitate the identification of small branching vessels.

MULTISLICE SPIRAL CT SCANNERS

In the early 1990s, the first multislice spiral CT scanner was developed, using two rows of detectors (ELSCINT, 1992). This scanner simply placed two single-row detectors side by side, doubling the rate of data acquisition. However, this architecture was not scalable to more than two channels of data acquisition. Multislice CT using more than two channels required the development of multidetector arrays.

The first four-channel multislice scanners were introduced in the late 1990s (11). The detector arrays on these scanners were segmented into multiple rows or arcs perpendicular to the longitudinal or z-axis. Although the detectors contained up to 32 elements in the z direction, the read-out electronics only permitted four channels of simultaneous data acquisition. Therefore, four of the central rows could be used to give maximum spatial resolution, or detector rows could be combined, decreasing spatial resolution but increasing the volume of tissue scanned per unit time. Along with improvements in the detector array, the rotational velocity of the gantry was increased from 1 second in single-slice spiral CT to 0.5 seconds in the fastest multislice spiral CT scanners. The combination of four read-out channels and twice the rotational speed increased the scanning speed by eight times over single-slice spiral CT equipment. In CTA, these improvements in data acquisition speed were used either to increase the volume of tissue scanned or to scan the same volume using thinner slices. The use of thinner slices decreased volume averaging and allowed the confident visualization of smaller vessels. It has been shown (17,18) that four-row multislice CT scanners can routinely identify subsegmental pulmonary artery segments. Faster gantry rotation time decreases the effect of cardiac motion on noncardiac gated acquisitions. Additionally, the combination of faster gantry rotation time, the simultaneous acquisition of the patient's electrocardiogram, and specialized reconstruction techniques can provide nearly motion- free images during cardiac systole or diastole (19). Cardiac gated images should allow the calculation of cardiac volumes and ejection fraction using conventional CT scanners. Cardiac gated reconstruction also improves image quality in the great vessels (20) and in structures bordering the heart, including the right middle lobe and lingula. Various manufacturers have taken different approaches to the spacing of rows within the multislice array. Some are equally spaced (General Electric Medical Systems, Milwaukee, Wisconsin) while others use rows of varying thickness (Siemens Medical Systems, Erlangen, Germany and Marconi Medical Systems, Cleveland, Ohio). The former is called a matrix detector while the latter is an adaptive detector. The detector array electronics can sample individual rows or combinations of rows to produce images with varying slice thickness or longitudinal spatial resolution. In addition, some manufacturers have employed post-patient collimation of the detector array to increase the number of available row widths (Siemens, Marconi).

Multislice technology also increases the efficiency of x-ray tube utilization. In comparison to single-slice spiral CT scanners, there is decreased x-ray tube loading for the same scanned volume. Therefore, multislice technology increases the volume that can be scanned before tube-cooling delays are required. Clinically, this feature improves the evaluation of trauma patients and increases scanner efficiency.

Pitch

Currently, there are two definitions of pitch in use for multislice CT. The first is the original definition of pitch used in single-slice CT and defines pitch as the table travel per 360-degree gantry rotation divided by the product of the number of detector rows and the detector aperture. In this definition of pitch, the segmentation of the detector into rows is not considered. One manufacturer (General Electric Medical Systems) has proposed a new definition of

pitch for multislice CT as the table travel per 360-degree gantry rotation divided by the detector aperture. The removal of the number of detector rows from the denominator increases the value of pitch by the number of slices obtained. For example, the acquisition of four 1.25-mm slices at a table speed of 12 mm per second in a 0.5-second scanner results in a pitch of 1 using the standard definition. However, using the same parameters but changing the denominator to the detector aperture increases the value of pitch to 4. We agree with others (10) that this new definition of pitch is artificial since it does not clearly demonstrate the relationship between radiation dose and x-ray beam overlap found in the original definition. For this reason, we believe that the original definition of pitch is preferable.

Interpolation Algorithm

Interpolation algorithms for multislice spiral CT differ from those used in single-slice scanners. Since multiple detector rows are available, the detector row closest to the plane of reconstruction can be used (21), decreasing helical artifact. In this fashion, table motion can be partially compensated for by reverse motion in the detector array (22) (Figure 1-3). However, multislice CT suffers from a new form of image distortion, cone beam artifact (23). In multislice spiral CT, the x-ray beam to the outer detectors is angled relative to the transverse reconstruction axis of the images. Therefore, the raw scan data attenuation measurements are not made in exactly the same plane as the reconstructed images, creating cone beam artifact. Current four-row multislice scanners have relatively narrow cone beam angles (e.g., 4×1.25-mm mode, cone beam angles of -0.20, -0.07, 0.07, and 0.20

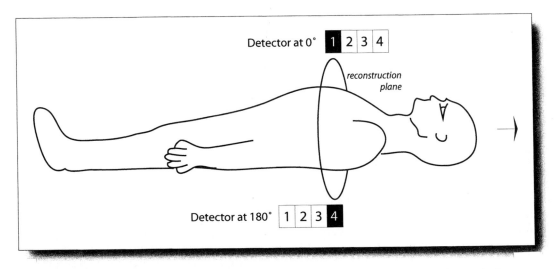

Detector at 0°   1 2 3 4

reconstruction plane

Detector at 180°   1 2 3 4

FIGURE 1-3. Line diagram showing the position of the reconstruction image plane relative to the detector array in a four-row multislice CT scanner at 0 degrees and 180 degrees. Using a multidetector array, the detector element closest to the plane of image reconstruction can be employed, decreasing helical artifact and improving z-axis spatial resolution.

degrees). These narrow cone beam angles only produce substantial distortion at the periphery of a large field of view (e.g., 50 cm). To our knowledge, cone beam artifact is not compensated for in currently used multislice reconstruction algorithms. Increasing the x-ray beam angle exacerbates image distortion caused by cone beam artifact. Larger beam angles are found in 16- and 32-track multislice scanner designs. In these proposed scanners, the cone beam angle will approximate 5 degrees and will likely have to be considered in the reconstruction algorithm. The effect of cone beam artifact can be minimized using a volumetric CT reconstruction technique instead of the currently used planar CT reconstruction. This modified reconstruction technique may be introduced with future 16- and 32-track multislice spiral CT scanners.

In the future, interpolation algorithms for multislice CT will likely use z-axis deconvolution to further improve longitudinal spatial resolution (8). In conjunction with narrow detector rows, z-axis deconvolution techniques can generate isometric submillimeter voxels, which provide true multiplanar images. Using these techniques there will be no loss of spatial resolution when volumetric CT image data sets are viewed in any orientation (coronal, sagittal, and oblique imaging planes).

Reconstruction Parameters

Using multislice spiral CT, the raw scan data can consist of thin slices that are averaged together to generate thicker slices for the initial reconstruction. These thicker slices have improved signal-to-noise ratio and contrast resolution over the acquired thinner slices, but are limited by inferior spatial resolution and associated volume averaging. Using this technique, once an abnormality is found using these thicker slices, a repeat reconstruction can be performed on the raw scan data. The repeated reconstruction is performed without averaging and produces thinner slices with improved spatial resolution. Initially viewing averaged thicker slices will decrease the number of images that must be screened by the radiologist, possibly increasing reader efficiency. The clinical utility of this approach requires further investigation.

The large number of possible reconstruction techniques (thick slice, thin slice, sagittal and coronal reformats) available with multislice spiral CT will generate a large number of images for each case, making review on the workstation and a PACS archive system essential. To facilitate this, all current multislice CT scanners are equipped with interfaces to the hospital information system and the radiology department information system (Hospital Information System-Radiology Information System interface). These interfaces also increase technologist efficiency and facilitate patient throughput.

Early developmental work is being performed on flat panel detectors, which may contain thousands of rows allowing the entire chest to be imaged with one gantry rotation. Such a system would provide new insights into cardiovascular and pulmonary function.

Summary

As further experience is gained with multislice CTA, the optimal technical parameters will be described. Similar to single-slice spiral CT, multislice CTA studies should be optimal when acquired using the narrowest detector width compatible with the scan volume, pitch, and contrast injection protocol employed.

RADIATION DOSE

Overview

It is widely accepted that the best measurement of radiation dose is the effective dose (24), which is the sum of the calculated absorbed doses to individual organs weighted for their radiation sensitivity. Effective dose has replaced surface dose because it provides a direct measurement of the risk factors for radiologic procedures. Effective dose can account for partial irradiation of organs from noncontiguous CT protocols and can be related to other forms of radiation exposure such as natural background. Using effective dose measurement techniques, the risk of fatal cancer is estimated to be 50 per million exposed to 1 mSv.

Although CT represents only 2% of radiographic examinations, it results in at least 20% of the effective radiation dose from medical procedures (25). In comparison to plain film studies, the relatively high CT radiation dose results from two unique characteristics of this technique (13). First, the ability to window or map the entire gray scale onto selected segments of the CT number scale enhances visualization of image noise. As a result, image degradation due to quantum noise is easily recognized with narrow window settings. Second, since CT is a digital technique, image acquisition and display are independent processes. Therefore, when CT radiation dose is excessive, the image does not become too dark but merely improves because of decreased image noise (26). As a result of these two effects, a desired CT image quality often results in high patient radiation exposure, which may not be recognized by the radiologist. Concern has been raised about radiation doses in chest CT (27–29) and radiation dose surveys have documented wide variation in radiation exposure between different sites and equipment. Therefore, serious consideration needs to be given to the optimization of CT exposures (24). As with all other radiologic imaging modalities, optimal CT exposure requires an appropriate balance between diagnostic image quality and radiation dose. Effective dose values for a variety of radiologic chest studies are shown in Table 1-2.

TABLE 1-2. COMPARISON OF EFFECTIVE DOSES

Procedure	Effective Dose (mSv)
PA chest radiograph	0.05[a]
Conventional CT	7.0[b]
Spiral CT pitch 1	7.0[b]
Spiral CT pitch 2	3.5[b]
HRCT 10-mm interslice gap	0.7[b]
HRCT 20-mm interslice gap	0.35[b]
Thin-section, low-dose HRCT	0.02[c]
Conventional pulmonary angiography	9.0[d]
Digital pulmonary angiography	6.0[d]
Conventional bronchoscopy	3.0[e]
Natural background radiation	2.5[a]

[a]UNSCEAR (1993) (49)
[b]NRP (1992) (50)
[c]Lee KS, Primack SL, Staples CA, et al. (1994) (51)
[d]Calculated using data from NRPB.(1994) Report R262 assuming pulmonary angiography with 5 minutes of fluoroscopy and the equivalent of 30 PA and 30 lateral views.
[e]Bronchography performed with the assumption of 2 minutes of fluoroscopy and six PA and six lateral views.
CT, computed tomography; HRCT, .

Scanner Radiation Efficiency

Optimally, the primary x-ray beam incident on the patient should exactly correspond to the sensitive regions of the CT detector array. Practically, this is not achieved because of imperfect collimation of the x-ray beam and physical gaps between individual elements in the detector array due to its construction. Physical separation of individual detector elements creates gaps or dead space resulting in small zones of undetected primary beam. This problem is greater in multislice spiral CT scanners due to the additional separation of the detector rows. The septa that separate detector elements in current single and multislice scanners measure approximately 0.06 mm in thickness. Depending on the detector configuration, these septa reduce the multislice detector efficiency by 2% to 4.5% (11).

Multislice spiral CT image quality is more sensitive to the alignment of the x-ray tube focal spot with the detector rows than single-slice spiral CT. In multislice scanners, the active detector elements must be irradiated by the umbra of the x-ray beam. If they are exposed to the reduced radiation of the penumbra, artifacts are seen in the reconstructed images. Excluding the penumbra represents wasted radiation exposure to the patient and decreases multislice scanner radiation efficiency. Accurate alignment of the umbra with the active rows in the detector improves both image quality and radiation dose efficiency. One manufacturer actively tracks the umbra with the detector array to minimize any misalignment (30). The sum of these effects determines the ratio of detected to incident primary beam photons and is known as the geometric scanner efficiency. The geometric efficiency can vary between different makes of scanners.

In all radiology studies scattered radiation is formed by the interaction of the primary beam with the patient. Scattered radiation exits in all directions and if detected, only contributes to noise in the image. In CT, extensive pre- and postpatient collimation reduce the scatter fraction to less than 10%, increasing the soft tissue contrast of CT over that of the plain radiograph. However, compromises in CT scanner design can increase the scatter fraction, decreasing image quality. Increased radiation dose may be used to compensate partially for increased scatter fraction in some scanners.

CT detectors vary in their overall ability to convert x-ray photons into electric signals that can be reconstructed by computers into images. The overall efficiency of this process depends on the individual efficiency of a number of steps. Initially, the detector must detect the incident x-ray photons. The solid state detectors used in current generation single- and multislice spiral CT scanners detect 90% to 95% of incident x-ray photons. The ratio of detected to incident photons is known as the quantum detection efficiency (QDE). The accuracy of conversion of the absorbed x-ray photons into an electric signal is known as the conversion efficiency. The QDE and the conversion efficiency determine the detector efficiency. The overall dose efficiency of the scanner is determined by the detector efficiency and the geometric efficiency (31).

In addition, the detected signal is degraded by noise, which is introduced by the electronics of the scanner data acquisition system. Differences in dose efficiency and electronic noise create the variation in image quality between scanners at the same patient radiation exposure. Increased radiation dose is often used to improve image quality in scanners with inferior dose efficiency and increased electronic noise. The combined effects of geometric efficiency, scanner dose efficiency, and electronic noise can be measured using standard phantoms. Imaging physicists typically perform these measurements when scanners are purchased and installed.

Summary

CT scanning now accounts for a substantial portion of the medically associated radiation dose to the population. This has spurred research into the relationship between radiation dose, image quality, and diagnostic accuracy in CT (32–34). This research should help establish appropriate radiation exposure parameters for CTA studies, which will uphold the World Health Organization's recommendation of As Low As Reasonably Achievable (ALARA). Once radiation dose and diagnostic accuracy issues are resolved, we believe that automatic exposure control will be developed for CT scanners.

CONTRAST ENHANCEMENT PROTOCOLS
Overview

Intravascular contrast enhancement is required for CTA as there is insufficient contrast between flowing blood, an intraluminal clot, and the vessel wall. Nonionic contrast media is preferred over ionic media as it is associated with a lower incidence of major and minor reactions (35,36). Iodinated contrast media freely exchanges between the vascular and extravascular space in all tissues except the brain. Since the extravascular space is many times larger than the intravascular space, there is rapid dilution of intravascular contrast media following its passage through the heart. This limits the time that large differences can be seen between contrast enhanced blood and clot or vessel wall. Therefore, optimal CT angiograms are acquired during the rapid injection of intravenous contrast media.

Adults with normal renal function tolerate 100 to 150 mL of 60% iodinated contrast media with few side effects. Eighteen- or 20-gauge intravenous catheters are easily placed in arm veins and permit injection of contrast media at 2 to 5 mL per second. In most cases the contrast media is injected into a medially located antecubital veins in either arm, but other venous access sites can be used depending on the clinical setting. The use of other vascular access sites requires modification of the scan protocol (injection rate, scan delay). In our experience, we have found placing the injected arm by the patient's side does not substantially degrade chest images and improves contrast delivery by minimizing compression on the subclavian vein as it passes through the thoracobrachial junction (Figure 1-4).

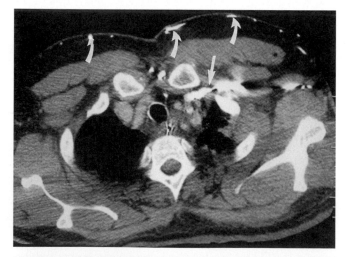

FIGURE 1-4. Contrast enhanced transverse CT image through the subclavian vein in a patient scanned with the left arm elevated above the head. A focal narrowing is seen in the subclavian vein as it passes under the clavicle (*arrow*). This causes relative obstruction with filling of collateral veins over the anterior chest wall (*curved arrows*). This effect was transient and resolved with positioning of the arm by the side.

Contrast Media and Injection Site

For pulmonary arterial studies there has been debate regarding the optimal rate of injection and the concentration of contrast media. Relatively low iodine concentration contrast media with a high injection rate was initially proposed, using 120 mg per mL iodine concentration and injection rates of 7 mL per second. This protocol resulted in a high degree of vascular opacification in most cases (74%) (7), allowing a confident diagnosis of central pulmonary emboli. However, this protocol gave suboptimal contrast enhancement in segmental and subsegmental vessels, limiting the diagnostic accuracy in these vessels. Currently, higher iodine concentration contrast media and lower injection rate techniques are used, using 120 to 140 mL of 240 to 300 mg per mL iodine concentration injected at 3 to 5 mL per second (16). This technique usually provides greater than 200 Hounsfield unit (HU) enhancement in the central pulmonary arteries and gives reliable depiction of segmental and proximal subsegmental pulmonary arteries. This injection protocol also provides excellent enhancement of the cardiac chambers and systemic arteries (see Appendix A for injection and scan protocols). In the pulmonary vasculature, maximal enhancement occurs while the contrast is being injected, making it essential to initiate scanning as soon as the bolus arrives in the target vessels and imaging the complete target volume before the contrast injection ends. Therefore, the contrast injection determines the time available for scan acquisition, which influences the choice of pitch and slice collimation.

Scan Delay

The delay between the start of the contrast injection and the start of the scan data acquisition is known as the scan delay. This delay allows the injected contrast media to flow from the injection site to the target vessels. If scanning starts before the contrast arrives, there is inadequate contrast enhancement. Alternately, if too long a scan delay is used, contrast is wasted and there is the possibility that the contrast injection will end before the target volume is completely imaged. This can lead to inadequate contrast enhancement at the end of the scan. To address this problem, most scanners come equipped with programs that allow continuous monitoring of the attenuation within a large target vessel (e.g., pulmonary artery, aorta). When a set level of contrast enhancement is reached within a region of interest placed in the target vessel, the diagnostic scan is automatically initiated. Alternately, a timing bolus of contrast media can be given, using the same injection parameters for contrast delivery as the diagnostic scan. The timing bolus is usually 20 mL and serial scans are performed at one level every 2 to 4 seconds. A region of interest (ROI) is placed in the target vessel and the time-density curve is mapped out. The scan delay is set to coincide with the peak of the timing bolus time-density curve.

Another approach to scan delay timing is to use an operator-selected delay. Typically, these scan delays are set at 10 to 20 seconds based on the experience of the radiologist. Shorter delays are used in younger patients with high cardiac outputs, with longer delays used in older patients or those with impaired cardiac function. The scan delay should be shortened when examining systemic veins and extended for systemic arteries. Additionally, operator determined scan delay times must be adjusted to compensate for the relative position of the contrast injection site and the target vessels of the examination.

Contrast-Related Artifacts

Streak artifacts arising from the subclavian or brachiocephalic veins and superior vena cava (Figure 1-5) can degrade CT angiograms that use high iodine concentration (320 mg per mL) contrast media injected through the upper arm veins. These artifacts are caused by photon starvation, beam hardening, and object motion in projections that traverse a segment of undiluted contrast media. This artifact is not seen in the lower chest since the contrast media is diluted in the right atrium by nonenhanced blood from the inferior vena cava. The impact of this artifact can be minimized by reducing the iodine concentration of the contrast media (37), viewing overlapping reconstructed images with widened window settings, or using a biphasic contrast media injection technique (38). Further research is necessary to determine which of these techniques provides optimal images.

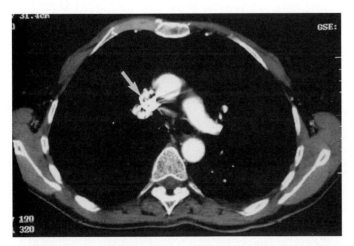

FIGURE 1-5. Transverse section through the superior vena cava (*arrow*) showing high and low signal intensity streak artifacts arising from high iodine concentration (320 mg per mL) contrast media. Beam hardening, photon starvation, and motion generate this artifact which degrades the image.

REFORMATTING AND VOLUME RENDERING TECHNIQUES

Overview

Using a computer graphic technique, stacks of transverse CT images can be analyzed as a volumetric data set using a number of approaches (39). Most simply, the volume data set can be reformatted and viewed in coronal, sagittal, or oblique imaging planes. Alternately, the volumetric data set can be interrogated for the maximum or minimum HU attenuation values. Using this approach, the attenuation values associated with certain anatomic features (e.g., contrast-enhanced vessels, airways) can be identified and these tissues either segmented out (surface-shaded display) or highlighted (volume rendering) within the data set. Viewing the data set in this fashion can both improve and speed up our three-dimensional understanding of the acquired transverse images. However, all of these image-processing techniques require high-quality transverse images, which are spatially registered and artifact-free. These volume-imaging techniques work best when the transverse images are acquired using narrow collimation and have nearly isometric voxels.

Unfortunately, single-slice spiral CT scanners can only scan small volumes with narrow collimation (1 mm) due to their slow rate of data acquisition. If thicker slices are used the resulting volumetric images are blurred in the z-axis, limiting their diagnostic value. However, even these limited images may be useful to demonstrate anatomic relationships (Figure 1-6).

Volumetric techniques are greatly improved by multi-slice spiral CT scanners that can scan large volumes with narrow slice collimation. These new scanners promise to increase the diagnostic accuracy and clinical indications for volumetric image display. Real-time volumetric displays may improve the efficiency of scan interpretation in the future.

Multiplanar Reformatting

Multiplanar reformatting creates sagittal, coronal, oblique, or curved imaging planes providing unique displays for the transverse images. It has been shown that two-dimensional reformations improve the diagnostic accuracy in interpreting CT angiograms for pulmonary embolism when compared to review of the transverse images (Figure 1-7) (40). This study showed improved detection of clot burden in cases of proven pulmonary embolism and more confident exclusion of a clot in cases without pulmonary embolism. Although this approach was useful when scanning patients with a nominal section thickness of 5 mm, the current availability of thin-collimation for scanning the entire thorax has limited the indications of two-dimensional reformations in the diagnostic approach of acute pulmonary embolism.

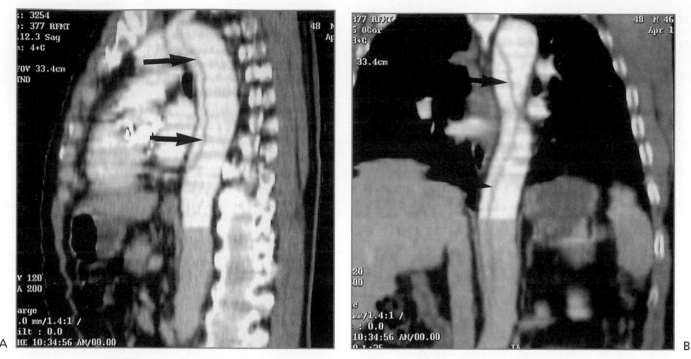

FIGURE 1-6. Sagittal (**A**) and coronal (**B**) reformatted images generated from a single-section spiral CT acquisition in a patient with a type B aortic dissection. An extensive dissection flap (*arrows*) is identified originating distal to the left subclavian artery and extending into the abdominal aorta.

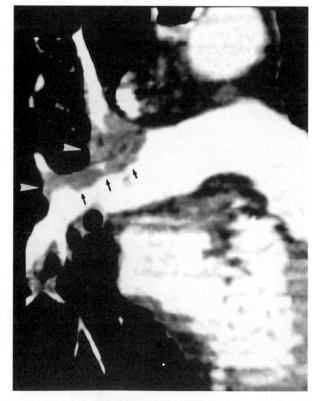

FIGURE 1-7. Coronal oblique reformation obtained along the main axis of the right pulmonary artery enables simultaneous recognition of complete filling defects at the level of the right upper lobe segmental arteries (*arrowheads*) and precise delineation of a mural clot (*arrows*).

Currently, most imaging workstations provide these reformations in real time, which allows the radiologist to view the volume data set from a number of angles. Standard angiographic projections (e.g., left anterior oblique view of the thoracic aorta) are easily generated and may be very useful for surgical planning. However, it should be noted that artifactual stenosis can be introduced into tortuous vessels by the limited width of the reformatted image plane. Patient movement during acquisition of the stack of transverse images can also cause artifactual stenosis or dilation of vessels. Close inspection of the acquired transverse images is often useful to fully understand the appearance of the reformations.

Shaded Surface Displays

This technique works best on structures that have large contrast differences with surrounding tissues, such as airways, vessels, or bones. A range of attenuation values is selected that identifies the target tissue (e.g., −500 to −700 HU for pulmonary arteriovenous malformations [PAVM]) and the remaining image data is discarded (Figure 1-8). A meshlike representation of the external surface of the target tissue is generated which can then be illuminated or shaded to provide depth cues to the observer. The object can be rotated and tipped to provide multiple viewing angles. Therefore, insights into the vascular anatomy of lesions can be obtained with these displays that are not possible using pul-

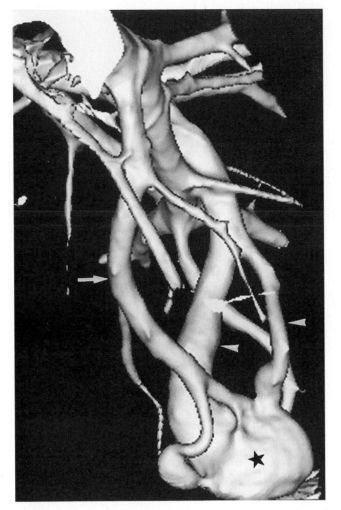

FIGURE 1-8. Shaded surface display of a left lower lobe pulmonary arteriovenous malformation showing the feeding artery (*arrow*), the aneurysmal sac (*star*), and the two draining veins (*arrowheads*).

visualization of small vessels and airways and introduce false contour artifacts. Therefore, to ensure accurate diagnosis, surface-shaded displays should be interpreted with reference to the original transverse images.

Volume Rendering

Volume-rendering techniques address some of the limitations of surface-shaded display techniques. The most commonly employed volume-rendering technique projects a series of rays through the object and extracts out the pixels with either maximum intensity projection (MIP)(42) or minimum intensity projection (MINIP). Since the pixel attenuation values are retained, relative attenuation values within the target tissue are displayed in the final image. Therefore, vessels of varying sizes, wall calcification, and stents can be seen in the extracted image using the appropriate display parameters (window and level). Similar to surface-shaded displays, volume averaging may limit the detection of small vessels and airways. Typically, a number MIP images are created, providing viewing angles that rotate around the object. These images are then displayed in a cine format which provides a three-dimensional understanding of the vessels or airways. MIP volume rendering can be performed in any axis if the base images are composed of isometric voxels. However, if the voxels are not isometric (e.g., single-slice spiral CT), complex blurring patterns result when the MIP volume renderings are viewed in coronal, sagittal, or oblique imaging planes. MIP images generated from nonisometric source data sets are best viewed in the transverse plane. This limitation will be removed using multislice spiral CT base images, which generate isometric voxels.

MIP imaging was first applied to bright blood three-dimensional magnetic resonance angiograms (MRA), where the MR pulse sequence provided high signal intensity isometric voxels in regions with flowing blood (43). The application of MIP volume-rendering techniques to CT angiograms is more complicated since the surrounding bones are detected and may obscure the contrast-enhanced vessels. The surrounding bony structures can either be edited out prior to performing the MIP operation or a connectivity algorithm can be applied to a seed point placed within a vessel by the operator. Connectivity algorithms may have difficulty excluding bones that are in contact with vessels (e.g., thoracic vertebral bodies adjacent to the descending thoracic aorta). Once surrounding bony structures have been removed, contrast-enhanced vessels can be easily visualized (44).

MIP rendering can be applied to either the entire imaged volume or can be targeted to a thin slab of tissue. This thin slab can then be shifted through the imaged volume, a technique known as sliding thin slab maximum intensity projection (STS-MIP) (45). STS-MIP or STS-MINIP images are usually viewed in the transverse plane to eliminate the

monary angiography. If smaller vessels need to be seen, the surface rendering can be repeated using a lower threshold value (e.g., −850 HU). Unfortunately, within the lung, the profusion of vessels seen with the lower threshold value can obscure the object of interest (e.g., the aneurysm of a PAVM). Review of these images prior to therapeutic angiography can facilitate the procedure by suggesting the optimal angiographic views to visualize feeding and draining vessels. The combined interpretation of surface-shaded display images and the original transverse slices has been shown to provide complete pretherapeutic evaluation of PAVMs in 95% of cases (41).

Since the pixel classification scheme used in surface-shaded displays results in a large amount of the data being discarded, these programs can be implemented on relatively unsophisticated workstations and run very quickly. However, volume averaging effects may obscure the interface between the target and surrounding tissues, which can limit effects of nonisometric voxels and resultant image blurring. Additionally, this orientation is computationally simple; therefore, images can be generated fast enough to allow the viewer to scroll the slab through the imaged volume providing an optimal assessment of the vasculature. This technique has been applied to pulmonary vessels (Figure 1-9) and nodules. The minimum intensity application of the same technique can be used to image airways and detect emphysema (46).

More sophisticated volume-rendering techniques address the major limitation of MIP and MINIP imaging, the inability to maintain the three-dimensional structural relationships inherent in the data set. These new volume-rendering techniques allow colors and opacity values to be applied to all the pixel values encountered by the viewing ray. Using these techniques, it is possible to display all organs within the imaged volume in a semitransparent fashion (Figure 1-10) (47). Additionally, the data set can be viewed from within as well as externally. These techniques can allow the user to "fly" through the airways or vasculature while seeing through the walls into the surrounding mediastinum or lung. These methods have been named vir-

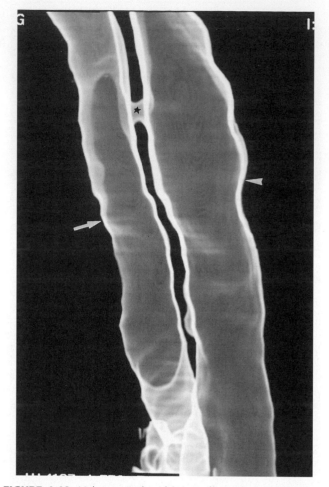

FIGURE 1-10. Volume-rendered image (*lateral view*) of a congenital tracheoesophageal fistula (*star*) responsible for abnormal dilation of the esophagus (*arrowhead*). The arrow points to the tracheal lumen.

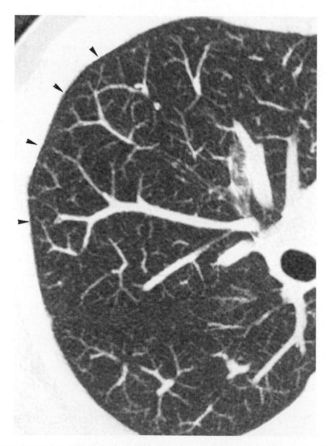

FIGURE 1-9. Sliding thin slab maximum intensity projection of the lung parenchyma obtained by stacking eight 1-mm thick transverse CT scans. Note the precise delineation of pulmonary vessels down to lobular divisions in the right upper lobe (*arrowheads*).

tual bronchoscopy, colonoscopy, or angioscopy (48) and may enhance our ability to detect subtle pathology. However, at this time, these complex three-dimensional rendering techniques require advanced computer workstations to generate these interactive images. Further research is required to determine the clinical utility of these advanced viewing capabilities.

Summary

Improvements in computer technology and graphic display algorithms will further improve the speed and quality of three-dimensional display techniques in the future. All reformatting and volume-rendering techniques provide optimal results when applied to motion-free, three-dimensional data sets composed of isometric voxels. Current multislice spiral CT scanners can provide three-dimensional data sets for this type of display. Further research is required to determine the clinical utility of these advanced display techniques.

REFERENCES

1. Petasnick JP. Radiologic evaluation of aortic dissection. *Radiology* 1991;180:297–305.
2. Demos TC, Posniak HV, Marsan RE. CT of aortic dissection. *Semin Roentgenol* 1989;24:22–37.
3. Kazerooni EA, Bree RL, Williams DM. Penetrating atherosclerotic ulcers of the descending thoracic aorta: evaluation with CT and distinction from aortic dissection. *Radiology* 1992;183:759–765.
4. Kalender WA, Seissler W, Klotz E, et al. Spiral volumetric CT with single-breath-hold technique, continuous transport, and continuous scanner rotation. *Radiology* 1990;176:181–183.
5. Costello P, Anderson W, Blume D. Pulmonary nodule: evaluation with spiral volumetric CT. *Radiology* 1991;179:875–876.
6. Remy-Jardin M, Remy J, Giraud F, et al. Pulmonary nodules: detection with thick-section spiral CT versus conventional CT. *Radiology* 1993;187:513–520.
7. Remy-Jardin M, Remy J, Wattinne L, et al. Central pulmonary thromboembolism: diagnosis with spiral volumetric CT with the single-breath-hold technique. Comparison with pulmonary angiography. *Radiology* 1992;185:381–387.
8. Wang G, Vannier MW. Longitudinal resolution in volumetric x-ray computerized tomography—analytical comparison between conventional and helical computerized tomography. *Med Phys* 1994;21:429–433.
9. Kalender WA, Polacin A, Suss C. A comparison of conventional and spiral CT: an experimental study on the detection of spherical lesions. *J Comput Assist Tomogr* 1994;18:167–176.
10. McCollough CH, Zink FE. Performance evaluation of a multislice CT system. *Med Phys* 1999;26:2223–2230.
11. Rydberg J, Buckwalter KA, Caldemeyer KS, et al. Multisection CT: scanning techniques and clinical applications. *Radiographics* 2000;20:1787–1806.
12. Kachelriess M, Kalender WA. ECG-correlated image reconstruction from subsecond spiral CT scans of the heart. *Med Phys* 1998;25:2417–2431.
13. Sprawls P Jr. *Physical principles of medical imaging*, 2nd ed. Gaithersburg, MD: Aspen Publications, 1993:361–369.
14. Polacin A, Kalender WA, Marchal G. Evaluation of section sensitivity profiles and image noise in spiral CT. *Radiology* 1992;185:29–35.
15. Kalender WA, Fuchs TOJ. Principles and performance of single- and multislice spiral CT. In: Goldman LW, ed. RSNA Categorical Course in Diagnostic Radiology Physics: CT and US Cross-Sectional Imaging 2000:127–142.
16. Remy Jardin M, Remy J, Petyt L, et al. Diagnosis of acute pulmonary embolism with spiral CT: comparison with pulmonary angiography and scintigraphy. *Radiology* 1996;200:699–706.
17. Ghaye B, Szapiro D, Delannoy V, et al. How far does multidetector CT allow the analysis of peripheral pulmonary arteries? A comparative study with thin collimation single detector CT. *Radiology* 2000;217(P):508.
18. Schoepf UO, Holzknecht NG, Helmberger TK, et al. Segmental and subsegmental pulmonary embolism (PE): improved detection with thin-slice multi-detector array spiral CT (MDCT). *Radiology* 2000;217(P):509.
19. Ohnesorge B, Flohr T, Becker C, et al. Cardiac imaging by means of electrocardiographical gated multisection spiral CT: initial experience. *Radiology* 2000;217:564–571.
20. Roos J, Willmann JK, Lachat M, et al. Comparison of ECG-Triggert and non-Triggert multi-slice CT in thoracic aortic disease. *Radiology* 2000;217(P):467.
21. Hu H. Multi-slice helical CT: scan and reconstruction. *Med Phys* 1999;26:1–18.
22. Hsieh J. CT image reconstruction. In: Goldman LW, ed. RSNA Categorical Course in Diagnostic Radiology Physics: CT and US Cross-Sectional Imaging. Chicago: 2000, 53–64.
23. Hsieh J. Image Artifacts in CT. In: Goldman LW, ed. RSNA Categorical Course in Diagnostic Radiology Physics: CT and US Cross-Sectional Imaging. Chicago: 2000, 97–115.
24. ICRP-60. *Recommendations of the International Commission on Radiological Protection*. Oxford: Pergamon Press, 1991.
25. NRPB. Documents of the National Radiological Protection Board. Chilton, Didcot, Oxon, UK. 1992;3(4):1–16.
26. Rothenberg LN, Pentlow KS. Radiation dose in CT. *Radiographics* 1992;12:1225–1243.
27. Di Marco AF, Briones B. Is chest CT performed too often? *Chest* 1993;103:985–986.
28. Naidich DP, Pizzarello D, Garay SM, et al. Is thoracic CT performed often enough? *Chest* 1994;106:331–332.
29. Di Marco AF, Renston JP. In search of the appropriate use of chest computed tomography. *Chest* 1994;106:332–333.
30. Toth TL, Bromberg NB, Pan T-S, et al. A dose reduction x-ray beam positioned system for high-speed multislice CT scanners. *Med Phys* 2000;27(12):2659–2668.
31. Cunningham IA. Computed tomography: instrumentation. In: Bronzino JE, ed. *The biomedical engineering handbook*. Boca Raton, FL: CRC Press, 1995:990–1002.
32. Lee KS, Primack SL, Staples CA, et al. Chronic infiltrative lung disease: comparison of diagnostic accuracies of radiography and low- and conventional-dose thin-section CT. *Radiology* 1994;191:669–673.
33. Mayo JR, Jackson SA, Müller NL. High-resolution CT of the chest: radiation dose. *Am J Roentgenol* 1993;160:479–481.
34. Mayo JR, Hartman TE, Lee KS, et al. CT of the chest: minimal tube current required for good image quality with the least radiation dose. *Am J Roentgenol* 1995;164:603–607.
35. Bettmann MA, Heeren T, Greenfield A, et al. Adverse events with radiographic contrast agents: results of the SCVIR contrast agent registry. *Radiology* 1997;203:611–620.
36. Lasser EC, Lyon SG, Berry CC. Reports on contrast media reactions: analysis of data from reports to the U.S. Food and Drug Administration. *Radiology* 1997;203:605–610.
37. Rubin GD, Lane MJ, Bloch DA, et al. Optimization of thoracic spiral CT: effects of iodinated contrast medium concentration. *Radiology* 1996;201:785–791.
38. Saremi F, Wilcox A, Palmer S. Biphasic contrast administration: a new injection protocol to reduce flow related artifacts and optimize the image quality in computed tomography pulmonary angiography. *Radiology* 2000;217(P):509.
39. Fishman E, Magid D, Nay DR, et al. Three dimensional imaging. *Radiology* 1991;181:321–337.
40. Remy-Jardin M, Remy J, Cauvain O, et al. Diagnosis of central pulmonary embolism with helical CT: role of two dimensional multiplanar reformations. *Am J Roentgenol* 1995;165:1131–1138.
41. Remy J, Remy-Jardin M, Giraud F, et al. Angioarchitecture of pulmonary arteriovenous malformations: clinical utility of three-dimensional helical CT. *Radiology* 1994;191:657–664.
42. Napel S, Marks N, Rubin G, et al. CT angiography with spiral CT and maximum intensity projection. *Radiology* 1992;185:607–610.
43. Laub G, Kaiser W. MR angiography with gradient motion refocusing. *J Comput Assist Tomogr* 1988;12:377–382.
44. Rubin G, Dake M, Napel SCM, et al. Three dimensional spiral CT angiography of the abdomen: initial clinical experience. *Radiology* 1993;186:147–152.
45. Napel S, Rubin GD, Jeffrey RB Jr. STS-MIP: a new reconstruction technique for CT of the chest. *J Comput Assist Tomogr* 1993;17(5):832–838.
46. Remy-Jardin M, Remy J, Gosselin B, et al. Sliding thin slab, minimum intensity projection technique in the diagnosis of emphy-

sema: histopathologic–CT correlation. *Radiology* 1996;200(3): 665–671.

47. Remy-Jardin M, Remy J, Artaud D, et al. Tracheobronchial tree: assessment with volume rendering—technical aspects. *Radiology* 1998;208(2):393–398.

48. Hopper K, Tunc-Iyriboz A, Wise S, et al. Mucosal detail at CT virtual reality: surface versus volume rendering. *Radiology* 2000; 214:517–522.

49. USCEAR. Report to the General Assembly, with Scientific Annexes. United Nations, New York, 1993.

50. NRPB. Documents of the NRPB 3:4:1–16 National Radiation Protection Board, Chilton, Didcot Oxon, UK, 1992.

51. Lee KS, Primack SL, Staples CA, et al. Chronic infiltrative lung disease: comparison of diagnostic accuracies of radiography low and conventional dose thin section CT. *Radiology* 1994;191: 669–673.

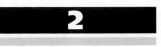

ANATOMY AND NORMAL VARIANTS

PULMONARY ARTERIES
Central Pulmonary Arteries
Branching Patterns in the Right and Left Lung
Right Pulmonary Arteries
Left Pulmonary Arteries

PULMONARY VEINS
Prevailing Pulmonary Venous Patterns
Pulmonary Venous Variants

SYSTEMIC VESSELS
Bronchial Arteries
Thoracic Outlet

PULMONARY ARTERIES

Central Pulmonary Arteries

The pulmonary trunk (or main pulmonary artery) arises from the base of the right ventricle and courses cranially and dorsally, contained within the pericardium. On transverse CT scan images, the pulmonary trunk is recognized as the most anterior vascular structure arising from the heart, measuring up to 28 mm in diameter in normal subjects.

In the concavity of the aortic arch, it divides into the right and left pulmonary arteries which are nearly equal in size at their origin (1) (Figure 2-1). The right pulmonary artery, slightly longer and larger than the left, runs horizontally to the right, behind the ascending aorta, superior vena cava, and right upper pulmonary vein to the root of the right lung where it divides into two branches. The upper and smaller of these is an ascending trunk (truncus anterior) which accompanies the upper lobe bronchus; the lower and larger is a descending trunk (interlobar pulmonary artery), distributed to the right middle and lower lobes. The left pulmonary artery, a little shorter and smaller than the right, courses over the left main bronchus and penetrates the root of the left lung where it divides into two branches, one for each lobe of the lung.

Branching Patterns In the Right and Left Lung

In each lung, the common branching patterns usually consist of lobar, segmental, and subsegmental arteries. Standard nomenclature taken from Boyden (2) and Jackson and Huber (3) is commonly used to identify the segmental and subsegmental structures. According to the prevailing patterns described in three major anatomic textbooks (2–4), there are 10 segmental and 20 subsegmental pulmonary arteries per lung (Tables 2-1 and 2-2). The segmental arteries (i.e., third-order pulmonary arteries) are always seen near the accompanying branches of the bronchial tree and are situated either medially (in the upper lobes) or laterally (in the middle lobe and lingula and the lower lobes). The subsegmental arteries (i.e., fourth-order pulmonary arteries) are easily recognized as dichotomous divisions of the corresponding segmental artery. To provide readers with a practical means of identification of these branches on transverse CT images, slight modifications are made to the naming of a few subsegmental arteries in the right and left upper lobes. The modified naming conforms to the classic descriptions while attempting to name the subsegmental arteries on the basis of the respective orientations of the vessels on transverse CT scans. The fifth-order pulmonary arteries can be recognized as symmetric dichotomous divisions of the corresponding subsegmental branch. The sixth-order pulmonary arteries are then similarly identified as symmetric dichotomous divisions of the corresponding fifth-order pulmonary artery. To identify peripheral pulmonary arterial sections with confidence on transverse CT scans, lung and mediastinal images must be analyzed simultaneously. Multislice CT technology has considerably improved the analysis of peripheral pulmonary arteries on CT scans. Using 1-mm thick reconstructed scans, Ghaye and colleagues have

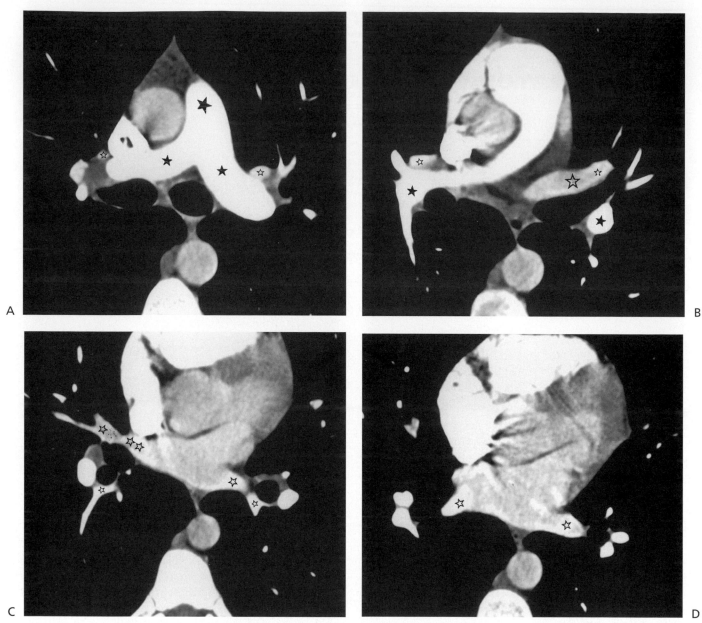

FIGURE 2-1. Cross-sectional anatomy of central vessels. **A:** CT scan at the level of the right and left main bronchi. Bifurcation of the pulmonary trunk (*large plain star*) into the right and left pulmonary arteries (*small plain stars*). The right and left open stars point to anterior segmental pulmonary veins. **B:** CT scan at the level of the right bronchus intermedius shows the right and left interlobar pulmonary arteries (*plain stars*). The open star on the right side points to the pulmonary venous return of the right upper lobe (RV1+2+3). The open stars on the left side point to the pulmonary venous return of the left upper lobe (*small open star*) and to the left superior pulmonary vein (*large open star*) at its junction with the left atrium. **C:** CT scan at the level of the upper part of the left atrium. On the right side, the large single star points to the venous drainage of the right middle lobe and the double large star to the right superior pulmonary vein entering the left atrium. On the left side, the large open star points to the left inferior pulmonary vein. Note the concurrent identification of the pulmonary veins draining the apical segments of the right and left lower lobes (RV6 and LV6, *small open stars on both sides*). **D:** CT scan at the level of the lower lobes shows the right and left inferior pulmonary veins (*open stars*) entering the left atrium.

TABLE 2-1. NOMENCLATURE OF BRONCHOPULMONARY SEGMENTAL ANATOMY

Jackson and Huber Systematization (3)	Boyden's Nomenclature (2)			
	Segments	Bronchi	Arteries	Veins
■ **Right upper lobe**				
Apical	S1	B1	A1	V1
Anterior	S2	B2	A2	V2
Posterior	S3	B3	A3	V3
■ **Right middle lobe**				
Lateral	S4	B4	A4	V4
Medial	S5	B5	A5	V5
■ **Right lower lobe**				
Superior (apical)	S6	B6	A6	V6
Medial basal (paracardiac)	S7	B7	A7	V7
Anterior basal	S8	B8	A8	V8
Lateral basal	S9	B9	A9	V9
Posterior basal	S10	B10	A10	V10
LEFT UPPER LOBE				
■ **Upper division**				
Apicoposterior	S1+3	B1+3	A1+3	V1+3
Anterior	S2	B2	A2	V2
■ **Lower (lingular) division**				
Superior lingular	S4	B4	A4	V4
Inferior lingular	S5	B5	A5	V5
■ **Left lower lobe**				
Superior (apical)	S6	B6	A6	V6
Anteromedial basal	S7+8	B7+8	A7+8	V7+8
Lateral basal	S9	B9	A9	V9
Posterior basal	S10	B10	A10	V10

demonstrated that 98% of subsegmental arteries were adequately analyzed (5). In addition, these authors showed that 74% of fifth-order branches and 35% of sixth-order branches could be confidently analyzed on CT angiograms.

Right Pulmonary Arteries

Right Upper Lobe

The prevailing pattern of the right upper lobe pulmonary arteries consists of an upper trunk (i.e., the truncus anterior), giving rise to the apical (RA1) and anterior (RA2) segmental arteries, and an ascending artery supplying the posterior segment (RA3), originating from the interlobar pulmonary artery (Figure 2-2). Each segmental artery then bifurcates into two subsegmental branches. RA1 usually divides into two branches, an apical ramus (RA1a) and an anterior ramus (RA1b). Owing to the posterior location of RA1a relative to RA1b on transverse CT sections, we can record RA1a as a posterior ramus whereas RA1b may remain recorded as the anterior ramus. RA2 usually gives rise to an anterior ramus (RA2b) and a posterior ramus (RA2a). Owing to the lateral location of RA2a relative to RA2b, the former branch can be recorded as a lateral ramus whereas RA2b can remain recorded as the anterior ramus.

RA3 usually splits into two branches, an apical ramus (RA3a) and a posterior ramus (RA3b). Owing to the lateral orientation of RA3a relative to RA3b, RA3a is recorded as the lateral ramus whereas RA3b remains recorded as the posterior ramus.

Right Middle Lobe

The right middle lobe arteries arise from the right interlobar pulmonary artery, either as a large artery (i.e., the right middle lobe artery) or as two smaller rami (i.e., the lateral [RA4] and medial [RA5] segmental arteries) (Figure 2-3). These branches are usually seen slightly above the level of the apical segmental artery of the right lower lobe (RA6). Each segmental artery divides into two subsegmental branches. RA4 gives rises to a posterior (RA4a) and an anterior ramus (RA4b). RA5 divides into a superior (RA5a) and an inferior ramus (RA5b).

Right Lower Lobe

After giving rise to the right middle lobe pulmonary arteries, the right interlobar pulmonary artery continues as the lower lobe pulmonary artery, coursing dorsally along the

TABLE 2-2. NOMENCLATURE OF SEGMENTAL AND SUBSEGMENTAL ANATOMY

| Jackson and Huber Systematization (3) Arteries | Boyden's Nomenclature (2) | | |
	Segments	Segment Arteries	Subsegment
■ **Right upper lobe**			
Apical	S1	RA1	RA1a (posterior)[a]
			RA1b (anterior)
Anterior	S2	RA2	RA2a (lateral)[a]
			RA2b (anterior)
Posterior	S3	RA3	RA3a (lateral)[a]
			RA3b (posterior)
■ **Right middle lobe**			
Lateral	S4	RA4	RA4a (posterior)
			RA4b (anterior)
Medial	S5	RA5	RA5a (superior)
			RA5b (inferior)
■ **Right lower lobe**			
Superior (apical)	S6	RA6	RA6a+b (superomedial)
			RA6c (lateral)
Medial basal (paracardiac)	S7	RA7	RA7a (anterolateral)
			RA7b (anteromedial)
Anterior basal	S8	RA8	RA8a (lateral)
			RA8b (basal)
Lateral basal	S9	RA9	RA9a (lateral)
			RA9b (basal)
Posterior basal	S10	RA10	RA10a (laterobasal)
			RA10b (mediobasal)
LEFT UPPER LOBE			
■ **Upper division**			
Apicoposterior	S1+3	LA1	LA1a (posterior)[a]
			LA1b (anterior)[a]
		LA3	LA3a (lateral)[a]
			LA3b (posterior)[a]
Anterior	S2	LA2	LA2a (lateral)[a]
			LA2b (anterior)[a]
■ **Lower (lingular) division**			
Superior lingular	S4	LA4	LA4a (posterior)
			LA4b (anterior)
Inferior lingular	S5	LA5	LA5a (superior)
			LA5b (inferior)
■ **Left lower lobe**			
Superior (apical)	S6	LA6	LA6a+b +(superomedial)
			LA6c (lateral)
Anteromedial basal	S7+8	LA7+8	LA7 a (anterior)
			LA7b (medial)
			LA8a (lateral)
			LA8b (basal)
Lateral basal	S9	LA9	LA9a (lateral)
			LA9b (basal)
Posterior basal	S10	LA10	LA10a (laterobasal)
			LA10b (mediobasal)

[a]Naming slightly modified for the purpose of CT interpretation.

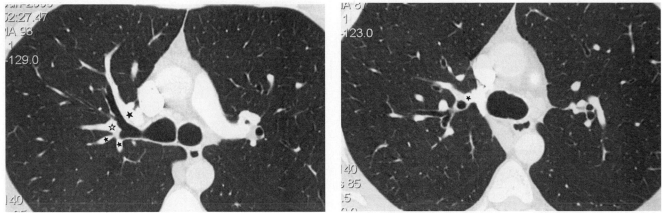

FIGURE 2-2. Right upper lobe segmental vessels. **A:** CT scan at the level of the right upper lobe bronchus and its anterior (RB2) and posterior (RB3) divisions. The anterior plain star points to the anterior segmental artery (RA2), giving rise to its anterior ramus (RA2b). The posterior plain stars point to the divisions of the posterior segmental artery (RA3), namely its lateral (RA3a) and posterior (RA3b) rami. The open star points to RV3, the segmental vein draining the posterior segment of the right upper lobe. **B:** CT scan obtained 10 mm above (**A**) shows the medial location of the apical segmental artery (*plain star*) relative to its accompanying bronchus.

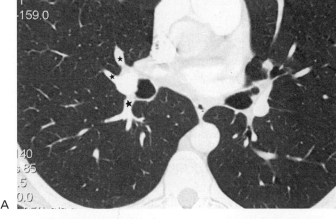

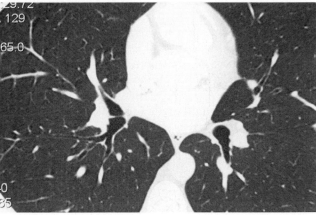

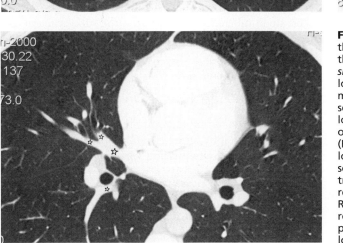

FIGURE 2-3. Right middle lobe segmental vessels. **A:** CT scan at the level of the origin of the right middle lobe bronchus shows the lateral (RA4, *small anterior plain star*) and medial (RA5, *small anterior plain star*) segmental arteries of the right middle lobe, originating as separate rami from the right interlobar pulmonary artery. Note the concurrent identification of the apical segmental artery (RA6, *large posterior plain star*) of the right lower lobe dividing into three subsegmental rami. **B:** CT scan obtained 10 mm below **A** shows the right middle lobe bronchus (RB4+5) and the apical segmental bronchus (RB6) of the right lower lobe, coursing below their corresponding arteries. **C:** CT scan obtained 10 mm below **B** shows the pulmonary venous trunk draining the right middle lobe (RV4+5, *large open star*), resulting from the confluence of two segmental veins (RV4 and RV5, *small anterior open stars*), both coursing below their corresponding bronchi. Note the concurrent identification of the pulmonary vein draining the apical segment of the right lower lobe (RV6, *small posterior open star*).

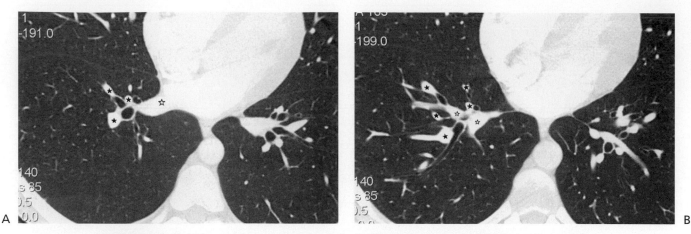

FIGURE 2-4. Right lower lobe segmental vessels. **A:** CT scan at the level of the lower lung zones shows the right lower lobe segmental arteries (*plain stars*), namely the paracardiac artery (RA7), the anterior basal artery (RA8), and a common trunk for the lateral basal and posterior basal segmental arteries (RA9+10), easily recognized by means of their lateral location relative to their accompanying bronchi. Note the concurrent identification of the right inferior pulmonary vein (*open star*) entering the left atrium. **B:** CT scan obtained 10 mm below (**A**) shows subsegmental arterial rami (*anterior plain stars*) in the paracardiac, anterior, and lateral segments and the origin of the posterior segmental artery (*posterior plain star*). Open stars point to segmental tributaries of the common basal vein of the right lower lobe (RV8, *lateral open star*; RV9+10, *medial open star*).

posterolateral aspect of the right lower lobe bronchus. Almost immediately, it gives off the segmental artery to the superior segment (RA6) which arises posteriorly, and then continues as a common trunk (i.e., the common basal artery) which supplies the basal segments. In the apical segment, the prevailing pattern is a bifurcation of the single RA6 into combined medial and superior rami (RA6a+b) and a lateral ramus (RA6c) (Figure 2-3).

The distribution of arteries to the medial basal (RA7) and anterior basal (RA8) segments follows the bronchial divisions (Figure 2-4). RA7 bifurcates into subsegmental anterolateral (RA7a) and subsegmental anteromedial (RA7b) rami. RA8 most often arises as a single branch of the basal artery, then giving rise to lateral (RA8a) and basal (RA8b) rami. The basal artery terminates normally by bifurcating into a lateral basal segmental artery (RA9) and a posterior basal (RA10) segmental artery. RA9 divides into lateral (RA9a) and basal (RA9b) subsegmental arteries. RA10 splits into two subsegmental rami, RA10a (laterobasal ramus) and RA10b (mediobasal ramus).

Left Pulmonary Arteries

Left Upper Lobe (Upper Division)

Whereas the segmental arterial pattern of the left upper lobe resembles that of the right lung (LA1, LA2, LA3), the chief difference lies in the greater number of separate subsegmental arteries. In most cases, the pulmonary artery arch gives off anterior arteries to the upper division bronchi (i.e.,

LA1, LA2, and LA3) together with an ascending subsegmental branch for the posterior segment (Figure 2-5). For practical purposes, we propose a slightly modified nomenclature for the anterior segment: the lateral and anterior subsegmental arteries of the upper division of the left upper lobe can be coded as LA2a and LA2b, respectively. In contrast to the common origin of the bronchial trunk for the apical and posterior segments of the upper lobe, the apical (LA1) and posterior (LA3) arteries usually arise independently of each other. This justifies the attribution of two separate numbers to those arteries; the subsegmental arteries are coded in a manner similar to that of the right upper lobe.

Left Upper Lobe (Lower Division)

After giving rise to branches supplying the upper division of the left upper lobe, the left pulmonary artery gives off branches to the lower division (or lingula). The prevailing pattern is a single lingular artery supplying both lingular segments via two separate segmental arteries (Figure 2-6). The superior lingular artery (LA4) divides into two subsegmental branches, a posterior ramus (LA4a) and an anterior ramus (LA4b). The inferior lingular artery (LA5) divides into a superior ramus (LA5a) and an inferior ramus (LA5b).

Left Lower Lobe

As on the right side, the left lower lobe pulmonary artery finally descends along the posterolateral side of the left

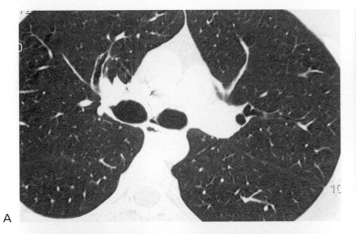

A

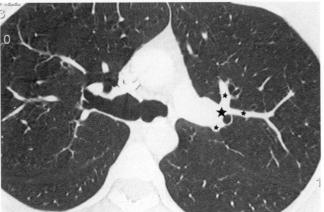

B

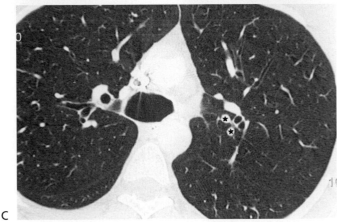

C

FIGURE 2-5. Left upper lobe (upper division) segmental vessels. **A:** CT scan at the level of the left main bronchus shows the origin of the segmental bronchi, namely a common trunk for the apical and posterior segments (LB1+3) and the anterior segmental bronchus (LB2) dividing into two subsegmental branches. **B:** CT scan obtained 10 mm above **A** shows the anterior segmental artery (LA2, *large plain star*) dividing into two subsegmental rami (*small anterior plain stars*) above their corresponding bronchi, and the origin of a common trunk for the apical and posterior segments (LA1+3, *small posterior star*) seen posterior to LB1+3. **C:** CT scan obtained 10 mm above **B** shows the medial location of the apical (LA1, *anterior plain star*) and posterior (LA3, *posterior plain star*) segmental arteries of the left upper lobe relative to their accompanying bronchi.

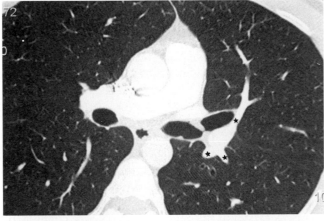

A

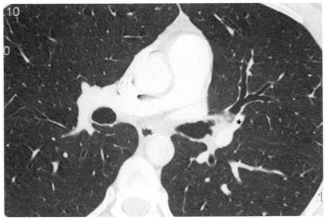

B

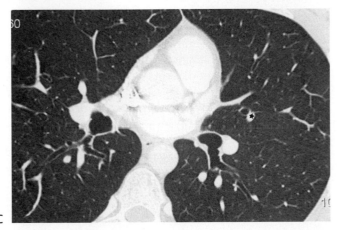

C

FIGURE 2-6. Left upper lobe (lower division) segmental vessels. **A:** CT scan at the level of the left upper lobe bronchus shows the superolateral location of the superior lingular artery (LA4) relative to its accompanying bronchus, seen 10 mm below on **B**. Note the identification of the origin of the inferior lingular artery (**B**, *plain star*) coursing lateral to its accompanying bronchus (**C**, *plain star*). The posterior plain stars on **A** point to two subsegmental rami of the apical segmental artery (LA6) of the left lower lobe.

21

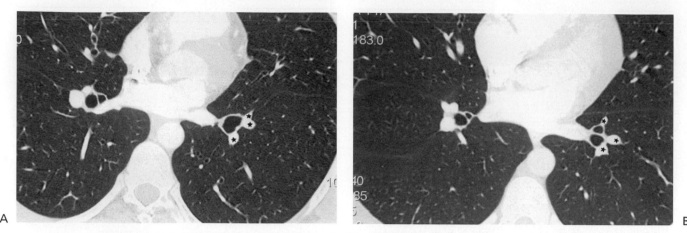

FIGURE 2-7. Left lower lobe segmental vessels. CT scans at the level of the common basal trunk dividing into the anteromedial basal bronchus (LB7+8) and a common trunk for the lateral basal and posterior basal bronchi (LB9+10) (**A** and **B**). Note the lateral position of the accompanying arteries, namely the paracardiac and anterior (LA7 and LA8, *anterior plain stars* on **A** and **B**) segmental arteries and the common trunk for the lateral basal and posterior basal segmental arteries (LA9+10, *posterior plain stars* on **A** and **B**) of the left lower lobe.

lower lobe bronchus. The first artery to the lower lobe, LA6, arises from its posterior wall above the level of the lingular branches (Figure 2-6). LA6 usually bifurcates into LA6a+b, a superomedial ramus, and LA6c, a lateral ramus. In the medial and anterior segments of the left lower lobe, two segmental branches (LA7 and LA8) usually arise from a common trunk (LA7+8) with two subsequent subsegmental branches (Figure 2-7). LA7 divides into an anterior ramus (LA7a) and a medial ramus (LA7b); LA8 divides into a lateral ramus (LA8a) and a basal ramus (LA8b). The artery to the lateral basal segment (LA9) most often originates from a common trunk with the artery of the posterior basal segment (LA10) (Figure 2-7). Each of these segmental arteries divides into a lateral ramus (LA9a, LA10a) and a basal ramus (LA9b, LA10b).

PULMONARY VEINS

According to Boyden (2), the naming of the veins attempts to relate the vein name to that of adjacent bronchi and arteries, thus indicating the segmental portions of the lung which are drained by a given vein (Table 2-1). While bronchi and arteries are adjacent to each other throughout the lungs, veins are located within intersegmental planes until they reach the hila. Arising from alveolar capillaries, pulmonary veins are first seen at the periphery of the secondary pulmonary lobule, while pulmonary arteries and bronchioles lie in the center of these units. They are then seen at the periphery of subsegments, segments, and lobes before reaching the left atrium.

In both lungs, there are two superior and inferior pulmonary veins. On the right, the superior pulmonary vein drains the upper and middle lobe while on the left, this vein drains the upper and lower divisions of the left upper lobe. The right and left inferior pulmonary veins drain the lower lobes. On each side, two veins are seen entering the left atrium.

Prevailing Pulmonary Venous Patterns

As the distribution of veins in the two lungs are similar, the description of the prevailing patterns will be limited to that of the right lung.

Right Upper Lobe

Three major veins are usually recognized, namely V1, the apical; V2, the anterior; and V3, the posterior. In most of the cases, V1 descends superficially beneath the pleura of the mediastinal surface of the right upper lobe. Its apical ramus (V1a) drains the apex while its anterior ramus (V1b) is intersegmental, separating the apical from the anterior segment. V2 is formed by the confluence of two mediastinal veins, a superior ramus (V2a), and an inferior ramus (V2b). The latter lies inferior to B2 and is intersegmental when the upper and middle lobes are fused. The largest segmental vein is V3, emerging at the angle of bifurcation between B2 and B3 before joining a superficial vein draining the interlobar aspect of this lobe (Figure 2-2). V1, V2, and V3 join to form a large vein (V1+2+3) in front of the right interlobar pulmonary artery. This vein represents the most anterior vascular structure of the right hilum (Figure 2-1).

Right Middle Lobe

The venous drainage of the right middle lobe is usually composed of a single trunk, V4+5, resulting from the confluence of V4 (the lateral vein) and V5 (the medial vein). This trunk courses below the right middle lobe bronchus before joining the superior pulmonary vein on the medial side of the right middle lobe bronchus (Figures 2-1 and 2-3). It should be noted that in approximately half of the cases, the right middle lobe is drained by two or more veins that terminate separately.

Right Lower Lobe

The right inferior pulmonary vein has two principal tributaries, a superior vein (V6) draining the apical segment of the lower lobe, and a common basal vein (V7+8+9+10) draining the basal segments (Figures 2-3 and 2-4). V6 runs caudad to B6 and cephalad and lateral to the posterior wall of the common basal bronchus before entering the right inferior pulmonary vein at a lower level on the medial side of B7. V6 is recognized in its intersegmental course as a tubular structure. Its medial part is seen as an oval or tubular density. The other tributaries of the common basal vein are usually easily identified, except for V7 because of its small size. V8 and V9 lie medial and behind B8 and B9, and V10 lies anterior to B10.

Pulmonary Venous Variants

Anatomic variants of the pulmonary venous return are more common than pulmonary artery variants. Their recognition is important because they can mimic a variety of congenital and acquired disorders and because their presence may be surgically relevant. These variants are related to an abnormal course of a pulmonary vein within the lung parenchyma and/or an unusual branching pattern when reaching the left atrium. Their hallmark is a normal drainage into the left atrium and thus, the absence of a left-to-right shunt.

Abnormal Course

1. The most common finding is a focal nodularity in close contact with the posterior wall of the bronchus intermedius, caused by a branch of the draining vein from the posterior segment of the right upper lobe (i.e., RV3) (6). Instead of running with RV1 between RB2 and RB3 near their origin, this branch runs behind the right bronchus intermedius before ending into the right inferior pulmonary vein or, less commonly, the right superior pulmonary vein or directly into the left atrium. A second cause of nodularity in the posterior wall of the bronchus intermedius can be a branch of the draining vein of the superior segment of the right lower lobe (RA6) (6). This normal nodularity should not be confused with expansive or infiltrative processes of the anatomic structures in close contact with the posterior wall of bronchus intermedius, such as abnormal thickening of peribronchovascular interstitium, neoplasms, or lymphadenopathy.

2. A right-sided pulmonary vein may have an abnormal course within the lung parenchyma mimicking a scimitar vein (i.e., an anomalous right-sided pulmonary venous drainage into the inferior vena cava) (see Chapter 7). The pseudoscimitar vein corresponds to an abnormally large pulmonary vein, producing a curved vascular shadow along the right-heart border on the chest radiograph, otherwise draining normally into the left atrium. This abnormal course can be isolated (7,8) or associated with various anomalies such as an azygos continuation of the inferior vena cava (9), a small-sized right lung (10), and a systemic arterial supply to the right lung (11). A pseudoscimitar vein can also be seen on the left side. Apart from the vertically oriented pseudoscimitar vein, a variety of sinuous pulmonary venous pathways can be seen on imaging studies (Figure 2-8).

Unusual Branching Patterns

1. The usual pulmonary venous return of the right middle lobe consists of one or two intersegmental veins, occasionally three, emptying into the superior pulmonary vein on the inferomedial side of the right middle lobe bronchus. According to Yamashita (4), in 4.8% of individuals, the right middle lobe pulmonary venous drainage empties into the right inferior pulmonary vein (Figure 2-9). When performing a right lower lobectomy, surgeons usually ligate and divide the right inferior pulmonary vein without exposure of its tributaries (12). This procedure can cause blockage of venous return from the middle lobe vein in patients who have this anatomic variation of middle lobe drainage, leading to severe pulmonary edema. This surgically significant variation also exits in the left lung, in which the lingular segment vein can empty into the left inferior pulmonary vein, a finding seen in 2.5% of subjects (4).

2. A single left (or less frequent, right) pulmonary vein may mimic pulmonary arteriovenous fistula, anomalous systemic arterial supply, or lung nodules on chest radiographs. CT angiography (CTA) allows noninvasive recognition of this silent anomaly, characterized by a large and tortuous pulmonary vein entering the left atrium in the conventional location of the superior (13) or inferior (14) pulmonary vein.

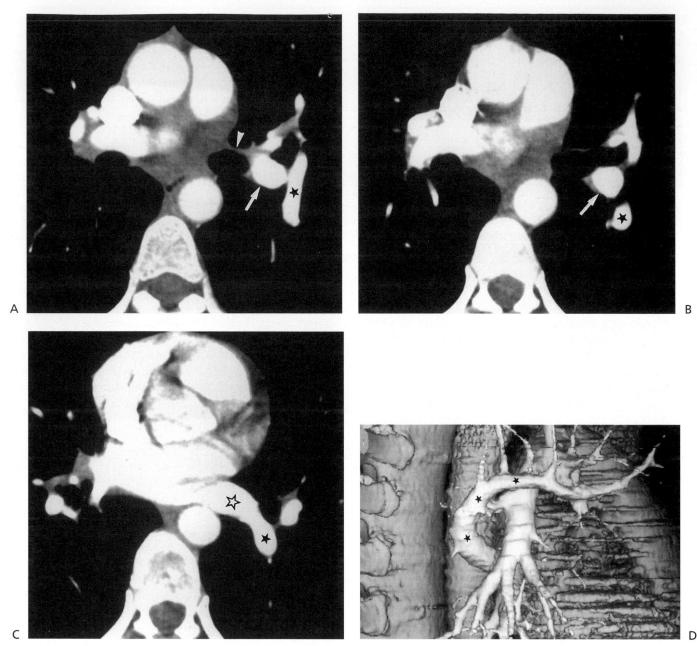

FIGURE 2-8. Abnormal course of the left superior pulmonary vein on cross-sectional images (**A**, **B**, and **C**) and three-dimensional, shaded-surface display (**D**) of the left pulmonary vasculature. Note the horizontal (**A** and **D**, *plain star*), then vertical (**B**, **C**, and **D**, *plain star*) course of the left superior pulmonary vein, in close contact with the left interlobar pulmonary artery (**A** and **B**, *arrow*) before joining the left inferior pulmonary vein (**C**, *open star*). The arrowhead on **A** points to the lack of a venous section in front of the left upper lobe bronchus, a CT feature highly suggestive of an abnormal course of the corresponding vessel.

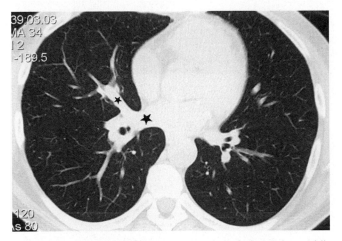

FIGURE 2-9. Unusual branching pattern of the right middle lobe venous return (*small plain star*), emptying into the right inferior pulmonary vein (*large plain star*).

SYSTEMIC VESSELS

Bronchial Arteries

The normal bronchial artery is a small vessel (2 mm or less in diameter) that arises directly from the descending thoracic aorta and supplies the airways, the esophagus, and lymph nodes (15,16). Recognition of bronchial arteries on CT scans requires enlargement of these vessels which occurs in a variety of cardiovascular and pulmonary diseases, such as acute or chronic pulmonary infections, pulmonary thromboembolism, and chronic obstructive lung disease (17,18). Awareness of the normal anatomy and course of the bronchial arteries allows recognition of hypertrophied bronchial arteries on CT. This recognition can be valuable information to the bronchoscopist prior to a planned transbronchial needle aspiration or biopsy, and to the interventional radiologist prior to embolization procedures in the clinical context of hemoptysis.

The most common anatomic presentation of the bronchial circulation consists of a single right bronchial artery arising from an intercostobronchial trunk and two left bronchial arteries. Bronchial arteries usually originate from the descending aorta at the level of the left main bronchus. The right intercostobronchial trunk arises from the medial, anteromedial, or posteromedial aortic wall. The left bronchial arteries arise from the anterior, anteromedial, or anterolateral aortic wall. However, atherosclerosis results in medial rotation of the descending thoracic aorta. Therefore in older individuals, the left bronchial artery ostia can be displaced medially and the right bronchial artery ostia can be displaced posteriorly.

The right intercostobronchial trunk commonly takes an initial vertical or oblique course cephalad and to the right after it arises in the retroesophageal space within the mediastinum after it arises from the aorta. The right bronchial artery often makes a hairpin turn at the aortic arch level and is directed caudally toward the right hilar area, coursing behind the posterior wall of the right main bronchus and the bronchus intermedius. The most common locations of hypertrophied right bronchial arteries are the retrotracheal area, the retroesophageal area, and the posterior walls of the right main bronchus and bronchus intermedius where they can be observed as dots or lines of increased attenuation on CT angiograms (18). Two left-sided bronchial arteries are commonly observed. Near their origin, they are situated in the aorticopulmonary window. The upper left bronchial artery has a more horizontal course within the mediastinum, as it passes forward beside the lateral wall of the esophagus and crosses the peribronchial space from the left main bronchus level toward the left hilum. Hypertrophied left bronchial arteries are often found in the aorticopulmonary window and the anterior and posterior walls of the left main bronchus.

CTA can also help demonstrate a common trunk to the right and left bronchial arteries arising from the anterior wall of the descending thoracic aorta as well as an ectopic origin of the bronchial arteries, seen in 10% of subjects. The most common abnormal origins of the bronchial arteries are concavity of the aortic arch, the subclavian arteries, or the brachiocephalic trunk.

Thoracic Outlet Vessels

CTA has become a valuable tool for the diagnosis of arterial and venous compression at the level of the thoracic outlet. A precise knowledge of the normal CT anatomy of this region and its modification with hyperabduction of the arm is essential for proper interpretation of CT findings in these syndromes (19–21) (Figures 2-10 and 2-11).

The subclavian vein is always situated anterior to the subclavian artery. On CT, the venous sections are consistently of greater diameter (average, 12 mm) than the arterial sections (average, 7 mm). In the neutral position, the subclavian vein is the only vascular structure present at the level of the largest portion of the costoclavicular space, identified in only 12% to 17% of female subjects and 7% to 11% of male subjects. After the postural maneuver, spiral CT enables the demonstration of a posteroanterior displacement of the subclavian vascular bundle, identified in the costoclavicular space in 75% of female subjects and 71% of male subjects. It is noteworthy that the subclavian artery and vein are identified in the costosubclavian space in 83% and 67% of females, respectively, and in 79% of males (19). These anatomic findings allow understanding of the potential pathophysiologic importance of the subclavius muscle in vascular compression at the level of the costoclavicular space. At the level of the subcoracoid tunnel, the neurovascular bundle passes beneath the coracoid process deep to the tendon of the smaller pectoral muscle in patients in the neutral position. During hyperabduction, the costocoracoid ligament restricts the space anteriorly,

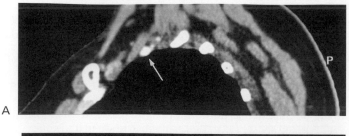

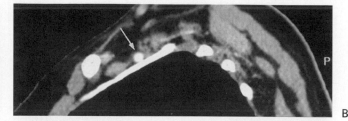

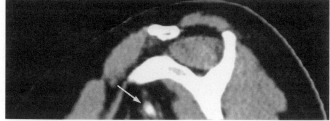

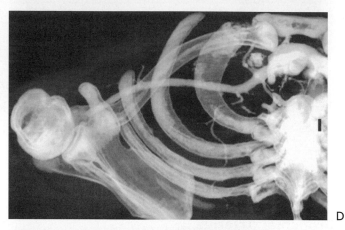

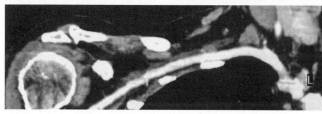

FIGURE 2-10. CT angiography (CTA) of the right thoracic outlet illustrating a normal CT angiogram in the neutral position. **A, B,** and **C:** Sagittal reformations, spaced 7 mm apart, depict the right subclavian artery behind the anterior scalene muscle (**A**, *arrow*) at the level of the costoclavicular space (**B**, *arrow*) and at the level of the subcoracoid tunnel (**C**, *arrow*). **D:** Volume-rendered image (vertical view) of the right thoracic outlet enables the concurrent depiction of arterial and bony structures. The transparency given to the bony structures allows an accurate analysis of the diameter of the subclavian and axillary arteries along their length. **E:** Curved reformation obtained along the main axis of the subclavian and axillary arteries demonstrating their normal caliber.

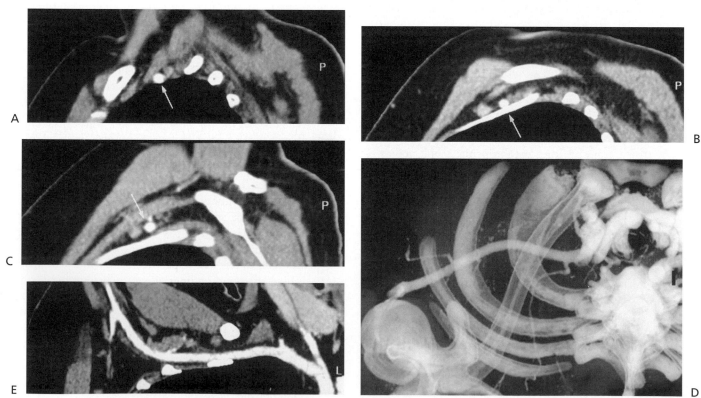

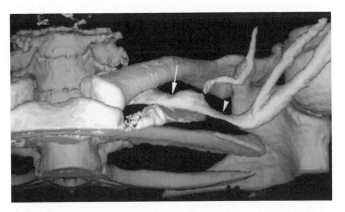

FIGURE 2-12. CT venogram of the left thoracic outlet illustrating dynamically-induced venous flattening at the level of the costoclavicular space (*arrow*) and subcoracoid tunnel (*arrowhead*) in an asymptomatic subject.

and the vascular bundle is reported to be bowed around the coracoid process, a statement contradicted by CT findings showing the vascular bundle located 20 to 40 mm below the anterior extremity of the coracoid process (19,22). The role of hypertrophied muscles enclosing the vascular bundle at the level of the subcoracoid tunnel can be suggested by the CT demonstration of narrow spaces between the posterior border of the smaller pectoral muscle and the anterosuperior chest wall (19). These findings could help account for the high frequency of false-positive results reported in healthy subjects after postural maneuvers (23–27).

Understanding of dynamically induced thoracic outlet venous flattening is also essential for confident assessment of abnormal venous compression in symptomatic patients. In 43 subjects referred for suspicion of unilateral thoracic venous compression, functional anatomy of the asymptomatic side was evaluated on contiguous sagittal reformations and volume-rendered images (21). In the neutral position, venous flattening was depicted at the level of the prescalenic space in 9% of cases, in the costoclavicular space in 30% of cases, and in the subcoracoid tunnel in 11% of cases. After postural maneuver, venous flattening was found in 81% of cases in the prescalenic space, 91% of cases in the costoclavicular space, and 19% of cases in the subcoracoid tunnel in the absence of abnormal narrowness of these anatomic compartments. These findings led the authors to suggest that venous flattening is a frequent finding on

dynamic spiral CT venograms of the thoracic outlet in asymptomatic subjects (Figure 2-12). In addition, they represent strong arguments in favor of the administration of contrast material with the patient's arm alongside the body in order to obtain high-quality CT angiograms.

REFERENCES

1. Williams PL, Warwick R, eds. *Gray's anatomy*, 36th ed. London: Churchill Livingstone, 1980:667.
2. Boyden EA. *Segmental anatomy of the lungs*. New York: McGraw-Hill, 1955.
3. Jackson CL, Huber JF. Correlated applied anatomy of the bronchial tree and lungs with a system of nomenclature. *Dis Chest* 1943;9:319–326.
4. Yamashita H. *Roentgenologic anatomy of the lung*. Stuttgart: Thieme and Tokyo: Igaku-Shoin Ltd., 1978.
5. Ghaye B, Szapiro D, Delannoy V, et al. How far does multidetector CT allow analysis of peripheral pulmonary arteries? *Radiology* 2001;219:629–636.
6. Kim JS, Choi D, Lee KS. CT of the bronchus intermedius: frequency and cause of a nodule in the posterior wall on normal scans. *Am J Roentgenol* 1995;165:1349–1352.
7. Takeda SI, Imachi T, Arimitsu K, et al. Two cases of scimitar variant. *Chest* 1994;105:292–293.
8. Alfke H, Wagner HJ, Klose KJ. A case of an anomalous pulmonary vein of the right middle lobe. *Cardiovasc Intervent Radiol* 1995;18:406–409.
9. Herer B, Jaubert F, Delaisements C, et al. Scimitar sign with normal pulmonary venous drainage and anomalous inferior vena cava. *Thorax* 1988;43:651–652.
10. Goodman LR, Jamshidi A, Hipona FA. Meandering right pulmonary vein simulating the scimitar syndrome. *Chest* 1972;64:510–512.
11. Cukier A, Kavakama J, Ribeiro Teixeira L, et al. Scimitar sign with normal pulmonary venous drainage and systemic arterial supply. Scimitar syndrome or bronchopulmonary sequestration? *Chest* 1994;105:294–295.
12. Sugimoto S, Izumiyama O, Yamashita A, et al. Anatomy of inferior pulmonary vein should be clarified in lower lobectomy. *Ann Thorac Surg* 1998;66:1799–1800.
13. Tretheway DG, Francis GS, MacNeil DJ, et al. Single left pulmonary vein with normal pulmonary venous drainage: a roentgenographic curiosity. *Am J Cardiol* 1974;34:237–239.
14. Benfield JR, Gots RE, Mills D. Anomalous single left pulmonary vein mimicking a parenchymal nodule. *Chest* 1971;59:101–103.
15. Butler J. *The bronchial circulation*. New York: Marcel Dekker Inc, 1992.
16. Sjoerd A, Botenga J. *Selective bronchial and intercostal arteriography*. HE Stenfert Kroese NV, Leiden, 1970.
17. Furuse M, Saito K, Kunieda E, et al. Bronchial arteries: CT

FIGURE 2-11. CT angiography (CTA) of the right thoracic outlet illustrating a normal CT angiogram after postural maneuver (same patient as shown in Figure 2-10). **A, B,** and **C:** Sagittal reformations, spaced 7 mm apart, depict the right subclavian artery behind the anterior scalene muscle (**A,** *arrow*) at the level of the costoclavicular space (B, *arrow*) and at the level of the subcoracoid tunnel (C, *arrow*). **D:** Volume-rendered image (vertical view) of the right thoracic outlet enables assessment of normal caliber of the right subclavian and axillary arteries. Note the modification in the arterial curvature after postural maneuver, compared with Figure 2-10D. **E:** Curved reformation obtained along the main axis of the subclavian and axillary arteries demonstrating their normal caliber after postural maneuver.

demonstration with arteriographic correlation. *Radiology* 1987; 162:393–398.

18. Song JW, Im JG, Shim YS, et al. Hypertrophied bronchial artery at thin-section CT in patients with bronchiectasis: correlation with CT angiographic findings. *Radiology* 1998; 208:187–191.

19. Remy-Jardin M, Doyen J, Remy J, et al. Functional anatomy of the thoracic outlet: evaluation with spiral CT. *Radiology* 1997; 205:843–851.

20. Matsumura JS, Rilling WS, Pearce WH, et al. Helical computed tomography of the normal thoracic outlet. *J Vasc Surg* 1997;26: 776–783.

21. Mastora I, Masson P, Delannoy V, et al. Thoracic outlet venous compression during postural maneuver: prevalence in asymptomatic subjects on spiral CT venograms. *Eur Radiol* 2001;11(S): 155.

22. Luoma A, Nelems B. Thoracic outlet syndrome: thoracic surgery perspective. *Neurosurg Clin North Am* 1991;2:187–226.

23. Falconer MA, Weddell G. Costoclavicular compression of the subclavius artery and vein: relation to the scalenus anticus syndrome. *Lancet* 1983;2:539–545.

24. Telford ED, Mottershead S. Pressure at the cervicobrachial junction. *J Bone Joint Surg* 1948;30:249.

25. Serratrice B, Schiano A. Sur la valeur de certaines manoeuvres d'exploration clinique du hile neurovasculaire du membre supérieur. *N Presse Med* 1978;43:3932–3933.

26. Gergoudis R, Barnes RM. Thoracic outlet arterial compression: prevalence in normal persons. *Angiology* 1980;31:538–541.

27. Hachulla E, Camillieri G, Fournier C, et al. Etude clinique, vélocimétrique et radiologique de la traversée thoracobrachiale chez 95 sujets témoins: limites physiologiques et incidences pratiques. *Rev Med Int* 1990;11:19–24.

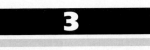

THORACIC AORTA

CONGENITAL ANOMALIES

Aberrant Right Subclavian Artery
Right Aortic Arch
Double Aortic Arch
Coarctation
Pseudocoarctation

ANEURYSM AND PSEUDOANEURYSM

Atherosclerotic Aortic Aneurysm
Medial Degeneration
Mycotic Aneurysm

AORTIC DISSECTION

INTRAMURAL HEMATOMA

PENETRATING ATHEROSCLEROTIC ULCER

AORTITIS

Infectious Aortitis
Takayasu's Arteritis
Giant Cell Arteritis

TRAUMA

POSTOPERATIVE EVALUATION

AORTIC ENDOVASCULAR STENT GRAFTS

CONGENITAL ANOMALIES

Congenital anomalies of the aorta and great vessels occur in 0.5% to 3% of the population (1). The most common anomalies seen in adults are a left aortic arch with aberrant right subclavian artery, right aortic arch, double aortic arch, coarctation, and pseudocoarctation.

Aberrant Right Subclavian Artery

This is the most common congenital abnormality of the aortic arch vessels being seen in 0.4% to 2.3% of the population (2,3). The aberrant right subclavian artery originates not as the first branch of the aortic arch, as is normally the case, but as the last branch, distal to the left subclavian artery. It courses cephalad from left to right obliquely across the mediastinum posterior to the trachea and esophagus. In up to 60% of cases, the proximal portion of the aberrant subclavian artery is associated with an outpouching at its origin, a finding known as the diverticulum of Kommerell (2,4). The size and configuration of this diverticulum are variable (2). Occasionally, the diameter of the diverticulum may approximate the diameter of the aortic arch (5). Ath-

erosclerotic changes and intramural thrombus formation within the diverticulum are relatively common in older adults (Figure 3-1). Aneurysm formation can also occur (Figure 3-2).

The aberrant subclavian artery seldom causes clinical symptoms. Occasionally, it may result in compression of the esophagus and trachea leading to dysphagia and dyspnea. Compression of adjacent structures occurs most commonly in older adults when the aberrant subclavian artery becomes tortuous and ectatic (1). Symptoms also occur when there is an associated right rather than a left ligamentum arteriosum resulting in a vascular ring. In the latter circumstance, the trachea is encircled by the retroesophageal aberrant subclavian artery, right ligamentum arteriosum, left aortic arch, and right and main pulmonary arteries. The diagnosis of aberrant subclavian artery can be readily made on CT (Figures 3-1 and 3-2).

Right Aortic Arch

A right aortic arch occurs in approximately 0.1% to 0.2% of the population (6). There are two main types of right aortic arch anomaly: right arch with mirror-image branch-

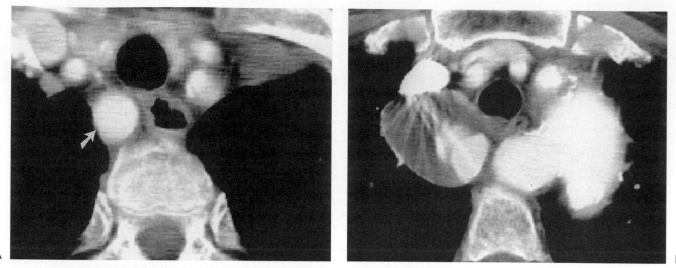

A   B

FIGURE 3-1. Aneurysmal dilation of an aberrant right subclavian artery. CT angiogram image (**A**) shows ectatic aberrant right subclavian artery (*arrow*) in a 74-year-old woman. CT angiogram image at the level of the aortic arch (**B**) shows diverticulum of Kommerell and aberrant right sub-clavian artery coursing from left to right behind the esophagus and trachea. Note calcification in the wall of the aorta and diverticulum of Kommerell (*curved arrows*). Moderate intramural thrombus is seen along the wall of the aberrant subclavian artery.

ing and right arch with aberrant left subclavian artery (Box 3-1).

The right aortic arch with mirror-image branching is the anatomic counterpart of the left aortic arch. In this anomaly, the great arteries originate from the right aortic arch in the following order: left innominate, right carotid, and right subclavian. The descending aorta is usually right-sided (1). Over 96% of patients with this anomaly have associated congenital heart disease, usually cyanotic (1). The most common types of congenital heart disease associated with a right aortic arch and mirror-image branching are tetralogy of Fallot, persistent truncus arteriosus, pulmonary artery atresia with ventricular septal defect (VSD), double outlet right ventricle, and transposition of the great arteries (7,8).

The right aortic arch with mirror-image branching is the most common right arch anomaly seen in children (1). Because of the associated cardiac disease, the diagnosis is usually made in infancy or early childhood. Adults present-

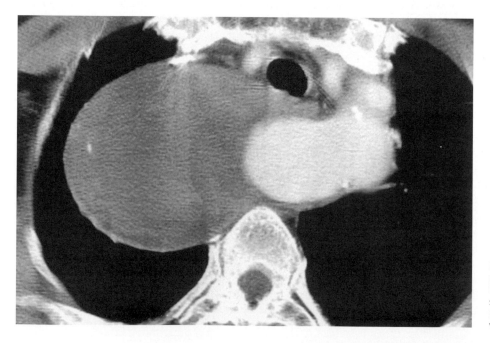

FIGURE 3-2. Aneurysm of aberrant right subclavian artery. CT angiogram image shows aneurysm of aberrant right subclavian artery with a large amount of intramural thrombus in a 75-year-old woman.

BOX 3-1. RIGHT AORTIC ARCH

A. Mirror-image branching
- 96% have congenital heart disease
- Tetralogy, truncus, pulmonary atresia, double-outlet ventricle, transposition
- Seen most commonly in children

B. Right arch with aberrant left subclavian artery
- 12% have congenital heart disease
- Most commonly tetralogy of Fallot
- May result in a vascular ring
- Seen most commonly in adults
- Usually asymptomatic in adults

ing with this anomaly usually have no associated congenital heart disease (1).

The most common right aortic arch anomaly seen in adults is the right arch with aberrant left subclavian artery (Figure 3-3). In this anomaly, the great arteries originate from the right aortic arch in the following order: left carotid, right carotid, right subclavian, and aberrant left subclavian. The aberrant left subclavian artery is often associated with a diverticulum of Kommerell. The majority of patients are asymptomatic. Approximately 12% of patients have associated congenital heart disease, most commonly

tetralogy of Fallot (1,7). In the majority of cases, the ligamentum arteriosum is on the right. A left ligamentum arteriosum results in a vascular ring, the trachea being encircled by the ligamentum, left pulmonary artery, aberrant left subclavian artery, and right aortic arch. The diagnosis of the various forms of right aortic arch can be readily made on contrast-enhanced spiral CT.

Double Aortic Arch

A double aortic arch occurs in 0.05% to 0.3% of the population (1,9). In this anomaly, both right and left aortic arches are present. Usually both arches are patent, the right arch giving rise to the right carotid and subclavian arteries and the left arch giving rise to the left carotid and subclavian arteries (10). Occasionally, a portion of the left arch is atretic. The arches may be symmetric but usually the right is larger and extends more cephalad and posteriorly than the left. The aorta usually descends on the left side and the ductus is on the left as well (9).

A double aortic arch is the most common cause of complete vascular ring (9). The symptoms are due to tracheal and esophageal compression and depend on the tightness of the vascular ring. The majority of patients present with stridor or dysphagia and are diagnosed within the first 6

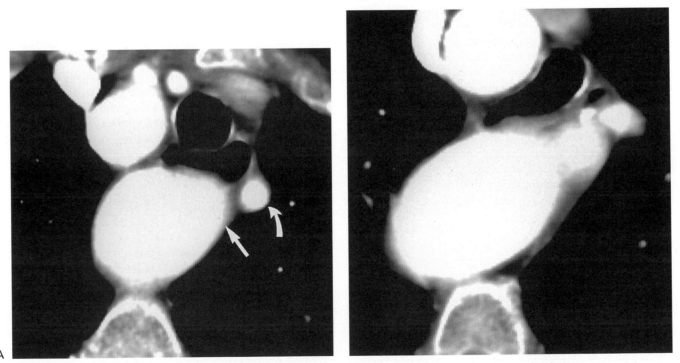

A   B

FIGURE 3-3. Right aortic arch with aberrant left subclavian artery. **A:** CT angiography demonstrates right aortic arch and a focal outpouching (diverticulum of Kommerell) (*straight arrow*) at the origin of the aberrant left subclavian artery (*curved arrow*). Also note extrinsic compression of the trachea and esophagus between the ectatic right aortic arch and the aberrant right subclavian artery and dilation of the esophagus above the level of the diverticulum of Kommerell. **B:** Image immediately caudad to **A** demonstrates continuity between the diverticulum of Kommerell and the aberrant left subclavian artery.

months of life (9). Occasionally, the abnormality is found incidentally in an asymptomatic adult.

In the vast majority of cases, CT angiography (CTA) allows diagnosis of a double aortic arch and distinction from other congenital arch anomalies. However, it may be difficult or impossible to distinguish a double aortic arch with an atretic segment between the left common carotid and subclavian arteries from a right aortic arch with an aberrant left subclavian artery and left ligamentum arteriosum (9,11).

Coarctation

Coarctation of the aorta is a malformation characterized by focal narrowing of the aorta, usually at or below the region of the ligamentum or ductus arteriosus. It can be classified into two main types: infantile and adult (Box 3-2).

The infantile type of coarctation is associated with tubular hypoplasia of the aortic arch or descending aorta. This form is often associated with congenital heart disease, the most common associated abnormalities consisting of patent ductus arteriosus, VSD, hypoplastic left heart, and transposition of the great vessels (12,13). The infantile type usually presents in the first 6 months of life (1).

The adult type of coarctation typically presents later in life, although it may also be seen in infants and children (1). It is often discovered during diagnostic evaluation of hypertension or of a coexistent cardiac anomaly, the most common being a bicuspid aortic valve (14). The characteristic clinical finding of coarctation consists of increased blood pressure in the upper extremities and decreased pressure in the lower extremities. In patients with an aberrant right subclavian artery (3% to 4% of cases), the right arm pressure may be lower than the left (1).

In patients with the adult type of coarctation, the ascending aorta is often enlarged and the descending aorta immediately distal to the coarctation shows poststenotic dilation. This results in a characteristic contour abnormality on the chest radiograph, known as the "3 sign," the indentation corresponding to focal narrowing at the level of

the ligamentum arteriosum (1). Scalloping of the undersurface of the ribs (rib notching) is usually present in adults. Rib notching in coarctation is bilateral and involves the inferior aspects of the third to ninth ribs. The notching is due to erosion by the intercostal arteries, which have increased pulsation and are dilated secondary to collateral circulation.

The diagnosis of coarctation, identification of the site, and severity of coarctation and tubular hypoplasia, can be readily made with CTA, particularly with the use of surface shading and maximum intensity projection (MIP) three-dimensional reconstructions (1). Becker and colleagues assessed the reliability of CTA in the assessment of 18 patients with suspected or surgically proven coarctation (15). The patients ranged from 4 months to 20 years of age (mean, 12 years). In addition to the transverse sections, three-dimensional reconstructions such as shaded-surface display (SSD) and MIP were used to determine the diameters of the coarctation, pre- and poststenotic aorta and to visualize the collateral vessels. There was no significant difference between the diameters derived from CTA and angiography in the three aortic regions. However, the degree of aortic stenosis as measured from the MIP images correlated poorly with the blood pressure gradient across the stenosis. SSD images allowed visualization of the collateral vessels in the majority of cases. The internal mammary arteries were seen on SSD images in 16 of the 18 patients and the posterior intercostal arteries and their communication with the descending aorta in 13 patients. The authors concluded that CTA with three-dimensional reconstruction allows reliable noninvasive assessment of the severity of coarctation and the visualization of collateral vessels. An advantage of CTA over angiography is that it can be performed following a single bolus injection of contrast medium while several injections are required for angiography. However, angiography allows acquisition of additional information such as pressure gradient and oxygen saturation data (15).

Pseudocoarctation

Pseudocoarctation is a localized kink in the proximal descending aorta that results from a congenital elongation of the aortic arch and resultant redundancy (16). Occasionally, a similar appearance may be seen in older adult patients with an ectatic, tortuous aortic arch (17). Unlike coarctation, pseudocoarctation does not result in any demonstrable obstruction (18). The arterial pressures in the arms and legs are similar (less than 25 mm Hg difference) (19).

Pseudocoarctation is usually asymptomatic. Occasionally, it may result in aneurysm formation or dissection and may rupture (1,20,21).

The radiologic appearance consists of an elongated aortic arch associated with a kink in the proximal descending aorta. The configuration resembles the "3 sign" of coarctation.

BOX 3-2. COARCTATION

A. Infantile form
- Tubular hypoplasia of arch or descending aorta
- Often associated with congenital heart disease
- Patent ductus arteriousus, VSD, hypoplastic left heart
- Usually presents in early infancy

B. Adult form
- Focal narrowing at level of ligamentum arteriousum
- Seldom associated with congenital heart disease
- Usually seen in older children and young adults
- Hypertension in upper extremities
- Decreased pressure and pulses in lower extremities
- Diagnosis readily confirmed with CT angiography

VSD, ventricular septal defect.

Although pseudocoarctation is usually an isolated finding, it is associated with a slightly increased incidence of congenital heart disease, particularly patent ductus arteriosus, VSD, and bicuspid aortic valve (1,22,23). Occasionally, patients may have the kink of pseudocoarctation, focal narrowing, and collateral vessels (i.e., features of both pseudocoarctation and coarctation) (24). Because pseudocoarctation and coarctation involve similar portions of the aorta and are associated with similar congenital cardiac malformations, it is controversial whether they are distinct entities or represent different degrees of severity of the same process (1).

ANEURYSM AND PSEUDOANEURYSM

Aortic aneurysm is defined as irreversible dilation of the aorta to twice its normal diameter with all components of the aortic wall being present in the dilated segment (25,26). Pseudoaneurysm (false aneurysm) is a focal dilation of the aorta that does not contain one of the layers, usually the media.

The average diameter of the proximal ascending aorta in normal individuals is 3.6 cm (range, 2.4 to 4.7 cm), the proximal descending aorta is 2.6 cm (range, 1.6 to 3.7 cm), and the distal descending aorta is 2.4 cm (range, 1.4 to 3.3 cm) (27). Aortic diameters are larger in men than women and increase with age (26). Because of the variable size of the aorta and because surgery is seldom contemplated for aortas of smaller size, for practical purposes, an aortic aneurysm may be considered present when the aorta measures 5 cm or more in diameter (17).

By far the most common cause of aortic aneurysm is atherosclerosis (28,29). Other causes include cystic medial necrosis (as seen in Marfan's disease and Ehlers-Danlos syndrome), aortitis (infective and inflammatory), previous surgery, hemodynamic alterations (from aortic stenosis or regurgitation), and trauma (17,26). Although trauma can result in true aneurysms, usually it results in pseudoaneurysm formation. Similarly, surgery and aortitis may result in true or false aneurysm formation. Other causes of pseudoaneurysm are infection and penetrating atherosclerotic ulcers (26).

Atherosclerotic Aortic Aneurysm

The majority of thoracic aortic aneurysms due to atherosclerosis are located in the distal arch or descending thoracic aorta (Box 3-3). However, aneurysmal involvement is often diffuse or multifocal. Close to 30% of patients with thoracic aneurysms have concomitant aneurysm of the infrarenal abdominal aorta (25,26). The average age at presentation is 60 years and there is a 3-to-1 male preponderance (17,28).

In one investigation of 230 patients with thoracic aortic aneurysms, the average diameter at presentation was 5.2 cm

---

BOX 3-3. ATHEROSCLEROTIC AORTIC ANEURYSM

- Diameter of aorta greater than 5 cm
- Usually involves distal arch or descending aorta
- Usually fusiform
- Average growth rate 0.42 cm/y
- Surgery recommended for ascending aortic aneurysms greater than 5.5 cm and descending aneurysms greater than 6.5 cm
- *Complications:* Rupture, dissection, aortic regurgitation, distal embolization, compression of adjacent structures, erosion into lungs, bronchi, or esophagus
- Diagnosis readily made on spiral CT or CT angiography

---

and the median diameter at time of dissection or rupture was 6.0 cm for ascending and 7.2 cm for descending aortic aneurysms (30). In a longitudinal study of 82 thoracic aneurysms, the average growth rate was 0.42 cm per year (31). Approximately 40% to 75% of individuals with untreated aortic aneurysms die from aortic rupture (17,32). The 5-year survival rate of patients with aortic aneurysms who do not undergo surgical repair is approximately 20% compared to a survival of approximately 60% for surgically treated patients (17,33). In one investigation of 136 patients who underwent surgical repair of thoracic aortic aneurysms, the mortality rate for elective surgery was 9% and that for emergency surgery 22% (30). Because the risk of rupture increases with size and because of the high mortality rate associated with rupture, surgery is recommended for ascending aortic aneurysms measuring 5.5 cm or more in diameter and aneurysms of the descending aorta measuring 6.5 cm or more in diameter (30).

Other complications of aortic aneurysm include aortic dissection, aortic regurgitation, distal embolization, compression of adjacent structures, and, occasionally, erosion into the lungs, bronchi, or esophagus. Compression of the left recurrent laryngeal nerve can result in vocal cord paresis or paralysis. Compression of the left main bronchus can cause wheezing, recurrent infection, or atelectasis of the left lower lobe or the entire left lung. Aneurysms not compressing adjacent structures are often asymptomatic or associated with nonspecific symptoms such as vague chest pain, transient ischemic attacks, and syncope. Rupture results in chest and/or back pain and hypotension.

Atherosclerotic aortic aneurysms are usually fusiform in shape, contain a mural thrombus, and approximately 85% have foci of calcification in the thrombus or aortic wall (Figure 3-4) (26,34,35). Occasionally, atherosclerotic aneurysms can be focal and mimic a posttraumatic or mycotic aneurysm or pseudoaneurysm (Figure 3-5) Evaluation of the presence of focal or diffuse aortic dilation and length of aneurysm can be readily made on unenhanced CT scans (36). Unenhanced scans are required for assessment of the presence and extent of mural calcification (36). However, intravenous contrast is usually

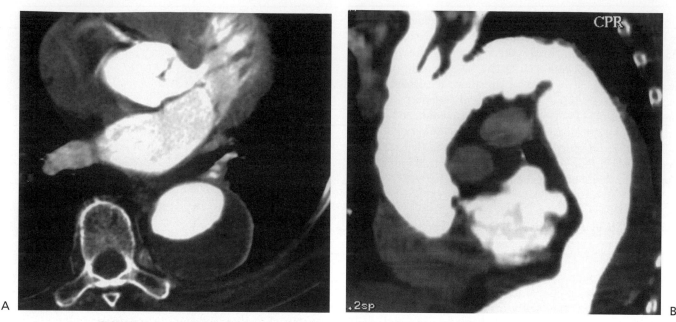

FIGURE 3-4. Atherosclerotic aortic aneurysm. Transverse (**A**) and sagittal reformatted (**B**) CT angiogram images demonstrate fusiform aneurysm of the descending thoracic aorta containing a large intramural thrombus in an 87-year-old woman. (Case courtesy of Dr. Ann Leung, Stanford University School of Medicine, Palo Alto, CA.)

required to differentiate between the patent lumen and a mural thrombus (36).

CTA allows assessment of aortic size, proximal and distal extent of an aortic aneurysm, and presence of a thrombus or other mural abnormalities and is usually the only imaging modality required prior to surgery (Figures 3-4 through 3-6). Techniques of reconstruction include multi-

planar reconstruction (MPR) images, angiographic projection MIP images, CT angioscopy, and true three-dimensional SSD images (37–39). Quint and colleagues assessed the diagnostic accuracy of CTA with and without multiplanar reconstructions in 49 patients with thoracic aortic disease (36 aneurysms, 6 penetrating ulcers, 5 dissections, and 2 pseudoaneurysms) (38). The overall diagnostic accuracy

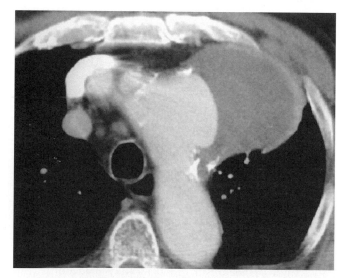

FIGURE 3-5. Atherosclerotic aortic aneurysm. CT angiogram image shows saccular aneurysm of the aortic arch. The aneurysm contains a large intramural thrombus. The patient was an 87-year-old man.

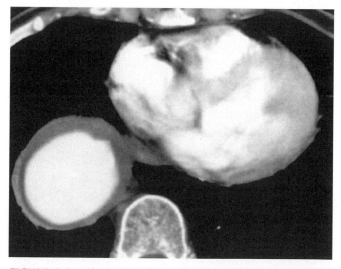

FIGURE 3-6. Atherosclerotic aortic aneurysm. CT angiography demonstrates aneurysm of the descending thoracic aorta. Note extensive intramural thrombus formation. The aorta was tortuous and elongated leading to displacement of the descending aorta to the right of the lower thoracic spine.

of CTA was 92% (45 of 49 patients). In all patients, aortic aneurysms were correctly identified on the transverse CT images. Multiplanar reconstructions did not change the diagnosis in any patient, but allowed better assessment of aneurysmal extension into the arch in two patients. Furthermore, multiplanar reconstructions allow depiction of the extent of aneurysms in a format that is more familiar to the surgeon (38). Kimura and associates have shown that CTA with SSD and, particularly, CT angioscopy, are superior to conventional axial images for assessing the relationship of aortic aneurysms to the origin of arch vessels (39). In a study of 12 patients with distal arch aneurysms, these authors found that the relationship between the aneurysm and the origin of the left subclavian artery was correctly identified on transverse images in 5 (42%) patients, on three-dimensional reconstructions in 9 patients (75%), and on three-dimensional endoscopic renderings in 11 (92%) patients (39).

CTA data allow accurate objective measurement of aortic cross-sectional and longitudinal dimensions and of aortic curvature (40). Objective measurements may prove to be particularly helpful in planning for endovascular stent-graft placement, a technique that is being increasingly used in the treatment of patients who have high surgical risk (41). The main limitations of CTA are the inability to adequately image the origin of the coronary arteries and the intercostal arteries that supply the spinal cord (T8-L1) (26).

Acute or impending contained rupture results in a high attenuation crescent of blood within a mural thrombus ("crescent sign") (42,43). Another CT finding of a contained rupture is the "draped aorta" sign (44). This sign is considered present when the posterior aspect of the aortic wall cannot be identified and the aorta follows the vertebral contour (44). Rupture can result in mediastinal hematoma, hemopericardium, and hemothorax. CTA may also demonstrate deformities of the enhanced lumen, and, occasionally, active extravasation of contrast (26).

Medial Degeneration

Medial degeneration, as the name implies, is an entity characterized by degenerative changes of the elastic tissue and smooth muscle of the aortic media (Box 3-4). Degeneration of the media is the most common cause of aneurysm of the ascending aorta (36,45). It can occur in association with

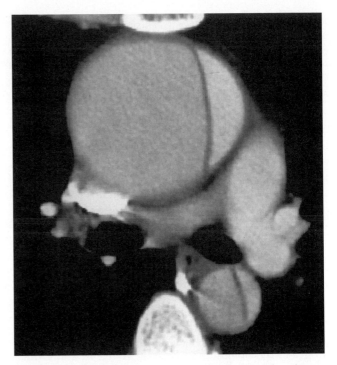

FIGURE 3-7. Medial degeneration. CT angiography demonstrates aneurysmal dilation of the ascending aorta and an intimal flap in the ascending and descending aorta. Note decreased enhancement of the false lumen. The patient was a 42-year-old man with idiopathic medial degeneration of the aorta.

genetically transmitted disorders, such as Marfan's syndrome or Ehlers-Danlos syndrome, or it may be idiopathic. In patients with genetically transmitted disorders, the onset of medial degeneration occurs earlier in life and progresses more rapidly than in the idiopathic form (36).

Cardiovascular abnormalities occur in the vast majority of patients with Marfan's syndrome and account for more than 90% of deaths (46). The most common abnormalities are aortic aneurysm, aortic dissection, and aortic and mitral regurgitation (Figure 3-7). The aneurysmal dilation typically involves mainly the aortic root and decreases at higher levels of the ascending aorta; the aortic arch is usually normal (36). Aortic valve regurgitation occurs in approximately 80% of patients with an aortic root diameter greater than 5 cm and in 100% of patients with a diameter greater than 6 cm (36).

Mycotic Aneurysm

A mycotic aneurysm is an aneurysm caused by nonsyphilitic infection of the arterial wall (36). The term is misleading because the infection is rarely fungal in etiology. Furthermore, infectious aortitis does not necessarily lead to aneurysm formation (see "Aortitis," later in this chapter). The most common causes of mycotic aneurysm are nonhemolytic streptococcus, *Streptococcus pneumoniae*, and

---

BOX 3-4. MEDIAL DEGENERATION

- Degenerative changes of elastic tissue and smooth muscle of aortic media
- Associated with Marfan's and Ehlers-Danlos syndromes
- May be idiopathic
- *Complications:* Aortic aneurysm, dissection, aortic regurgitation, mitral regurgitation
- Most common cause of aneurysm of ascending aorta

staphylococcus organisms (36). The infection usually is secondary to hematogenous spread; however contiguous extension may occur. The latter may be seen in bacterial endocarditis and in tuberculosis, which can extend from the adjacent spine or lymph nodes (36,47).

Factors that predispose to the development of mycotic aneurysms include atherosclerosis, intravenous drug abuse, trauma, surgical manipulation, arterial catheterization, bacterial endocarditis, and impaired immunity (36,48). The majority of mycotic aneurysms are true aneurysms, although false aneurysms can occur (36).

Mycotic aneurysms most commonly are saccular and involve the ascending aorta (36). Symptoms are nonspecific and include fever and back pain (17). If left untreated, they lead to sepsis and aortic rupture(36).

AORTIC DISSECTION

Aortic dissection is an abnormality characterized by longitudinal cleavage of the aortic media by a stream of blood (Box 3-5). The longitudinal cleavage results in a false lumen that may remain contained or propagate distally or, less commonly, proximally, and reenter the true lumen (49,50). The false lumen usually is located in the anterolateral aspect of the ascending aorta, the superior aspect of the arch, and the left posterolateral aspect of the descending aorta (51). In the majority of cases, the initiating event is believed to be a tear of the intima through which blood surges into the media (49). A second proposed mechanism is bleeding into the media from the vasa vasorum and secondary tear of the intima (52). Many patients have underlying medial degeneration (49).

Aortic dissections most commonly originate in the ascending aorta within a few centimeters of the aortic valve (49). The second most common site of origin is in the descending thoracic aorta immediately distal to the origin of the left subclavian artery. Because of the more lethal nature of dissections involving the ascending aorta, these dissections are seen more commonly in autopsy series than in clinical studies (49).

BOX 3-5. AORTIC DISSECTION

- Longitudinal cleavage of aortic media by blood
- Usually due to tear of intima
- 70%–90% of patients have arterial hypertension
- Many patients have medial degeneration
- Type A is most common, involves ascending aorta
- Type B spares ascending aorta
- Type B usually originates just distal to left subclavian artery
- Diagnosis readily made on contrast-enhanced spiral CT
- Characteristic finding: intimal flap
- Ancillary finding: differential flow between true and false lumens

The most important predisposing factor for the development of aortic dissection is systemic arterial hypertension, a finding present in 70% to 90% of cases (49). Other predisposing conditions include Marfan's syndrome, Ehlers-Danlos syndrome, congenital bicuspid aortic valve, and aortic coarctation (49,53). Dissection may also be caused by surgical incision or manipulation (aortic cross clamping), cannulation or catheterization of the aorta, and placement of intraaortic balloon pumps (32,49).

Dissections occur three times more commonly in males than in females (49). Approximately 50% of aortic dissections in women under the age of 40 occur during pregnancy, usually in the third trimester (49,54).

The characteristic clinical presentation of acute aortic dissection consists of severe chest pain, a finding present in 90% of patients (55). The pain is often described as "tearing" or "ripping" and tends to migrate as the dissection extends along the aorta (49). The pain is felt in the substernal region in dissections involving the ascending aorta and in the left shoulder or back in descending aortic dissections. Less common manifestations include stroke, paraparesis or paraplegia due to compromise of blood supply to the spinal cord, and syncope due to cardiac tamponade (49). Approximately two-thirds of patients develop aortic insufficiency due to compression and displacement of the valve leaflets by the false channel or disruption of the structure of the annulus (49). Occasionally, patients may have minimal or no symptoms (56).

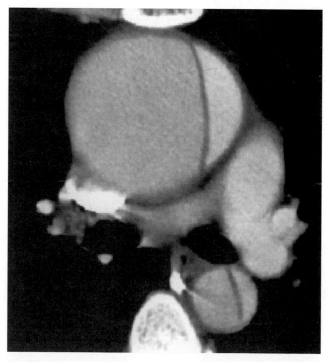

FIGURE 3-8. Type A dissection. CT angiography demonstrates aneurysmal dilation of the ascending aorta and an intimal flap in the ascending and descending aorta. Note slightly decreased enhancement of the false lumen.

Untreated aortic dissection has a poor prognosis, with a 36% to 72% mortality within 48 hours, 62% to 91% mortality within the first week, and 91% to 95% mortality within 1 year (49,57). With treatment, the overall 10-year actuarial survival is approximately 40%, while the 10-year actuarial survival of patients who leave the hospital is approximately 60% (49).

The two most widely used classification systems for aortic dissection are the DeBakey and the Stanford classifications. DeBakey recognized three types of dissection: type I which involves the ascending aorta, arch, and descending aorta; type II which involves only the ascending aorta; and type III which involves only the descending aorta (58). A more pragmatic and currently favored approach is the Stanford classification, which divides dissections into those that involve the ascending aorta (type A) (Figure 3-8) and those that affect only the descending aorta (type B) (Figure 3-9) (59). Type A dissections usually require urgent surgery while type B dissections can usually be successfully managed with medical treatment. Surgery consists of obliteration of the false channel proximally and distally and reconstitution of the aorta, usually by interposing a synthetic sleeve graft. Aortic valve repair or replacement may be required. Medical treatment consists of lowering the arterial blood pressure and reducing the velocity of ventricular contraction with beta-adrenergic receptor blockers (49).

The chest radiograph plays a limited role in the diagnosis of dissection. Although the aorta is often enlarged, it is seldom aneurysmal (49). Suggestive findings include progressive enlargement of the aorta on serial radiographs, a double contour of the aortic arch, and a greater than 6-mm displacement of intimal calcification (60).

Contrast-enhanced CT is currently the most widely used imaging modality in the diagnosis of acute dissection. It is rapid, relatively noninvasive, readily available, highly sensitive, and specific. The diagnostic feature of aortic dissection consists of an intimal flap separating the true and false lumens (Figures 3-7 through 3-9). Ancillary findings include differential flow between the true and false lumens and compression or irregularity of the true lumen (Figure 3-10).

A large number of studies have assessed the role and accuracy of contrast-enhanced conventional CT in the diagnosis of aortic dissections. A review of the studies published prior to 1993 revealed that the sensitivity of CT ranged form 83% to 100% and the specificity from 90% to 100% (61). In an investigation published in 1993, the sensitivity of contrast-enhanced conventional CT in 110 patients with clinically suspected dissection was 94% and the specificity was 87% (62).

Only a small number of studies have assessed the diagnostic accuracy of CTA in the diagnosis of aortic dissection. Zeman and coworkers reported a diagnostic accuracy of 96% in 23 patients clinically suspected of having aortic dissection (63). Multiplanar reformations and three-dimensional renderings were superior to axial images in delineating the extent of the intimal flaps.

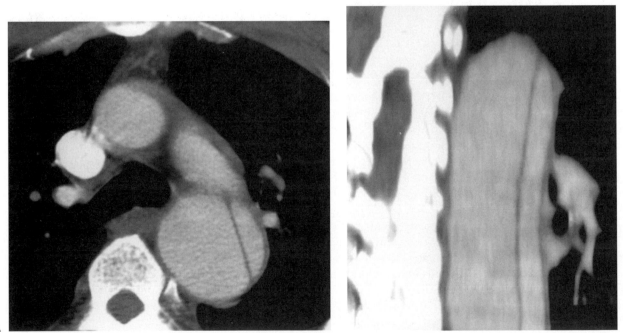

A   B

FIGURE 3-9. Type B dissection. Cross-sectional CT angiogram image (**A**) and coronal reconstruction (**B**) show aneurysm of the proximal descending aorta and intimal flap. Also noted is a focus of calcification in the ascending aorta. The ascending aorta is otherwise unremarkable.

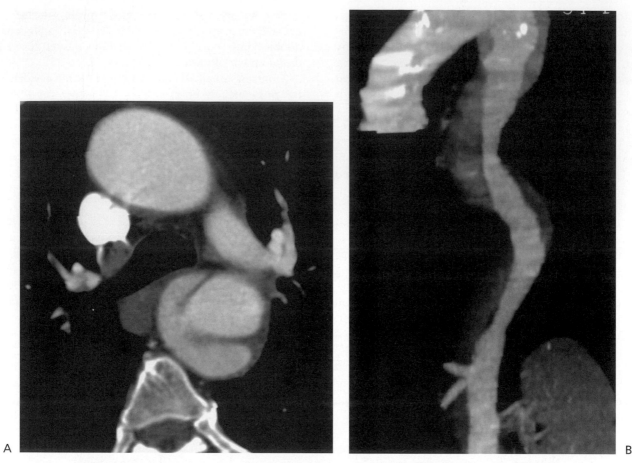

FIGURE 3-10. Type B dissection. Cross-sectional CT angiogram image (**A**) shows aneurysmal dilation of the descending thoracic aorta and intimal flap. Sagittal reconstruction (**B**) demonstrates decreased attenuation of the false lumen and compression and distortion of the true lumen. (Case courtesy of Dr. Ann Leung, Stanford University School of Medicine, Palo Alto, CA.)

Chung and colleagues reported a 100% accuracy of CTA in 49 patients with suspected aortic dissection (37). Sommer and associates compared CTA, transesophageal echocardiography, and magnetic resonance imaging (MRI) in 49 symptomatic patients with clinically suspected aortic dissection (64). All techniques had a sensitivity of 100%. The specificity was 100% for CTA, 94% for transesophageal echocardiography, and 94% for MRI. CTA was also superior in the assessment of aortic arch vessel involvement. The sensitivity of CTA for detecting arch vessel involvement was 93%, compared to 60% and 67% for echocardiography and MRI, respectively; the specificity was 97% compared to 85% and 88%, respectively (64). Multiplanar reconstructions were helpful in assessing the relationship between the dissection and the aortic arch vessels.

Although CTA has a high diagnostic accuracy in the diagnosis of aortic dissection, several pitfalls have been described that could potentially result in a false-negative or false-positive diagnosis (65). Of primary concern are insufficient vascular enhancement of the aortic lumen, streak artifacts, normal periaortic structures, aortic aneurysm with thrombus, and penetrating atherosclerotic ulcer. Periaortic structures that may mimic a false lumen include the superior pericardial recess, right atrial appendage, and residual thymus (65). The distinction between these structures can be readily made by analyzing sequential images. Aortic wall motion during systole and diastole results in curvilinear artifacts in the proximal ascending aorta or, occasionally, in a circle overlying the ascending aorta (Figure 3-11) (65,66). The artifact can be reduced by image reconstruction using a 180-degree linear interpolation algorithm (67). An aortic aneurysm with intraluminal thrombus may be difficult to distinguish from a dissection with a thrombosed false lumen (65). Findings suggestive of dissection include inward displacement of intimal calcification and high-attenuation of the thrombosed false lumen at unenhanced CT. The intimal calcification in aortic aneurysms is typically at the periphery of the aorta.

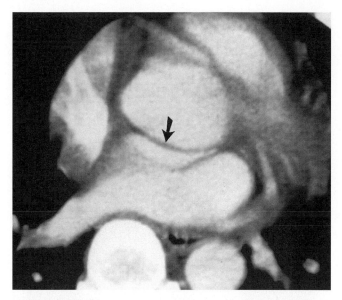

FIGURE 3-11. Motion artifact. CT angiography demonstrates curvilinear artifact (*arrow*) in the proximal ascending aorta mimicking a dissection. This artifact is caused by aortic wall motion and rotation of the aorta during systole and diastole.

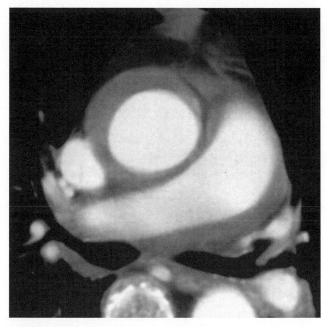

FIGURE 3-12. Intramural hematoma. CT angiography shows crescent of nonenhancing soft tissue attenuation in the wall of the ascending aorta.

INTRAMURAL HEMATOMA

Intramural hematoma, also known as aortic dissection without intimal flap, is defined as a hemorrhage confined to the aortic media (68,69). Several etiologic mechanisms have been proposed, including spontaneous rupture of the vasa vasorum, propagation of hemorrhage from an atherosclerotic ulcer, and complete thrombosis of the false lumen of an aortic dissection (68,70).

The clinical manifestations and the risk factors for the development of intramural hematomas are similar to those of classic aortic dissection (68). Similar to aortic dissection, intramural hematomas involving the ascending aorta usually require surgical repair whereas those confined to the descending aorta can be managed conservatively. In one study, four of five patients with intramural hematoma involving the ascending aorta who were treated conservatively died within 30 days of diagnosis, while all seven patients who underwent surgery survived (68). Patients with intramural hematoma confined to the descending thoracic aorta had no complications. In another study, four of five patients with intramural hematomas of the ascending aorta developed aortic dissection and required surgical intervention compared to only two of 17 patients with hematomas limited to the descending aorta (70). Complications of intramural hematomas involving the ascending aorta include aortic rupture and pericardial tamponade.

The imaging findings of intramural hematoma overlap with those of aortic dissection with thrombosed false lumen and those of penetrating atherosclerotic ulcer. However, in the vast majority of cases, CT allows accurate diagnosis of

contained intramural hematoma (71). The characteristic CTA finding of acute intramural hematoma consists of a crescent of nonenhancing soft tissue density (blood) involving the aorta (Figures 3-12 and 3-13). A helpful feature in differentiating intramural hematoma from aortic dissection with thrombosed lumen is the different relationship of the

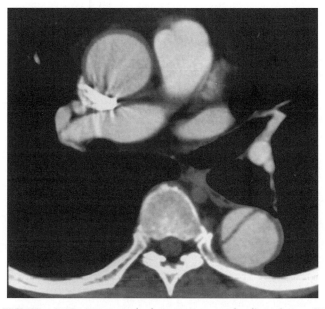

FIGURE 3-13. Intramural hematoma and dissection. CT angiogram image demonstrates intramural hematoma involving the ascending aorta and dissection involving the descending aorta. (Case courtesy of Dr. Ann Leung, Stanford University School of Medicine, Palo Alto, CA.)

abnormality with the aortic wall. Intramural hematoma tends to maintain a constant relationship with the aortic wall whereas the thrombosed false lumen of a dissection usually spirals longitudinally around the aorta (72). Patients with intramural hematoma may also demonstrate marked enhancement and thickening of the aortic wall adjacent to the hematoma, presumably due to inflammation of the adventitia (72).

Sueyoshi and coworkers performed CT and MR scans in 32 patients with intramural hematoma of the aorta (69). The patients had a mean age of 70 years and presented with acute chest or back pain. In 13 patients, the hematoma involved the ascending aorta or transverse arch and in 19, it was confined to the descending aorta. Serial examinations demonstrated that in all patients, the intramural hematoma decreased in size and in 13 of the 32 patients, it resolved completely without sequela. Penetrating atherosclerotic ulcers were seen at presentation in 6 patients and on follow-up exams, performed between 4 and 163 days later, in another 14 patients. Six patients developed fusiform aneurysms at 1 to 16 months follow-up. Two patients with intramural hematomas involving the ascending aorta developed classic type A dissection. Overall, 7 of 13 patients with intramural hematomas involving the ascending aorta survived without surgery (69).

PENETRATING ATHEROSCLEROTIC ULCER

Penetrating atherosclerotic ulcer is an atherosclerotic lesion that ulcerates through the intima of the aorta and allows hematoma formation within the media (Box 3-6) (73). The appearance resembles that of a peptic ulcer on a traditional upper gastrointestinal barium examination, a collection of contrast projecting beyond the lumen of the aorta (Figure 3-14). The majority of cases involve the descending thoracic aorta, although ulcers may also occur in the aortic arch and, occasionally, in the ascending aorta (26,74,75).

The ulcers may be asymptomatic or result in chest or back pain resembling that of aortic dissection (74,76). Occasionally, they may lead to distal embolism (76). The vast majority of patients are over 60 years of age and up to 90% are hypertensive (74,76).

CTA allows demonstration of the penetrating atherosclerotic ulcer, associated mural abnormalities, and com-

BOX 3-6. PENETRATING ATHEROSCLEROTIC ULCER

- Ulceration through intima with hematoma in media
- Patients over 60 years of age
- 90% have arterial hypertension
- Usually involves descending aorta
- *Complications:* Rupture, formation of pseudoaneurysm, saccular and fusiform aneurysm

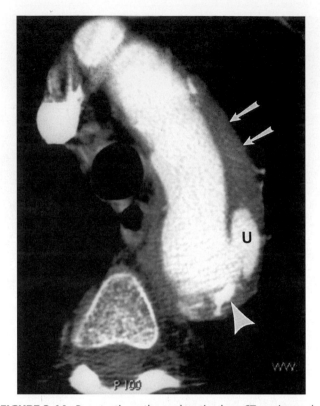

FIGURE 3-14. Penetrating atherosclerotic ulcer. CT angiography shows ulcerlike lesion (*U*) of the aorta with associated intramural hematoma (*arrows*). Also note displaced intimal calcifications (*arrowhead*). (From Quint LE, Williams DM, Francis IR, et al. Ulcerlike lesions of the aorta: Imaging features and natural history. *Radiology* 2001;218:719–723. With permission.) (Case courtesy of Dr. Leslie Quint, University of Michigan Medical Center, Ann Arbor, MI.)

plex spatial relationships with adjacent structures or great vessels (Figure 3-15) (37,77). The characteristic appearance of penetrating atherosclerotic ulcer consists of a focal collection of contrast projecting beyond the lumen of the aorta (Figures 3-14 through 3-16). There is often associated thickening or enhancement of the aortic wall (74,77). The atherosclerotic ulcers may have a wide or a narrow neck and range from a few millimeters to several centimeters in depth (74,76). They may be single (Figures 3-14 and 3-15) or multiple (Figure 3-16). Penetrating atherosclerotic ulcers can be readily distinguished from aortic dissection by their localized nature and lack of an intimal flap.

Kazerooni and coworkers reviewed the CT findings in 16 patients with penetrating atherosclerotic ulcers of the thoracic aorta (74). The patients ranged from 58 to 89 years of age (mean, 73 years). Fifteen patients had a solitary ulcer and one had multiple ulcers. All patients had intramural hematoma. In 13 of the 16 patients (81%), the hematoma could be clearly defined as subintimal on CT by the presence of displaced intimal calcification. Six patients (37%)

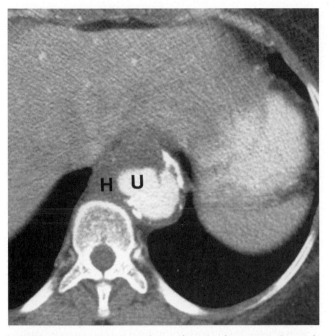

FIGURE 3-15. Penetrating atherosclerotic ulcer. CT angiography demonstrates ulcerlike lesion (*U*) of the aorta. Adjacent low attenuation material, consistent with hematoma (*H*), appears to lie within the aortic wall, partially within the aortic lumen, and possibly within mediastinal fat. (From Quint LE, Williams DM, Francis IR, et al. Ulcerlike lesions of the aorta: Imaging features and natural history. *Radiology* 2001;218:719–723. With permission.) (Case courtesy of Dr. Leslie Quint, University of Michigan Medical Center, Ann Arbor, MI.)

had thickening or enhancement of the aortic wall. One patient had a contained pseudoaneurysm. Mediastinal hemorrhage was present in four (25%) patients and hemorrhagic pleural fluid collections in two. Seven of the 16 patients underwent surgery because of imminent cardiovascular collapse, persistent or recurrent chest or back pain, or a focal pseudoaneurysm. One patient was not considered a surgical candidate. This patient underwent successful embolization of a 2-cm diameter ulcer in the descending thoracic aorta but died of pneumonia 6 days later. Eight patients were treated conservatively with antihypertensive therapy and did not experience another episode of chest or back pain during a median follow-up period of 9 months. The results of this study suggest that surgery is only required in patients with frank or contained aortic rupture, pseudoaneurysm formation, or persistent or recurrent pain despite antihypertensive therapy. In patients who are being treated conservatively, close follow-up is necessary because the ulcer may enlarge, progress to pseudoaneurysm formation, or be associated with development of saccular or fusiform aortic aneurysms (74-76).

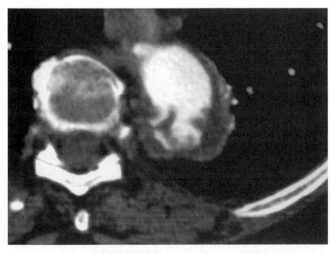

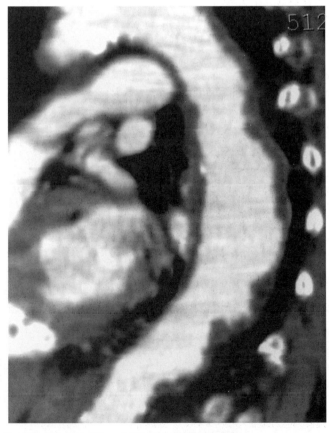

FIGURE 3-16. Multiple penetrating atherosclerotic ulcers. Cross-sectional (**A**) and sagittal (**B**) CT angiogram images demonstrate several atherosclerotic ulcers involving the descending thoracic aorta in a 69-year-old woman. (Case courtesy of Dr. Ann Leung, Stanford University School of Medicine, Palo Alto, CA.)

AORTITIS

Inflammation of the aortic wall may be of infectious or noninfectious etiology. As discussed previously (see page 35), although the term mycotic aneurysm is commonly used to refer to aortic infections, the term infectious aortitis is preferable because the vast majority of infections are of bacterial rather than fungal origin and because aortitis does not necessarily lead to aneurysm formation. In one review of 21 patients with bacterial aortitis, 13 had no previous aneurysm. In only six of these patients did serial CT scans demonstrate progressive enlargement of the aorta from a normal diameter to aneurysmal dilation. The two most important entities associated with noninfectious inflammation of the aortic wall are Takayasu's arteritis and giant cell arteritis.

Infectious Aortitis

The most common causes of infectious aortitis are non-hemolytic streptococcus, *Streptococcus pneumoniae*, and staphylococcus organisms (36). Other etiologies include tuberculosis, *Salmonella*, and syphilis (17,36,78).

Factors that predispose to the development of aortic wall infection include atherosclerosis, trauma, surgical manipulation, arterial catheterization, bacterial endocarditis, and impaired immunity (36,48). Clinical symptoms are nonspecific most commonly consisting of fever and back pain (17).

Findings on CT include aortic wall thickening, nodularity, periaortic haziness, presence of air in the aortic wall, aneurysm, and pseudoaneurysm formation (17,78,79).

Takayasu's Arteritis

Takayasu's arteritis is a chronic inflammatory disease of unknown etiology, which commonly affects the aorta and its major branches (Box 3-7) (80,81). The vast majority of cases occur in Asian countries. The estimated incidence in the Western Hemisphere is 2.6 cases per million population per year (80). It usually affects young women. In a review of 60 patients from the National Health Institutes (NIH),

BOX 3-7. TAKAYASU'S ARTERITIS

- Inflammatory disease of unknown etiology
- Most commonly seen in Asian countries
- 2.6 cases per million in Western Hemisphere
- 97% occur in women
- Median age 25 years
- Most commonly affects subclavian artery, common carotid artery, and aorta
- Long stenotic segments in 98% of patients
- Aneurysms may occur
- CT shows wall thickening
- Enhancement with intravenous contrast
- CT angiography accurately depicts luminal narrowing

97% were women; the median age was 25 years (range 7 to 64 years) (80).

In the NIH study, 43% of patients had constitutional symptoms, 53% had musculoskeletal symptoms, 57% had central nervous system symptoms, and 100% had vascular manifestations (80). The most common symptoms were claudication, fever, malaise, joint pain, and myalgia. Other manifestations included carotid bruit, diminished or absent pulses, hypertension, dizziness, visual abnormalities, stroke, and aortic regurgitation (80). Claudication and diminished or absent pulses were more common in the upper limbs than in the lower limbs. At angiography, the most common sites of abnormality were the subclavian artery (93% of patients), thoracic aorta (65%), common carotid artery (58%), renal artery (38%), vertebral artery (35%), innominate artery (27%), and axillary artery (20%). Arterial stenoses, typically involving long segments, were present in 98% of patients, irregularity of the vessel wall and poststenotic dilation in 33%, and aneurysms in 27% of patients (80). Involvement of the pulmonary arteries is common but is usually a late manifestation of the disease (see page 84).

The characteristic CTA findings consist of mural thickening and enhancement and long-segment stenosis of the aorta or great vessels (Figure 3-17). Several studies have demonstrated that CTA can accurately depict both the luminal and mural abnormalities of Takayasu's disease (37,81,82). Chung and colleagues evaluated the CTA findings in 12 patients, 8 with active disease and 4 with inactive disease (37). The precontrast CT images demonstrated high attenuation of the aortic wall in 10 (83%) and foci of intimal calcification in 9 (77%). Six of 8 (75%) with clinically active disease showed mural enhancement during the arterial phase of contrast injection. Mural enhancement was not seen in any of the patients with inactive disease. CT performed 7 minutes after the arterial phase showed mural enhancement in 8 patients, 7 of which had clinically active disease.

Yamada and colleagues assessed the CTA findings in 20 patients (81). The most common abnormalities consisted of mural thickening of the left common carotid artery (85% of patients), left subclavian artery (85%), brachiocephalic trunk (80%), right common carotid artery (80%), aortic arch (80%), descending thoracic aorta (75%), and ascending aorta (60%). Approximately 50% of patients had foci of mural calcification. The most common sites of stenosis were the left common carotid artery (40% of patients), left subclavian artery (40%), and descending aorta (30%). Only two patients had aneurysm formation, both of which involved the descending aorta. Vessel-by-vessel comparison of CTA with conventional angiography showed that CTA accurately depicted the luminal changes in 190 (95%) arteries. Overall, CTA was falsely interpreted as being normal in 2% of arteries that were shown to be stenotic or occluded at angiography, overestimated the extent of the stenotic lesions in 2%, and underestimated the extent in

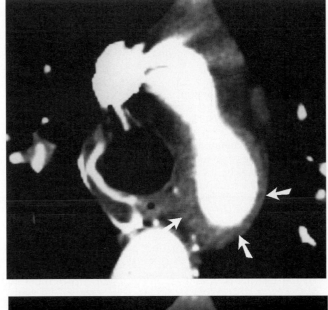
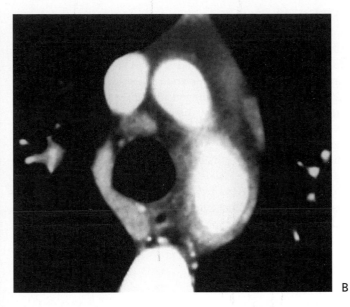

A

B

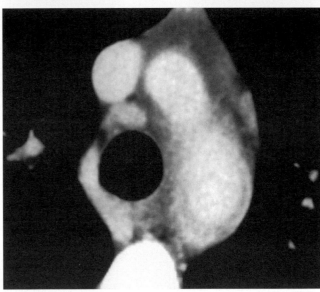

C

FIGURE 3-17. Takayasu's arteritis. CT angiogram image obtained during the early arterial phase **(A)** shows thickening of the wall of the distal aortic arch (*arrows*). CT angiogram image obtained 50 seconds later **(B)** demonstrates marked enhancement of the thickened aortic wall. CT angiogram image obtained 3 minutes after image **A (C)** demonstrates delayed enhancement of the aortic wall. The patient was a 13-year-old girl with active Takayasu's arteritis. (Case courtesy of Dr. Mitsuhiro Koyama, Department of Radiology, Osaka University Medical School, Osaka, Japan.)

2%. However, CT depicted mural changes, including wall thickening, calcification, and mural thrombi, which were not seen on conventional angiography (81).

Giant Cell Arteritis

Giant cell arteritis, also known as temporal arteritis, is an idiopathic vasculitis that affects persons over the age of 50 years (Box 3-8) (83,84). It is approximately three times more common in women than in men (83,84). The arteritis can be widespread but tends to predominantly involve the temporal arteries, aortic arch vessels, and extracranial carotid arteries.

The most common clinical manifestations include fever, malaise, headache, tenderness of the temporal artery, jaw claudication, scalp tenderness, and polymyalgia rheumatica (83). The diagnosis is made by biopsy of the temporal arter-

ies. Characteristic histologic findings consist of granulomatous inflammation, with histiocytes and multinucleated giant cells (83).

Approximately 10% of patients develop stenosis or occlusion of aortic arch vessels (aortic arch syndrome) (84).

BOX 3-8. GIANT CELL ARTERITIS

- Idiopathic granulomatous inflammation
- Patients 50 years or older
- 3 : 1 female-to-male ratio
- Involves predominantly temporal arteries, extracranial carotid arteries, and aortic arch vessels
- 10% develop stenosis or occlusion of arch vessels
- CT findings: thickening of aortic wall, periaortic edema, stenosis, dissection, aneurysm formation
- Diagnosis made by biopsy of temporal artery

Involvement of the aorta can result in weakening of the vessel wall leading to aneurysm formation, dissection, or rupture (84). Aortic involvement is usually a late manifestation. Evans and associates reported 41 patients with giant cell arteritis who had aneurysms and/or rupture of the thoracic aorta (84). The patients ranged from 52 to 88 years of age (median 67 years). Thirty-one were women and 10 were men. Three patients developed thoracic aortic aneurysm before the diagnosis of giant cell arteritis, 5 near the time of diagnosis, and 33 at a median of 7 years after the diagnosis of giant cell arteritis.

In patients with involvement of the aorta, the CT manifestations include thickening of the aortic wall, periaortic edema, stenosis, dissection, and aneurysm formation (17,84).

TRAUMA

Traumatic aortic rupture is a major cause of mortality following blunt chest trauma. Approximately 80% to 90% of cases are secondary to motor vehicle accidents, 5% to 10% are due to automobile–pedestrian accidents, and 5% to 10% are due to a fall from great height (85,86). In the majority of cases, rupture results in immediate death. With proper treatment, up to 80% of the patients who reach the hospital alive survive the injury (87).

In approximately 90% of the patients who survive the initial insult and are assessed radiologically, the injury involves the region of the aortic isthmus immediately distal to the left subclavian artery. Injuries to the ascending aorta, distal descending aorta, and aortic arch vessels are less frequent; 5% to 10% of patients have multilevel injuries (87,88).

The most widely accepted mechanism of injury is the development of deceleration-related shearing forces at the aortic isthmus caused by traction between the relatively mobile aortic arch and the fixed descending aorta (88). It has also been suggested that aortic laceration may be caused by an osseous pinch (89). According to this hypothesis, sudden chest compression depresses the anterior thoracic osseous structures pinching and shearing the aorta between the anterior chest wall and the spine.

Traumatic aortic injuries can range from focal intimal tears with medial hematomas to complete aortic ruptures or avulsion of arch vessels (88,90). Minor injuries such as a limited intimal flap or mural hematoma often regress spontaneously (88,91). Disruption of the intima and media results in pseudoaneurysm formation. The pseudoaneurysms usually enlarge over time, may serve as a nidus for distal embolization, and may rupture (88). Rupture of the aorta leads to immediate death in 75% to 90% of cases. In the remaining cases, the extravasation is contained by the periaortic hematoma and adjacent tissues (88).

The CT findings of aortic injury can be classified into direct and indirect signs (Box 3-9). Direct signs include contour abnormality, localized area of narrowing, intimal

BOX 3-9. TRAUMATIC AORTIC INJURY

A. Direct CT signs of injury
  ■ Contour abnormality
  ■ Localized area of narrowing
  ■ Intimal flap
  ■ Pseudoaneurysm
  ■ Contrast extravasation
  ■ Sensitivity of direct signs: 97–100%
  ■ Specificity: 96–99.8%
B. Indirect signs
  ■ Periaortic hematoma
  ■ Sensitivity: approximately 98–99%
  ■ Low specificity
  ■ Anterior mediastinal hematoma: not helpful

flap, pseudoaneurysm formation, and contrast extravasation (Figures 3-18 through 3-20) (92,93). The presence of a mediastinal hematoma is an indirect sign, which has a high sensitivity but a low specificity for the diagnosis of aortic injury.

A large number of studies have evaluated the diagnostic accuracy of contrast-enhanced CT in the diagnosis of aortic rupture. Mirvis and coworkers performed metaanalysis of the data from 15 studies published prior to 1996 and which included a total of 3,334 cases (92). The combination of mediastinal hematoma and presence of signs of direct injury on CT had a sensitivity of 99.3%, specificity of 87.1%, positive predictive value of 19.9%, and negative predictive value of 99.9% in the diagnosis of aortic injury. Direct signs analyzed in a total of 2,183 patients in two studies had a sensitivity of 97.0%, specificity of 99.8%,

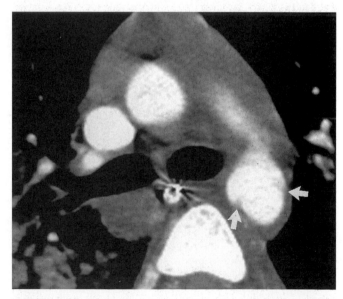

FIGURE 3-18. Traumatic aortic rupture. CT angiography demonstrates a pseudoaneurysm and intimal flap of the aortic wall (*arrows*) and extensive mediastinal hematoma. Also note consolidation of the right lung due to pulmonary contusion.

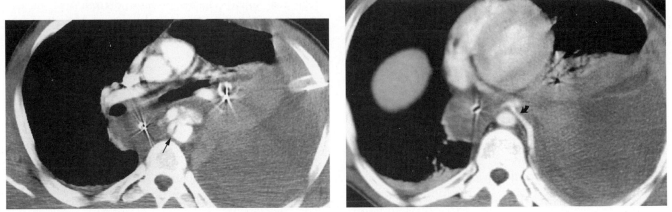

FIGURE 3-19. Traumatic aortic rupture. Contrast-enhanced CT image (**A**) shows marked irregularity of the descending thoracic aorta and an intimal flap (*straight arrow*). CT image at a lower level (**B**) shows extravasation of contrast (*curved arrow*) into the left pleural space. Also note mediastinal hematoma and large hemothorax. A left chest tube and a nasogastric tube are in place.

positive predictive value of 90.1%, and negative predictive value of 99.9% (92,93). The majority of these studies used conventional CT.

Dyer and coworkers assessed the value of CT in a retrospective study of 802 patients with suspected traumatic aortic injury (94). CT scans were considered abnormal if they showed any of the following findings: poorly defined fat planes, mediastinal hemorrhage, perivascular hemorrhage, periaortic hematoma, change in caliber of the aorta (i.e., acute coarctation), intimal flap, abnormal contour of the aorta, or abnormal contour of the proximal great vessels. Of the 802 patients, CT was normal in 638 (80%), abnormal in 152 (19%) and nondiagnostic in 12 (2%). Direct signs of aortic injury were observed on CT in 25 patients. Aortography was performed in 382 patients, including the 152 patients who had abnormal CT scans.

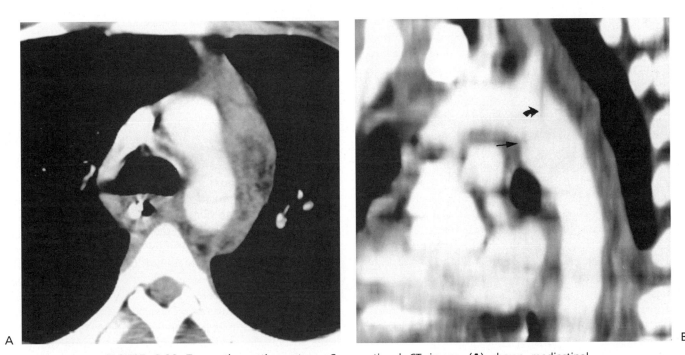

FIGURE 3-20. Traumatic aortic rupture. Cross-sectional CT image (**A**) shows mediastinal hematoma and questionable abnormality in the distal aortic arch. Sagittal reconstruction (**B**) demonstrates irregularity of the wall of the proximal descending aorta (*straight arrow*) and a traumatic intimal flap (*curved arrow*). (Case courtesy of Dr. Jim Barrie, University of Alberta Medical Centre, Edmonton, Alberta, Canada.)

Aortography demonstrated aortic injury in 10 patients, all of whom had direct signs of injury on CT. Therefore, when a positive CT was defined by the presence of any indirect or direct sign, the sensitivity was 100%, specificity 62%, positive predictive value 7%, and negative predictive value 100%. When a positive CT was defined as that demonstrating only a direct sign of aortic injury, the sensitivity and negative predictive value remained 100%, the specificity increased to 96%, and the positive predictive value increased to 40%. Cost analysis demonstrated that performing CT with follow-up aortography in patients with positive CT scans would have avoided 80% of aortograms, a considerable cost saving. Performing aortography only in patients with periaortic hematoma and direct signs of aortic injury on CT scans would have avoided 93% of aortograms while performing aortography only in patients with direct signs of aortic injury on CT would have avoided 96% of aortograms (94).

Gavant and coworkers assessed the efficacy of spiral CT as a screening imaging modality in 1,518 patients with nontrivial blunt chest trauma (93). In 92% of patients, the CT scans showed no mediastinal hematoma and no aortic abnormality, and no further investigation was undertaken. One hundred and twenty-seven patients (8%) had abnormal or indeterminate CT scans and underwent aortography. In 89 of these patients, CT demonstrated mediastinal hematoma but no aortic abnormality. In 85 of these 89 patients, aortography was normal, in three it was indeterminate or falsely positive because of the presence of prominent atherosclerotic plaques, and in one it was falsely positive because of a large ductus diverticulum proven at surgery. The remaining 38 patients with abnormal CT scans had either direct evidence of thoracic injury, indeterminate scans, or inadequate spiral CT scans. Seventeen of these patients had thoracic injury detected at aortography. In this study, therefore, spiral CT was more sensitive than aortography (100% versus 94%, respectively) but less specific (82% versus 96%, respectively) (93).

In a subsequent study, Gavant and coworkers evaluated the value of CTA in the diagnosis of aortic injury (95). CTA included two-dimensional multiplanar reconstructions and three-dimensional analysis based on MIP or shaded-surface display reconstructions. Of 3,229 patients with nontrivial blunt trauma included in the study, 36 had injuries of the aorta or great vessels. The extent of injury was identified in 100% of cases on standard axial spiral CT images, compared to 82% of cases on two-dimensional reconstructions, 82% on three-dimensional MIP images, 71% on three-dimensional surface shading reconstructions, and 88% on conventional aortography. CTA accurately demonstrated the presence and extent of aortic injuries when these were greater than 15 mm in length but was inferior to axial images for small tears. The authors concluded that axial spiral CT images allow detection of all aortic injuries and that CTA can replace conventional aortography except for small tears or indeterminate examinations (95).

The various studies demonstrate that spiral CT with or without CTA has a very high sensitivity and negative predictive value in the diagnosis of aortic injury. The results of some studies suggest that a normal aorta on spiral CT effectively excludes the possibility of aortic injury and that aortography is not necessary even in the presence of mediastinal hematoma (94,95). This is, however, controversial. The evidence in the literature indicates that aortography is not required in the presence of isolated anterior mediastinal hematoma (94,96). However, the majority of investigators recommend aortography in patients with periaortic hematoma (92,94,96,97). Aortography is also indicated in patients with equivocal signs of aortic injury on CT or suboptimal scans (94). Patients with unequivocal direct signs of aortic tear should proceed to immediate surgery.

POSTOPERATIVE EVALUATION

CTA is the imaging modality of choice for the assessment of complications following repair of aortic aneurysm or dissection and other acquired or congenital aortic abnormalities (Figure 3-21). It also allows excellent assessment of the aorta for perianastomotic complications following coronary artery bypass graft placement and placement of access cannulas for cardiopulmonary bypass (72).

Surgical repair of aortic aneurysm or dissection is usually performed using either an interposition graft or an inclusion graft (26). The interposition graft technique consists of excision of the abnormal portion of the aorta and interposition of a graft with end-to-end anastomosis. The graft inclusion technique consists of aortotomy, graft insertion, and enclosure of the graft within the remnant of the diseased aorta (aortic wrap).

In the graft inclusion technique there is a potential space between the graft and the aortic wrap. This potential space, known as the perigraft space may contain flowing blood, thrombus, or both (26,98). In patients with inclusion grafts, partial dehiscence of the proximal or distal anastomosis can result in persistent flow within the perigraft space or pseudoaneurysm formation (26). Persistent flow and pseudoaneurysm formation can also result from leakage through the needle holes.

When the aneurysm or dissection involves the aortic root, the patient may have graft placement, resuspension of the aortic valve, and reimplantation of the coronary arteries. Alternatively, surgery may involve placement of a composite graft that includes a prosthetic valve (Bentall procedure). The Cabrol graft consists of an ascending aortic graft,

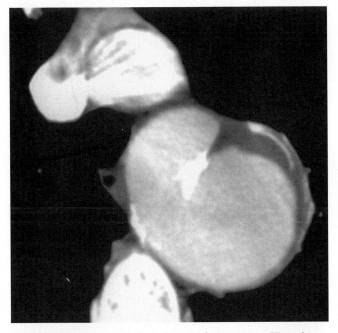

FIGURE 3-21. Postsurgical aortic pseudoaneurysm. CT angiography demonstrates pseudoaneurysm of the proximal descending thoracic aorta. The pseudoaneurysm developed following repair of coarctation of the aorta.

aortic valve, and a prosthetic conduit that is anastomosed directly to the main coronary arteries (99). On CTA or magnetic resonance angiography, this conduit may mimic a focal dissection of the aortic root (26,100). Complications following the various composite grafts include false aneurysm formation at the site of coronary anastomosis and pseudoaneurysms from dehiscence of the proximal or distal suture lines (26,101).

Routine postoperative CT examinations are important in the follow-up of patients with aortic grafts (102). On unenhanced CT images the prosthetic graft can often be visualized as a high attenuation ring contiguous with the aortic wall. Contrast-enhanced spiral CT allows reliable assessment of the perigraft space, distinction of perigraft flow from thrombus, and detection of pseudoaneurysm formation.

Rofsky and associates assessed the normal range of postoperative findings on contrast-enhanced conventional CT in 24 patients who underwent graft inclusion for repair of aortic aneurysms or dissections (98). The scans were performed 5 to 66 months after surgery (mean, 28 months). All patients were asymptomatic. Perigraft thickening was seen on 8 of the 24 patients (33%); thrombi outside the graft but contained within the aortic wrap were observed in 6 (25%); and flow outside the graft in 4 (17%). In the study by Pracki and colleagues, 2 of 39 patients developed pseudoaneurysms 3 or more months after composite graft

replacement of the ascending aorta with the graft inclusion technique (102).

Quint and coworkers performed serial spiral CT scans in 114 patients who had one or more thoracic aortic interposition grafts (103). The grafts were present in the ascending aorta in 93 patients, descending aorta in 25, and in the arch in 11. Sixty-eight patients had a composite interposition graft. Low-attenuation material was present adjacent to the ascending aortic graft in 55% to 82% of patients and adjacent to the descending graft in 60% to 79% of patients. The percentage of patients with low-attenuation material around the graft was greatest on CT scans performed within 1 to 6 months after surgery. Similarly, the thickness of the low-attenuation material decreased over time. The thickness of the low attenuation material around ascending aortic grafts ranged from 4 to 80 mm on CT scans performed within 1 to 6 months after surgery, 3 to 30 mm at 7 to 12 months, and 4 to 11 mm after 12 months. The thickness of low attenuation material around interposition grafts of the descending aorta ranged from 4 to 33 mm on CT scans performed 1 to 6 months after surgery, 4 to 10 mm at 7 to 12 months, and 4 to 9 mm after 12 months. A small percentage of patients had soft tissue attenuation or, occasionally, high attenuation material around the graft particularly in the first 6 months after surgery. CT scans in 4 of the 93 patients with ascending aortic grafts and one of 25 patients with descending aortic grafts demonstrated a pseudoaneurysm.

AORTIC ENDOVASCULAR STENT GRAFTS

Endovascular stent-graft implantation is a technique being used with increased frequency as an alternative to surgery for the treatment of aortic aneurysms, particularly in high-risk patients (104). Advantages of endovascular stent grafts over surgery include less blood loss, shorter stay in the intensive care unit, and quicker recovery (105). Complications following aortic endovascular stent-graft placement include leakage into the aneurysm, graft thrombosis, graft kinking, graft infection, graft occlusion, and shower embolism (104). The most common complication is leakage into the aneurysm, also known as endoleak. Endoleak can result from graft defects, retrograde blood flow via patent arteries, or incomplete fixation of the stent graft to the aortic wall (104).

CTA is the imaging modality of choice for the assessment of endoluminal stent grafts (Figure 3-22). It is superior to conventional aortography in ensuring that the stent graft has been optimally placed to completely exclude the aneurysm (72). It also allows detection of endoleaks in patients in whom aortography suggests optimal graft placement with complete exclusion of the aneurysm (72).

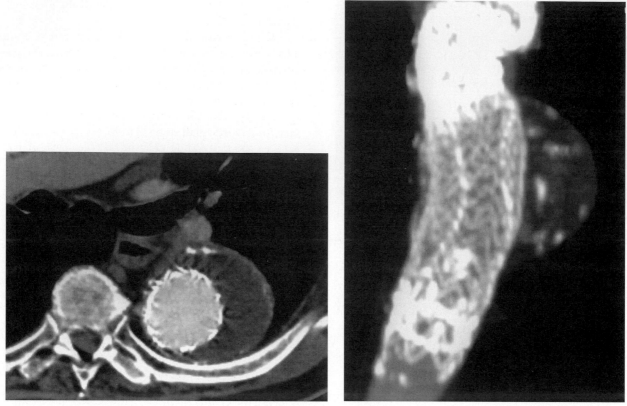

FIGURE 3-22. Endovascular stent graft. Cross-sectional (**A**) and coronal (**B**) CT angiogram images demonstrate endovascular stent-graft placement for treatment of saccular aneurysm of the descending thoracic aorta. (Case courtesy of Dr. Ann Leung, Stanford University School of Medicine, Palo Alto, CA.)

REFERENCES

1. VanDyke CW, White RD. Congenital abnormalities of the thoracic aorta presenting in the adult. *J Thorac Imaging* 1994;9: 230–245.
2. Salomonowitz E, Edwards JE, Hunter DW, et al. The three types of aortic diverticula. *AJR* 1984;142:673–679.
3. Proto AV, Cuthbert NW, Raider L. Aberrant right subclavian artery: further observations. *AJR* 1987;148:253–257.
4. Kommerell B. Verlagerung des oesophagus durch eine abnorm verlaufende arteria subclavia dextra (arteria lusoria). *Fortschr Geb Rontgenstr Nuklerarmed* 1936;54:590–595.
5. Blake HA, Manion WC. Thoracic arterial arch anomalies. *Circulation* 1962;26:251–265.
6. Raymond GS, Miller RM, Müller NL, et al. Congenital thoracic lesions that mimic neoplastic disease on chest radiographs of adults. *AJR* 1997;168:763–769.
7. Knight L, Edwards JE. Right aortic arch: types and associated cardiac anomalies. *Circulation* 1974;50:1047–1051.
8. Glew D, Hartnell GG. The right aortic arch revisited. *Clin Radiol* 1991;43:305–307.
9. Predey TS, McDonald V, Demos TC, et al. CT of congenital anomalies of the aortic arch. *Semin Roentgenol* 1989;14:96–111.
10. Shuford WH, Sybers RG, Weens HS. The angiographic features of double aortic arches. *AJR* 1972;116:125–140.
11. Hopkins KL, Patrick LE, Simoneaux SF, et al. Pediatric great vessel anomalies: initial clinical experience with spiral CT angiography. *Radiology* 1996;200:811–815.
12. Becker AE, Becker MJ, Edwards JE. Anomalies associated with coarctation of the aorta: particular reference to infancy. *Circulation* 1970;41:1067–1075.
13. Rosenberg HS. Coarctation as a deformation [Review]. *Pediatr Pathol* 1990;10:103–115.
14. Tawes RL, Berr CL. Congenital bicuspid aortic valves associated with coarctation of the aorta in children. *Br Heart J* 1969;31: 127–128.
15. Becker C, Soppa C, Fink U, et al. Spiral CT angiography and 3D reconstruction in patients with aortic coarctation. *Eur Radiol* 1997;7:1473–1477.
16. Soler R, Pombo F, Bargiela A, et al. MRI of pseudocoarctation of the aorta: morphological and cine-MRI findings. *Comput Med Imaging Graph* 1995;19:431–434.
17. VanDyke CV, Flamm SD, White RD. Diseases of the aorta. In: Freundlich IM, Bragg DG, eds. *A radiologic approach to diseases of the chest*. Baltimore: Williams & Wilkins, 1997:361–408.
18. Gay WA, Young WG. Pseudocoarctation of the aorta: a reappraisal. *J Thorac Cardiovasc Surg* 1969;58:739–745.
19. Dungan WT, Char F, Gerald BE, et al. Pseudocoarctation of the aorta in childhood. *Am J Dis Child* 1970;119:401–406.
20. LePage JR, Szechenyi E, Ross-Duggan JW. Pseudocoarctation of the aorta. *MRI* 1988;6:65–68.
21. Safir J, Kerr A, Morehouse H, et al. Magnetic resonance imaging of dissection in pseudocoarctation of the aorta. *Cardiovasc Intervent Radiol* 1993;16:180–182.
22. Young MW, Lau SH, Stein E, et al. Pseudocoarctation of the aorta. *Am Heart J* 1969;77:259–262.
23. Bilgic A, Ozer S, Atalay S. Pseudocoarctation of the aorta. *Jpn Heart J* 1990;31:875–879.

24. Lavin N, Mehta S, Liberson M, et al. Pseudocoarctation of the aorta: an unusual variant with coarctation. *Am J Cardiol* 1969;24:584–590.

25. Pressler V, McNamara JJ. Aneurysm of the thoracic aorta: review of 260 cases. *J Thorac Cardiovasc Surg* 1985;89:50–54.

26. Naidich DP, Webb WR, Müller NL, et al. *Computed tomography and magnetic resonance of the thorax*. Philadelphia: Lippincott-Raven, 1999:505–602.

27. Aronberg DJ, Glazer HS, Madsen K, et al. Normal thoracic aortic diameters by computed tomography. *J Comput Assist Tomogr* 1984;8:247–250.

28. Joyce JW, Fairbairn JFI, Kincaid OW, et al. Aneurysms of the thoracic aorta with special reference to prognosis. *Circulation* 1964;29:176–181.

29. Crawford ES, Crawford JL, Safi HJ, et al. Thoracoabdominal aortic aneurysms: preoperative and intraoperative factors determining immediate and long-term results of operations in 605 patients. *J Vasc Surg* 1986;3:389–404.

30. Coady MA, Rizzo JA, Hammond GL, et al. What is the appropriate size criterion for resection of thoracic aortic aneurysms? *J Thorac Cardiovasc Surg* 1997;113:476–491.

31. Hirose Y, Hamada S, Takamiya M, et al. Aortic aneurysms: growth rates measured with CT. *Radiology* 1992;185:249–252.

32. Kouchoukos NT, Dougenis D. Surgery of the thoracic aorta. *N Engl J Med* 1997;336:1876–1888.

33. Crawford ES, Svensson LG, Coselli JS, et al. Surgical treatment of aneurysm and/or dissection of the ascending aorta, transverse aortic arch, and ascending aorta and transverse aortic arch. Factors influencing survival in 717 patients. *J Thorac Cardiovasc Surg* 1989;98:659–673.

34. Torres WE, Maurer DE, Steinberg HV, et al. CT of aortic aneurysms: the distinction between mural and thrombus calcification. *AJR* 1988;150:1317–1319.

35. Heiberg E, Wolverson MK, Sundaram M, et al. CT characteristics of atherosclerotic aneurysm versus aortic dissection. *J Comput Assist Tomogr* 1985;91:78–83.

36. Posniak HV, Olson MC, Demos TC, et al. CT of thoracic aortic aneurysms. *Radiographics* 1990;10:839–855.

37. Chung JW, Park JH, Im JG, et al. Spiral CT angiography of the thoracic aorta. *Radiographics* 1996;16:811–824.

38. Quint LE, Francis IR, Williams DM, et al. Evaluation of thoracic aortic disease with the use of helical CT and multiplanar reconstructions: comparison with surgical findings. *Radiology* 1996;201:37–41.

39. Kimura F, Shen Y, Date S, et al. Thoracic aortic aneurysm and aortic dissection: new endoscopic mode for three-dimensional CT display of aorta. *Radiology* 1996;198:573–578.

40. Rubin GD, Paik DS, Johnston PC, et al. Measurement of the aorta and its branches with helical CT. *Radiology* 1998;206:823–829.

41. Jeffrey RB Jr. CT angiography of the abdominal and thoracic aorta. *Semin Ultrasound CT MRI* 1998;19:405–412.

42. Mehard WB, Heiken JP, Sicard GA. High-attenuating crescent in abdominal aortic aneurysm wall at CT: a sign of acute or impending rupture. *Radiology* 1994;192:359–362.

43. Arita T, Matsunaga N, Takano K, et al. Abdominal aortic aneurysms: rupture associated with the high-attenuating crescent sign. *Radiology* 1997;204:765–768.

44. Halliday KE, Al-Kutoubi A. Draped aorta: CT sign of contained leak of aortic aneurysms. *Radiology* 1996;199:41–43.

45. Frist WH, Miller DC. Aneurysms of ascending thoracic aorta and transverse aortic arch. *Cardiovasc Clin* 1987;17:263–287.

46. Murdoch JL, Walker BA, Halpern BL, et al. Life expectancy and causes of death in the Marfan syndrome. *N Engl J Med* 1972;286:804–808.

47. Felson B, Akers PV, Hall GS, et al. Mycotic tuberculous aneurysm of the thoracic aorta. *JAMA* 1977;237:1104–1108.

48. Johansen K, Devin J. Mycotic aortic aneurysms: a reappraisal. *Arch Surg* 1983;118:583–588.

49. DeSanctis RW, Doroghazi RM, Austen WG, et al. Aortic dissection. *N Engl J Med* 1987;317:1060–1067.

50. von Segesser LK, Killer I, Ziswiler M, et al. Dissection of the descending thoracic aorta extending into the ascending aorta: a therapeutic challenge. *J Thorac Cardiovasc Surg* 1994;108:755–761.

51. Roberts WC. Aortic dissection: anatomy, consequences, and causes. *Am Heart J* 1981;101:195–214.

52. Wilson SK, Hutchins GM. Aortic dissecting aneurysms: causative factors in 204 patients. *Arch Pathol Lab Med* 1982;106:175–180.

53. Larson EW, Edwards WD. Risk factors for aortic dissection: a necropsy study of 161 cases. *Am J Cardiol* 1984;53:849–855.

54. Pumphrey CW, Fay T, Weir I. Aortic dissection during pregnancy. *Br Heart J* 1986;55:106–108.

55. Slater EE, DeSanctis RW. The clinical recognition of dissecting aortic aneurysm. *Am J Med* 1976;60:625–633.

56. Spittell PC, Spittell JA Jr, Joyce JW, et al. Clinical features and differential diagnosis of aortic dissection: experience with 236 cases (1980 through 1990). *Mayo Clin Proc* 1993;68:642–651.

57. Anagnostopoulos CE, Prabhakar MJS, Kittle CF, et al. Aortic dissections and dissecting aneurysms. Am J Cardiol 1972;30:263–273.

58. DeBakey ME, Henly WS, Cooley DA, et al. Surgical management of dissecting aneurysms of the aorta. *J Thorac Cardiovasc Surg* 1965;49:130–149.

59. Daily PO, Trueblood W, Stinson EB, et al. Management of acute aortic dissections. *Ann Thorac Surg* 1970;10:237–247.

60. Chen JTT. Plain radiographic evaluation of the aorta. *J Thorac Imaging* 1990;5:1–17.

61. Cigarroa JE, Isselbacher EM, DeSanctis RW, et al. Diagnostic imaging in the evaluation of suspected aortic dissection: old standards and new directions. *AJR* 1993;161:485–493.

62. Nienaber CA, von Kodolitsch Y, Nicholas V, et al. The diagnosis of thoracic aortic dissection by noninvasive imaging. *N Engl J Med* 1993;328:1–9.

63. Zeman RK, Berman PM, Silverman PM, et al. Diagnosis of aortic dissection: value of helical CT with multiplanar reformation and three-dimensional rendering. *AJR* 1995;164:1375–1380.

64. Sommer T, Fehske W, Holzknecht N, et al. Aortic dissection: a comparative study of diagnosis with spiral CT, multiplanar transesophageal echocardiography, and MR imaging. *Radiology* 1996;199:347–352.

65. Batra P, Bigoni B, Manning J, et al. Pitfalls in the diagnosis of thoracic aortic dissections at CT angiography. *Radiographics* 2000;20:309–320.

66. Burns MA, Molina PL, Gutierrez FR, et al. Motion artifact simulating aortic dissection on CT. *AJR* 1991;157:465–467.

67. Loubeyre P, Angelie E, Grozel F, et al. Spiral CT artifact that simulates aortic dissection: image reconstruction with use of 180° and 360° linear-interpolation algorithms. *Radiology* 1997;205:153–157.

68. Nienaber CA, von Kodolitsch Y, Peterson B, et al. Intramural hemorrhage of the thoracic aorta: diagnostic and therapeutic implications. *Circulation* 1995;92:1465–1472.

69. Sueyoshi E, Matsuoka Y, Sakamoto I, et al. Fate of intramural hematoma of the aorta: CT evaluation. *J Comput Assist Tomogr* 1997;21:931–938.

70. Murray JG, Manisali M, Flamm SD, et al. Intramural hematoma of the thoracic aorta: MR image findings and their prognostic implications. *Radiology* 1997;204:349–355.

71. Patrick TO, Roman WD. Acute aortic dissection and its variants: toward a common diagnostic and therapeutic approach. *Circulation* 1995;92:1376–1378.

72. Rubin GF. Helical angiography of the thoracic aorta. *J Thorac Imaging* 1997;12:128–149.

73. Stanson AW, Kazmier FJ, Hollier LH, et al. Penetrating atherosclerotic ulcer of the thoracic aorta: natural history and clinicopathologic correlation. *Ann Vasc Surg* 1986;1:15–23.

74. Kazerooni EA, Bree RL, Williams DM. Penetrating atherosclerotic ulcers of the descending thoracic aorta: evaluation with CT and distinction from aortic dissection. *Radiology* 1992;183:759–765.

75. Quint LE, Williams DM, Francis IR, et al. Ulcerlike lesions of the aorta: Imaging features and natural history. *Radiology* 2001;218:719–723.

76. Harris JA, Bis KG, Glover JL, et al. Penetrating atherosclerotic ulcers of the aorta. *J Vasc Surg* 1994;19:90–98.

77. Hayashi H, Matsuoka Y, Sakamoto I, et al. Penetrating atherosclerotic ulcer of the aorta: imaging features and disease concept. *Radiographics* 2000;20:995–1005.

78. Oz MC, Brener BJ, Buda JA, et al. A ten-year experience with bacterial aortitis. *J Vasc Surg* 1989;10:439–449.

79. Gomez MN, Choyke PL. Infected aortic aneurysms: CT diagnosis. *J Cardiovasc Surg* 1992;33:684–689.

80. Kerr GS, Hallahan CW, Giordano J, et al. Takayasu arteritis. *Ann Intern Med* 1994;120:919–929.

81. Yamada I, Nakagawa T, Himeno Y, et al. Takayasu arteritis: evaluation of the thoracic aorta with CT angiography. *Radiology* 1998;209:103–109.

82. Park JH, Chung JW, Im J-G, et al. Takayasu arteritis: evaluation of mural changes in the aorta and pulmonary artery with CT angiography. *Radiology* 1995;196:89–93.

83. Hunder GG. Giant cell (temporal) arteritis. *Rheum Dis Clin North Am* 1990;16:399–409.

84. Evans JM, Bowles CA, Bjornsson J, et al. Thoracic aortic aneurysm and rupture in giant cell arteritis. *Arthritis Rheum* 1994;37:1539–1547.

85. Fisher RG, Chasen MH, Lamki N. Diagnosis of injuries of the aorta and brachiocephalic arteries caused by blunt chest trauma: CT vs aortography. *AJR* 1994;162:1047–1052.

86. Mirvis SE, Bidwell JK, Buddemeyer EU, et al. Value of chest radiography in excluding traumatic aortic rupture. *Radiology* 1987;163:487–493.

87. Groskin SA. Selected topics in chest trauma. *Semin Ultrasound CT MRI* 1996;17:119–141.

88. Prêtre R, Chilcott M. Blunt trauma to the heart and great vessels. *N Engl J Med* 1997;336:626–632.

89. Cohen AM, Crass JR, Thomas HA, et al. CT evidence for the "osseous pinch" mechanism of traumatic aortic injury. *AJR* 1992;159:271–274.

90. Parmley LF, Matingly TW, Manion WC, Jahnke EJ. Nonpenetrating traumatic injury of the aorta. *Circulation* 1958;17:1086–1101.

91. Frykberg ER, Crump JM, Dennis JW, et al. Non-operative observation of clinically occult arterial injuries: a prospective evaluation. *Surgery* 1991;109:85–96.

92. Mirvis SE, Shanmuganathan K, Miller BH, et al. Traumatic aortic injury: diagnosis with contrast-enhanced thoracic CT: five-year experience at a major trauma center. *Radiology* 1996;200:413–422.

93. Gavant ML, Menke PG, Fabian T, et al. Blunt traumatic aortic rupture: detection with helical CT of the chest. *Radiology* 1995;197:125–133.

94. Dyer DS, Moore EE, Mestek MF, et al. Can chest CT be used to exclude aortic injury? *Radiology* 1999;213:195–202.

95. Gavant ML, Flick P, Menke P, et al. CT aortography of thoracic aortic rupture. *AJR* 1996;166:955–961.

96. Wong Y-C, Wang L-J, Lim K-E, et al. Periaortic hematoma on helical CT of the chest: a criterion for predicting blunt traumatic aortic rupture. *AJR* 1998;170:1523–1525.

97. Van Hise ML, Primack SL, Israel RS, et al. CT in blunt chest trauma: indications and limitations. *Radiographics* 1998;18:1071–1084.

98. Rofsky NM, Weinreb JC, Grossi EA, et al. Aortic aneurysm and dissection: normal MR imaging and CT findings after surgical repair with the continuous-suture graft-inclusion technique. *Radiology* 1993;186:195–201.

99. Cabrol C, Pavie A, Mesnildrey P, et al. Long-term results with total replacement of the ascending aorta and reimplantation of the coronary arteries. *J Thorac Cardiovasc Surg* 1986;91:17–25.

100. Krinsky GA, Reuss P. MR angiography of the thoracic aorta. *MRI Clin North Am* 1998;6:293–320.

101. Gaubert J-Y, Moulin G, Thierry M, et al. Type A dissection of the thoracic aorta: use of MR imaging for long-term follow-up. *Radiology* 1995;196:363–369.

102. Pracki P, Petri D, Kellner H, et al. Composite graft (Medtronic-Hall) replacement of the ascending aorta and aortic valve in aortic aneurysms: what is adequate follow-up? *Thorac Cardiovasc Surg* 1995;43:104–107.

103. Quint LE, Francis IR, Williams DM, et al. Synthetic interposition grafts of the thoracic aorta: postoperative appearance on serial CT studies. *Radiology* 1999;211:317–324.

104. Mita T, Arita T, Matsunaga N, et al. Complications of endovascular repair for thoracic and abdominal aortic aneurysm: an imaging spectrum. *Radiographics* 2000;20:1263–1278.

105. Brewster D, Geller S, Kaufman J, et al. Initial experience with endovascular aneurysm repair: comparison of early results with outcome of conventional open repair. *J Vasc Surg* 1998;27:992–1005.

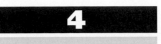

ACUTE PULMONARY EMBOLISM

BACKGROUND

Pulmonary embolism (PE) is a common condition with considerable morbidity and mortality (1). Prompt and accurate diagnosis is important because the mortality of untreated pulmonary embolism is high and serious complications can occur with its treatment, long-term anticoagulation (2). Because there are no specific signs or symptoms of this condition, the diagnosis relies on imaging tests. Until recently, nuclear medicine ventilation–perfusion scintigraphy, leg vein ultrasound, and pulmonary angiography were the main imaging techniques employed for the diagnosis of PE. However, despite the development of a variety of diagnostic algorithms, in many cases, a definitive diagnosis was not made due to limitations of these imaging tests (3).

The introduction of spiral CT angiography techniques in the early 1990s was quickly followed by their application to the diagnosis of PE (4). Spiral CT for PE has rapidly evolved in conjunction with advances in single slice and, more recently, multislice spiral CT scanners and is increasingly employed in the diagnostic algorithm for acute PE.

We will briefly review the strengths and limitations of the traditionally employed diagnostic tests for the diagnosis of acute PE (ventilation–perfusion lung scanning, Doppler ultrasound of the deep leg veins, and pulmonary angiography) and then follow with a discussion of spiral CT.

Ventilation–Perfusion Scintigraphy

Ventilation–perfusion (V/Q) lung scintigraphy is a safe, noninvasive technique to evaluate regional pulmonary perfusion and ventilation. It has been used extensively as the primary imaging modality for the assessment of patients suspected of having acute PE. The diagnosis of PE on scintigraphy is based on the presence of ventilation in the absence of perfusion (i.e., ventilation–perfusion mismatch distal to obstructing emboli). The combined findings on the ventilation and perfusion scintigrams are classified in terms of the probability of emboli being present, with the most commonly used reporting terms being: normal, near normal, low, intermediate, and high probability. A normal or near normal V/Q scan essentially rules out the presence of pulmonary emboli, and a high probability scan indicates PE. However, large studies such as the multicenter Prospective Investigation of Pulmonary Embolism Diagnosis (PIOPED) trial have shown that 60% to 70% of lung scans do not fall into these definitive categories (5). In the PIOPED study, the highest proportion of V/Q scans (40%) were interpreted as intermediate probability, followed by 34% low probability, 14% normal or near-normal, and 13% high probability. Pulmonary angiography confirmed PE in 88% of patients with a high probability scan. By comparison, angiographically proven PE was found in 33% of patients who had intermediate probability scans, 16% with low probability scans, and 9% of patients who had near-normal or normal ventilation–perfusion scans. Overall, the sensitivity, specificity, and positive predictive value of V/Q scanning for detecting acute PE were 41%, 52%, and 88%, respectively, in the PIOPED trial.

Although the use of revised criteria decreases the number of V/Q scans interpreted as intermediate probability and correctly classifies them as low probability, nondiagnostic studies remain the largest single category (6,7). Another major difficulty with scintigraphy is the lack of reproducibility that is most apparent in the low and intermediate probability scan categories. Although there is close agreement between observers in the classification of ventilation–perfusion scans that have a high or normal probability, there is a 25% to 30% interobserver disagreement in interpreting intermediate and low probability scans (5).

The results from the PIOPED study emphasized the importance of incorporating the pretest clinical likelihood of PE in the overall diagnostic evaluation. In patients who had a low or very low probability V/Q scan and no history of immobilization, recent surgery, trauma to the lower extremities, or central venous instrumentation, the prevalence of PE was only 4.5% (8). In patients who had scans which were interpreted as representing low or very low probability for PE and one risk factor, the prevalence of PE was 12% whereas for patients who had two or more risk factors, the prevalence was 21%. Despite the increased precision provided by the addition of clinical status, the largest proportion of patients in the PIOPED study had intermediate probability V/Q scans and an intermediate clinical likelihood of PE. For these patients, the combination of clinical assessment and interpretation of V/Q scan does not provide adequate information to accurately direct their management, and additional diagnostic tests are necessary.

Leg Vein Studies

The most common additional diagnostic test employed in the setting of a nondiagnostic lung scan is the noninvasive assessment of thrombosis in the deep veins of the legs. This is usually performed using ultrasound. Since deep venous thrombosis and PE are treated identically with long-term anticoagulation, these venous studies can direct patient management. However, deep venous thrombosis is found in less than one-half of patients with angiographically proven PE (9). Therefore, patients with nondiagnostic ventila-tion–perfusion scintigraphy and negative deep venous studies require additional diagnostic studies.

Pulmonary Angiography

In the past, pulmonary arteriography was been considered the most definitive technique for investigating suspected PE (5,8,10–12). At pulmonary angiography, a catheter is introduced transvenously into the proximal pulmonary arteries and contrast media is rapidly injected. This provides images of the pulmonary vasculature with high spatial and temporal resolution. Prior to the introduction of spiral CT angiography (CTA), pulmonary angiography was the only examination capable of directly imaging a clot in pulmonary vessels. However, pulmonary angiography is a technically challenging and invasive procedure. In the past, it has been associated with a 5% risk of cardiac or pulmonary complications and a 0.3% mortality (13). The introduction of soft pigtailed-shaped catheters (14) and the use of non-ionic contrast media have reduced both the morbidity and mortality of the procedure (15).

The introduction of digital subtraction angiography (DSA) was heralded as a potential advance for pulmonary angiography. The increased contrast sensitivity of the DSA technique allowed visualization of vessels with more dilute contrast media. As a result, peripheral or central venous injections of contrast media could visualize the pulmonary vessels, eliminating the potentially hazardous and technically difficult placement of a catheter across the right heart (16). Unfortunately, a number of studies showed that venous DSA was less sensitive and more difficult to interpret than classic pulmonary angiography (13,17). However, the technical specifications of DSA equipment are superior to cut-film equipment, imaging at up to 30 frames per second with exposure times as short as 5 milliseconds. Classic pulmonary angiograms obtained on DSA equipment have better image quality than film angiograms and therefore allow more confident detection of pulmonary emboli (18). For these reasons, most pulmonary angiograms are obtained using catheters placed in the pulmonary arteries and imaged using digital subtraction angiography units.

Pulmonary angiography has limitations, since it provides two-dimensional planar images of the complex three-dimensional branching pattern of the pulmonary vasculature. These images can be difficult to interpret because of vessel overlap. Additionally, the contrast sensitivity of pulmonary angiography is limited because of the large amount of scattered radiation present and the diversion of contrast away from vessels that harbor emboli. This causes difficulty in the reliable detection of small emboli in subsegmental-sized vessels (19–21). In a study investigating the reliability of selective pulmonary arteriography in 60 patients suspected of harboring PE, three angiographers reviewed the arteriograms retrospectively, independently, and without benefit of additional data (22). Although the agreement between observers was almost 100% for detecting emboli involving the main, lobar, and segmental vessels, it was only 13% for subsegmental emboli. In the PIOPED study, 1,111 patients underwent catheterization for pulmonary angiography (23). In this large group, 61% had negative angiograms and 35% had positive angiograms. The overall agreement between independent readers regarding the interpretation of angiograms as positive, negative, or nondiagnostic was 81%. However, when the agreement between observers was related to the size of the affected vessel, agreement was 98% for lobar vessels, 90% for segmental vessels, and only 66% for subsegmental vessels (23). Therefore, pulmonary angiography has limitations in the assessment of subsegmental pulmonary arteries.

Although pulmonary angiography is considered to be the gold standard for the diagnosis of PE, the procedure is only requested in a small percentage of patients who have clinically suspected emboli and nondiagnostic ventilation–perfusion scans and negative deep venous studies of the legs. For example, in one review of 316 consecutive cases of suspected PE in a large university medical center in the United States, only 17% of 141 patients who had indeterminate ventilation-perfusion scans underwent angiography (24). In a survey of 360 acute care hospitals in the United Kingdom, it was found that approximately 47,000 ventilation–perfusion lung scans had been obtained compared to only 490 pulmonary angiograms (25). Even if one postulates that only 20% of the scans were intermediate probability, in which angiography is indicated, approximately 9,000 angiograms should have been done. Part of the reluctance to request pulmonary angiography is due to the invasive nature of the examination and the concern about the perceived risks (15,26,27).

Summary

Imaging algorithms utilizing ventilation–perfusion scintigraphy, leg venous studies, and pulmonary angiography have substantial limitations, and often result in patients being treated on clinical grounds without a definitive diagnosis. For this reason, the introduction of spiral CT angiography of the pulmonary arteries has been greeted with enthusiasm.

TECHNIQUE OF SPIRAL CT ANGIOGRAPHY FOR ACUTE PULMONARY EMBOLISM

Equipment Factors

Initial studies assessing the potential role of CT in the diagnosis of pulmonary embolism used conventional stop-and-shoot CT scanners that required a 1- to 2-second breath-hold for each transverse slice and a 6- to 8-second delay between slices. The slow rate of scan acquisition made it impossible to cover the central, segmental, and subsegmental pulmonary arteries during the bolus phase of contrast enhancement. As

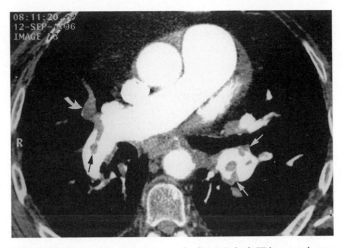

FIGURE 4-1. Acute pulmonary embolism. Spiral CT image shows several partial (*straight arrows*) filling defects and one complete (*curved arrow*) filling defect in the pulmonary arteries. The image was obtained using single-slice spiral CT and 2-mm collimation. Note enlarged pulmonary arteries consistent with pulmonary arterial hypertension.

a consequence, only large emboli in the main or interlobar pulmonary arteries could be seen (28–31).

The development of single-slice spiral CT made it possible to image the central, segmental, and subsegmental pulmonary arteries within the 40-second duration of a peripheral venous contrast media injection. This technique allowed the direct visualization of pulmonary emboli in central and segmental vessels (Figure 4-1). These early spiral CT scanners provided gantry rotation times of 1 second. Advances in spiral CT scanner technology have increased gantry rotation speed, initially to 0.75 seconds and more recently to 0.5 seconds. Faster gantry rotation has allowed the section collimation to be reduced from 5 mm to 2 mm while maintaining the same volume coverage. This change in scan acquisition decreased volume-averaging effects and has permitted the analysis of subsegmental pulmonary vessels. Image quality on thin-collimation, single-slice spiral CT examinations is sufficient to enable a debate in the literature regarding the relative diagnostic accuracy of spiral CT versus pulmonary angiography (32).

The introduction of four-row multislice scanners has allowed even thinner section collimation to be used (1.0 to 1.25 mm), providing improved images of subsegmental vessels (33). The improved diagnostic accuracy of this equipment in acute PE will require further patient studies.

Scanning Technique

Adequate screening for acute PE requires that the main, lobar, segmental, and subsegmental arteries of the upper, middle, and lower lobes be imaged. Because the acquisition protocol is directly dependent on the CT technology used, we will describe the optimal protocol for scanning patients with single-slice CT, and then summarize the modifications induced by the introduction of multislice CT.

CT Angiography Protocol With Single-Slice CT

Acquisition Parameters

CTA on single-slice spiral CT is usually preceded by a non-contrast examination over the entire thorax aimed at searching for pleural and parenchymal abnormalities associated with acute PE (i.e., lung infarction, pleural effusion, and additional abnormalities), sometimes unsuspected clinically and suggestive of an alternative diagnosis. Whereas this noncontrast examination can be obtained with a variety of protocols, we recommend scanning the entire thorax with a high-resolution CT technique, namely to obtain 1-mm thick sections at 10-mm intervals. This selection allows an accurate depiction of CT features of chronic PE, in particular mosaic perfusion and bronchial dilation, because some patients may present with acute PE superimposed on chronic PE. The second advantage of this thin-collimation protocol is to provide an insight into the patient's underlying respiratory disorders, such as chronic obstructive pulmonary disease (COPD).

CTA is performed over a region-of-interest of approximately 10 to 12 cm, extending from the aortic arch to 2 cm below the inferior pulmonary veins. This region must be covered during peak contrast enhancement and preferably with the patient motionless in suspended inspiration. The direction of scanning, cranial to caudal or caudal to cranial, appears not to be a major issue as various groups of investigators have reported comparable results with both techniques. The selection of the thinnest possible collimation (i.e., 3 or 2 mm), in conjunction with a pitch of 1.7 to 2.0 has been shown to optimize the visualization of distal segmental and subsegmental vessels (34). A narrow angle (e.g., 180 degrees) interpolation algorithm should be used to minimize the effective section thickness. In patients who cannot hold their breath for the duration of the scan, it is preferable to scan in quiet breathing than to attempt a breath-hold and have part of the scan degraded by gasping respiration. Scans at either full inspiration or near end expiration provide the highest pulmonary vascular resistance, which facilitates high quality pulmonary arterial opacification (35). Images should be reconstructed using the standard algorithm and a field of view appropriate to the patient size. Overlapping reconstruction is not routinely necessary for 2- and 3-mm collimation studies, except in regions of equivocal interpretation. Sagittal, coronal, and oblique reformations may be useful to differentiate endoluminal clot from arterial wall thickening and surrounding hilar lymph nodes (36).

Further discussion of contrast injection techniques, scan delay, and venous access sites can be found in Chapter 1. Specific scanning protocols are found in Appendix A.

Injection Parameters

The injection parameters depend on the site of administration of contrast material. When an antecubital vein is available, we favor the use of a 24% contrast agent administered at a rate of 4 mL per second. A start delay of 15 seconds is commonly chosen for patients with normal hemodynamic status, whereas it should be increased to 18 to 20 seconds in patients with known or suspected pulmonary hypertension and/or right heart failure. When a more peripheral venous access has to be used, it is necessary to reduce the rate of injection to avoid extravasation of contrast material. As a consequence, we commonly use a more concentrated contrast agent (i.e., a 30% contrast agent), and increase the start delay to allow the contrast material to opacify pulmonary arteries on the first levels imaged. With a central venous access the scan delay is shorter due to the location of the tip of the catheter in the superior vena cava or right atrium. Because of the high frequency of venous flattening after positioning the upper limb above the patient's head (see Chapter 2), we recommend the administration of contrast material with the ipsilateral arm positioned alongside the body.

CT Angiography Protocol With Multislice CT

On multislice CT scanners, depending on the patient's breath-hold capabilities, two protocols can be considered. In patients able to hold their breath, the entire thorax is scanned using 4× 1-mm collimation and a pitch of 2.0, requiring a breath-hold of 20 seconds or less. This acquisition is obtained during administration of contrast material. The injection parameters do not differ from those described for single-slice CT except an increase in the start delay, preferably chosen around 18 seconds to allow adequate enhancement of all visualized pulmonary arteries. If the patient is short of breath, we suggest following a protocol similar to that proposed with single-slice CT. This should be started with a noncontrast CT examination of the entire thorax obtained with a 4× 1-mm collimation and a pitch of 2.0 (breath-hold duration: 10 seconds maximum), then followed by a CT angiogram over the 10- to 12-cm region-of-interest, also obtained with a 4× 1-mm collimation and a pitch of 2.0 after selection of a start delay of 15 seconds in the absence of hemodynamic abnormalities. Although most of the injection parameters are similar to those recommended for single-slice CT, scanning the thorax with multislice CT allows the overall volume administered to the patient to be reduced by 30% (37). Whatever the protocol selected, all these examinations are reconstructed with 1-mm thick sections, enabling an accurate evaluation of peripheral pulmonary

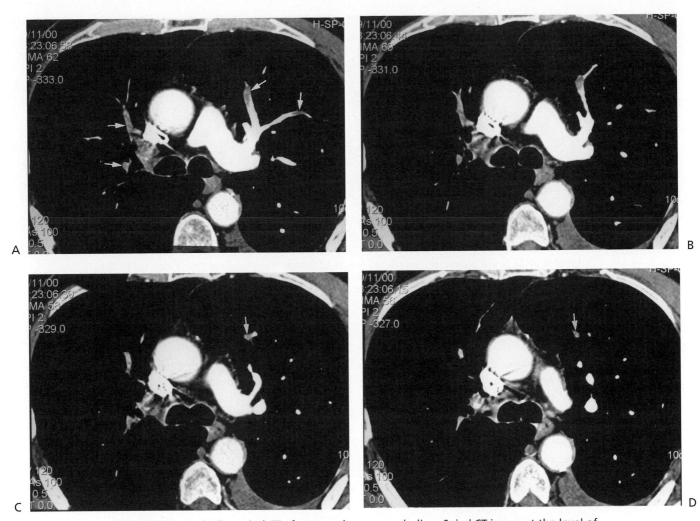

FIGURE 4-2. Multislice spiral CT of acute pulmonary embolism. Spiral CT image at the level of bifurcation of the anterior segmental artery of the left upper lobe (**A**) shows partial peripheral filling defects in the subsegmental branches (*arrows*). Also noted are complete filling defects in the apical and anterior segmental arteries of the right upper lobe (*arrows*). Image 2-mm caudad (**B**) essentially confirms the presence of multiple emboli. Image 2-mm caudad to **B** (**C**) shows filling defect in divisions of LA2 corresponding to a fifth-order arterial branch (*arrow*). Image 2-mm caudad to **C** (**D**) confirms the presence of the embolus. The images were obtained using multislice CT with ×4 1-mm collimation and 1.25-mm reconstructions.

arteries, including subsegmental and fifth-order arterial branches (Figure 4-2).

DIAGNOSTIC FINDINGS IN ACUTE PULMONARY EMBOLISM

The diagnosis of acute PE on contrast-enhanced spiral CT is based on the presence of partial or complete filling defects within the contrast-enhanced lumen of the pulmonary arteries (4,29) (Box 4-1). These signs are the spiral CT

BOX 4-1. SIGNS OF ACUTE PULMONARY EMBOLISM

Mediastinal windows
    Partial filling defects
        Central
        Marginal
    Complete filling defects
    Abrupt occlusion
Lung windows
    Wedge-shaped, pleural-based consolidation
    Dilated central or segmental pulmonary arteries

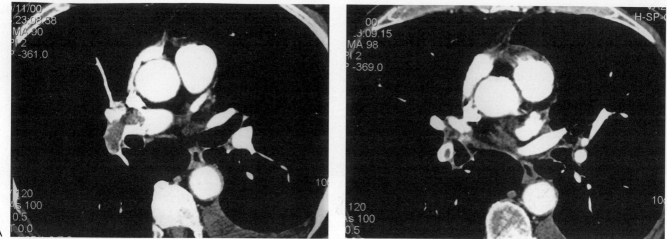

FIGURE 4-3. Acute pulmonary embolism. Spiral CT image shows partial filling defects in the right main, right interlobar (**A**), and right lower lobe (**B**) pulmonary arteries. Also noted is a small left pleural effusion. The image was obtained on a single-slice spiral CT scanner using 2-mm collimation.

equivalent of classic pulmonary angiographic signs of PE (i.e., the railway track sign and the abrupt vascular cutoff sign). Partial filling defects are defined as intravascular central or marginal areas of low attenuation surrounded by variable amounts of contrast material (Figure 4-3). Complete filling defects are defined as an intraluminal area of low attenuation that occupies the entire arterial section (i.e., the abrupt absence of contrast material in a previously contrast-enhanced vessel) (Figures 4-1 and 4-2). The most reli-

able signs of an acute embolism are a central filling defect or a marginal filling defect forming an acute angle with the vessel wall (Figures 4-1 and 4-3).

Most authors review transverse images at mediastinal (window width 450 HU, window level 35 HU) and lung (window width 1,500 HU, level −700 HU) settings. Review of both mediastinal and lung window settings is essential for distinction of pulmonary arteries from veins at the segmental and subsegmental levels (Figures 4-4 and 4-

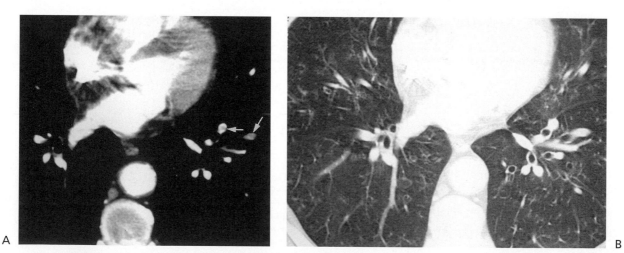

FIGURE 4-4. Acute pulmonary embolism: value of analysis of lung windows. Spiral CT images at the same anatomic level photographed using mediastinal (**A**) and lung (**B**) window settings. The presence of filling defects in the medial (LA7) and anterior (LA8) basal segmental arteries (*arrows*) of the left lower lobe can be recognized by analysis of both mediastinal and lung windows, which allow easy differentiation between pulmonary arteries and veins. The images were obtained on a single-detector spiral CT scanner using 2-mm collimation.

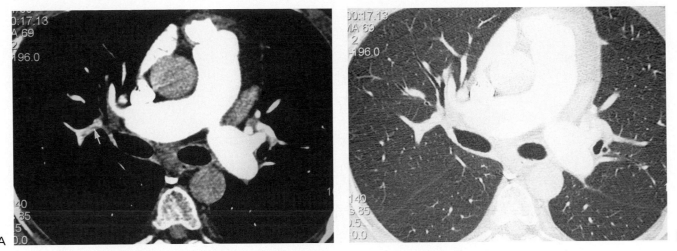

FIGURE 4-5. Pseudo-filling defect: value of analysis of lung windows. Spiral CT image photographed at mediastinal window settings (**A**) shows apparent filling defects (*arrow*). Image at the same anatomic level photographed at lung window settings (**B**) shows that the vessel is a vein, the posterior segmental vein of the right upper lobe (RV3). The images were obtained on a multislice CT scanner using ×4 1-mm collimation and 1.25-mm reconstructions.

5). It should be noted, however, that on conventional mediastinal window settings, partially occlusive thrombi may be obscured by high-density contrast material. Optimized window settings for the visualization of pulmonary emboli have been investigated in a porcine model (38). These window settings, which are wider than the conventional mediastinal settings, are further customized by referencing them to the actual attenuation in the right and left pulmonary arteries. In our experience, these optimized viewing parameters are most helpful in the analysis of subsegmental (fifth generation) vessels.

INTERPRETATIVE PITFALLS IN ACUTE PULMONARY EMBOLISM

A number of interpretative pitfalls exist in assessing contrast-enhanced spiral CT images, but their recognition becomes less problematic as experience is gained with this technique (Box 4-2). Pseudo-filling defects, which masquerade as pulmonary emboli, may arise from five major sources: motion artifact, partial volume averaging of vessels coursing in and out of the plane of section, suboptimal contrast injection technique, hilar lymph nodes, and asymmetric pulmonary vascular resistance. Respiratory and cardiac motion artifacts result in apparent termination of vessels or give rise to volume averaging with surrounding air-filled lung, mimicking intraluminal filling defects (Figure 4-6). Observing the chest wall for respiratory motion during cine viewing of the images on the workstation aids in the recognition of this artifact.

BOX 4-2. MIMICS OF ACUTE PULMONARY EMBOLISM ON SPIRAL CT

Technical factors
- Breathing artifacts
- Suboptimal enhancement
- Partial volume effect
- Streak artifacts around the superior vena cava mimicking a thrombus within RA1

Anatomy
- Hilar lymph nodes
- Poor venous enhancement

Pathophysiologic factors
- Unilateral increase in pulmonary vascular resistance
    Large pleural effusion
    Extensive lung consolidation
    Hyperinflation
    Hypoxic vasoconstriction
    Conditions with elevated venous pressure
- Left-to-right shunt: severe chronic inflammatory disease
- Right-to-left shunt: patent foramen ovale

Noncruoric emboli
- Septic
- Tumoral
    PA sarcomas
    Right heart myxoma
    Metastatic emboli
    Hepatic artery chemotherapy
- Embolic material
    Systemic AV fistula
    Varicoceles
    Esophageal varices
    Bullet trauma
- Hydatic emboli

AV, arteriovenous; PA, pulmonary artery; RA1, apical segmental artery of the right upper lobe.

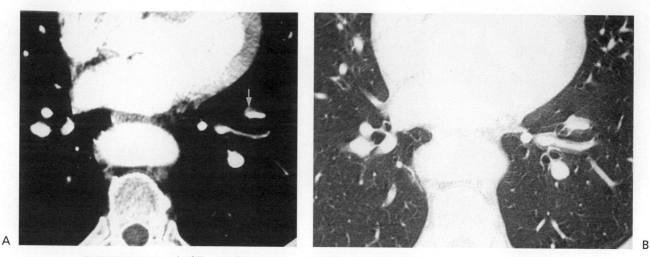

FIGURE 4-6. Pseudo-filling defect due to cardiac motion. Spiral CT images at the same anatomic level photographed at mediastinal (**A**) and lung (**B**) window settings. Image at mediastinal window settings (**A**) shows apparent filling defect (*arrow*) in the anteromedial basal segmental artery of the left lower lobe (LA8). Image at lung window settings (**B**) shows that the apparent filling defect is due to motion. Note blurring of the left lower lobe vessels due to cardiac motion. (From Remy-Jardin M, Baghaie F, Bonnel F, et al. Thoracic helical CT: influence of subsecond scan time and thin collimation on evaluation of peripheral pulmonary arteries. *Eur Radiol* 2000;10: 1297–1303, with permission)

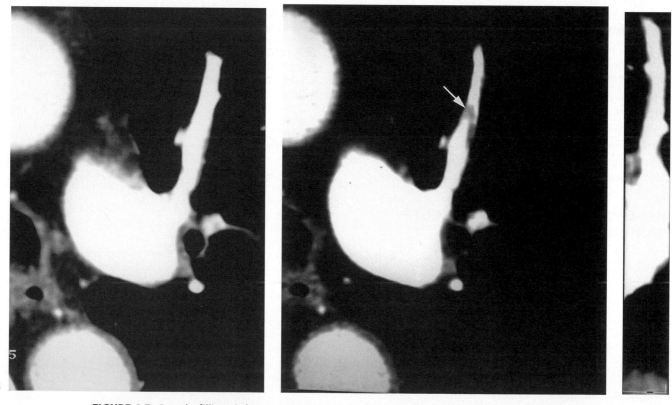

FIGURE 4-7. Pseudo-filling defect: value of two-dimensional reformation. Spiral CT image (**A**) at the level of the anterior segmental artery of the left upper lobe (LA2) is normal. Image immediately caudad (**B**) shows apparent filling defect (*arrow*). Two-dimensional reformatted image of the anterior segmental artery (**C**) is normal. The apparent filling defect seen in image **B** is due to partial volume averaging as the most inferior portion of the vessels courses in and out of the plane of section. The CT scan was obtained on a single-slice spiral scanner using 2-mm collimation and overlapping reconstructions at 0.5-mm intervals.

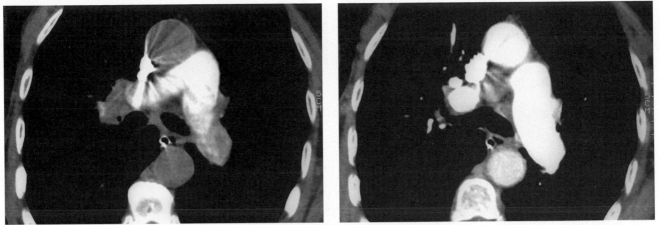

FIGURE 4-8. Pseudo-filling defect due to insufficient scan delay. Spiral CT image obtained 7 seconds after the start of intravenous injection of contrast (**A**) shows apparent filling defects in the pulmonary arteries. Spiral CT image obtained 8 seconds later (**B**) is normal. The apparent filling defects were due to too short a scan delay. The CT was performed on a single-slice spiral scanner using 3-mm collimation.

Pseudo-filling defects may also occur due to volume averaging of vessels coursing in and out of the plane of section (Figure 4-7). An inappropriate choice of scanning delay can result in inadequate contrast enhancement at either the beginning or the end of the scan (Figure 4-8). The occurrence of contrast delivery-related pseudo-emboli at the beginning of the scan acquisition can be minimized by the use of a timing bolus or automated scan initiation technique. Ensuring that the contrast bolus extends to the end of the scan acquisition can eliminate poor contrast enhancement at the end of the scan.

Knowledge of the size and location of pulmonary hilar lymph nodes is essential in the interpretation of spiral CT pulmonary angiograms (39). Normal and abnormal nodes are seen as low-density structures adjacent to vessels. They can appear as intraluminal defects when they are located at vessel bifurcations and can be mistaken for pulmonary emboli. Coronal and sagittal reformations may be helpful in differentiating nodes adjacent to vessels from emboli within vessels.

Asymmetry in pulmonary vascular resistance, which is usually due to extensive airspace consolidation and reactive pulmonary vascular vasoconstriction, can lead to the false positive diagnosis of PE (Box 4-2). These pulmonary vascular flow problems have been previously recognized with both pulmonary angiography and ventilation–perfusion scintigraphy (40,41). They arise from either: (a) "occult" pulmonary artery; (b) a unilateral pulmonary artery obstruction of extrinsic, mural, or endoluminal origin; (c) a unilateral increase in pulmonary vascular resistance secondary to airway obstruction, lung destruc-

tion or consolidation, pleural restriction, or elevated pulmonary venous pressure; or (d) congenital and acquired systemic-to-pulmonary shunting affecting one hemithorax (Figure 4-9). These flow-related causes of pseudo-emboli are best recognized through the use of a second contrast-enhanced spiral acquisition with an extended delay to allow visualization of delayed blood flow into the affected lung.

LUNG PARENCHYMAL FINDINGS IN ACUTE PULMONARY EMBOLISM

Spiral CT visualization of lung parenchymal and pleural abnormalities in patients with acute PE has been investigated in two studies. The first evaluated 88 patients with clinically suspected acute PE (42). This study found that wedge-shaped, pleural-based consolidation (Figure 4-9), linear bands, and dilated central or segmental pulmonary arteries (Figure 4-10) were statistically significantly associated with PE. Similar findings were reported in a second independent study of 92 patients (43). Of note, the presence of pleural effusion was not correlated with PE in either study. Although parenchymal and pleural findings have been shown to be of limited value, the identification of these features at CT may be useful to direct further investigations when there is suboptimal visualization of central or segmental vessels.

Recently, there has been interest in detection of pulmonary parenchymal blood flow using CT (Figure 4-11). Schoepf and colleagues used contrast-enhanced electron

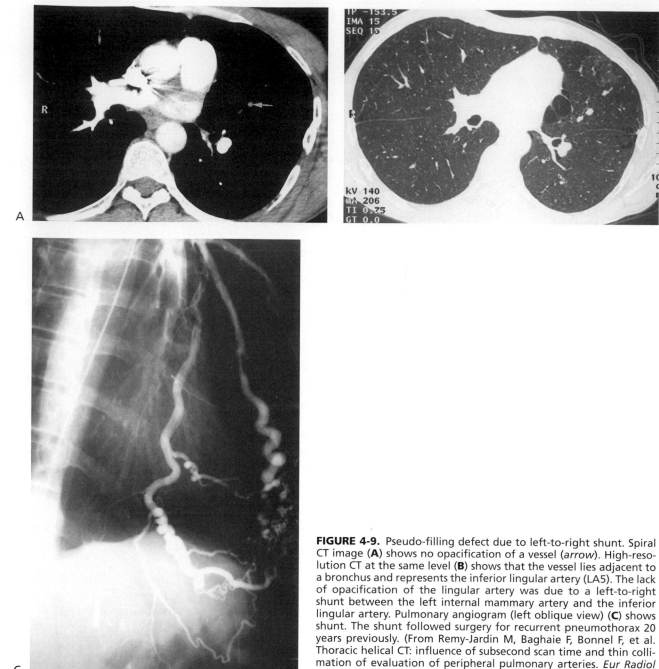

FIGURE 4-9. Pseudo-filling defect due to left-to-right shunt. Spiral CT image (**A**) shows no opacification of a vessel (*arrow*). High-resolution CT at the same level (**B**) shows that the vessel lies adjacent to a bronchus and represents the inferior lingular artery (LA5). The lack of opacification of the lingular artery was due to a left-to-right shunt between the left internal mammary artery and the inferior lingular artery. Pulmonary angiogram (left oblique view) (**C**) shows shunt. The shunt followed surgery for recurrent pneumothorax 20 years previously. (From Remy-Jardin M, Baghaie F, Bonnel F, et al. Thoracic helical CT: influence of subsecond scan time and thin collimation of evaluation of peripheral pulmonary arteries. *Eur Radiol* 1998;8:1376–1390, with permission.)

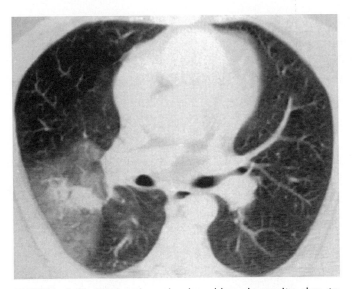

FIGURE 4-10. Wedge-shaped, pleural-based opacity due to occlusive embolus. Lung window settings (width 1500 HU, level −750 HU) in a patient with acute pulmonary embolism shows a wedge-shaped, pleural-based, ground-glass opacification and central consolidation in the posterior segment of the right upper lobe. An occlusive thrombus was present in the posterior segmental artery to the right upper lobe.

beam CT to measure blood flow in the pulmonary microcirculation in patients harboring segmental pulmonary emboli (44). The multislice mode of the scanner was used to obtain eight sections in a 7.6-cm volume at 20 consecutive time points during a contrast injection. This allowed them to monitor the passage of the contrast material bolus

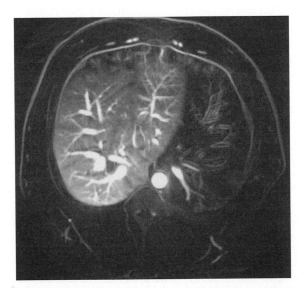

FIGURE 4-11. Absent perfusion due to vascular occlusion. Contrast-enhanced spiral CT through the lower lobes of a pig with balloon occlusion of the left lower lobe pulmonary artery. This enhanced image (peak attenuation change) demonstrates absent perfusion in the left lower lobe compared to the normal right lower lobe. Retrograde flow of contrast is seen in the left lower lobe pulmonary vein.

through the lung parenchyma. They found mean pulmonary blood flow of 0.63 mL per minute per mL in occluded segments compared to 2.27 mL per minute per mL in nonoccluded segments. Using spiral CT as the gold standard to identify occluded segmental arteries, they found the sensitivity and specificity of CT perfusion maps to be 75% and 82%. This study demonstrated the feasibility of using spiral CT to characterize blood flow in both the large conducting pulmonary vessels and in the microcirculation.

DIAGNOSTIC ACCURACY OF SPIRAL CT IN ACUTE PULMONARY EMBOLISM

Introduction

Initial studies using single-slice spiral CT showed high-sensitivity and specificity for pulmonary emboli in main, lobar, and segmental vessels (Table 4-1). More recent studies using improved techniques (thin collimation of 3 mm or less), single-slice spiral CT, or multislice spiral CT have extended these favorable results to subsegmental vessels. In published studies, the specificity of spiral CT in acute PE has been high, ranging from 78% to 100%. However, the sensitivity values have shown a larger variation, ranging from 53% to 100%. Most investigators have reported a 2% to 4% rate of suboptimal spiral CT examinations in acute PE (45), which is comparable to the 3% rate of suboptimal pulmonary angiograms reported in the PIOPED trial (5). Both spiral CT and pulmonary angiography produce suboptimal examinations most often in patients with severe dyspnea.

Debate over the of role of spiral CT in acute PE has centered around the sensitivity value. Authors reporting sensitivity values greater than 85% have recommended spiral CT as a screening study for acute PE (46,47). Conversely, those finding sensitivity values less than this value have recommended spiral CT as a confirmatory study (48). The cutoff value of 85% sensitivity arises from cost-effectiveness modeling studies of acute PE diagnostic algorithms (49). These statistical models have investigated algorithms utilizing ventilation–perfusion scanning, D-dimer analysis, pulmonary angiography, venous ultrasound, and spiral CT. In balancing cost-effectiveness and safety, these researchers found that the inclusion of spiral CT into the diagnostic algorithm improved patient outcome if the CT sensitivity was greater than 85%. Therefore, the substantial variation in the reported sensitivity values from different studies has fuelled the debate surrounding its place in the diagnostic algorithm. Review of the scan acquisition and interpretative techniques employed in the published studies indicates substantial evolution of spiral CT techniques since the initial study in 1992. This variation in technical factors, coupled with selection bias in the study populations, accounts for the range of reported sensitivity values. In the following

TABLE 4-1. ACCURACY OF SPIRAL CT IN THE DIAGNOSIS OF ACUTE PULMONARY EMBOLISM

Study	Year	No. of Patients in Study	Collimation (mm)	Lower Anatomic Level of Interpretation	Sensitivity (%)[a]	Specificity (%)[a]	k Value[a]
Remy-Jardin, et al. (4)	1992	42	5	Segmental	100	96	NC
Goodman, et al. (61)	1995	20	5	Segmental	86	92	NC
Senac, et al. (62)	1995	45	5	Segmental	86	100	NC
van Rossum, et al. (51)	1996	149	5	Segmental	82–90	93–96	0.774
Remy-Jardin, et al. (46)	1996	75	5, 3	Segmental	91	78	NC
Ferretti, et al. (55)	1997	164	5	Segmental	NC	NC	NC
Mayo, et al. (47)	1997	142	3	Segmental	87	95	0.85
van Rossum, et al. (63)	1998	123	5	Segmental	75	90	NC
Drucker, et al. (48)	1998	47	5	Segmental	53–60	81–97	NC
Herold, et al. (52)	1998	401	3	Subsegmental	88	94	0.72
Garg, et al. (64)	1998	54	3	Subsegmental	67	100	NC
Baghaie, et al. (65)	1998	370	3, 2	Subsegmental	96	100	0.87
Kim, et al. (54)	1999	110	3	Segmental	92	96	NC
Qanadli, et al. (50)	2000	157	2.5, dual section	Subsegmental	90	94	0.86

[a]NC, not calculated in that study.

paragraphs, we will briefly review some the studies of spiral CT for acute PE.

Comparison With Pulmonary Angiography

The first blinded prospective study comparing spiral CT to pulmonary angiography for the detection of acute PE was performed by Remy-Jardin and colleagues (4). This study included 24 patients without embolism and 18 who had angiographically proven disease. Spiral CT was correctly interpreted as positive in all 18 patients who had angiographically proven embolism (sensitivity 100%) and as negative in 23 of 24 patients without embolism (specificity 96%). In this study, the 112 central emboli (8 involving the main pulmonary arteries, 28 the lobar, and 76 the segmental) that were identified on spiral CT corresponded exactly to the angiographic findings; however, 9 intersegmental lymph nodes were erroneously interpreted as filling defects. This study, which constitutes a proof of concept study, excluded inconclusive CT studies and had a lower mean age (34 years) than other studies. These study conditions may have contributed to the high accuracy of spiral CT. The same group performed a follow-up prospective study comparing spiral CT to pulmonary angiography and ventilation–perfusion scintigraphy in 1996. They studied 75 patients and reported a sensitivity of 91% and a specificity of 100% for spiral CT (46). Again, pulmonary angiography was the gold standard examination for this trial.

Drucker and coworkers reported lower sensitivity and specificity values in a study comparing spiral CT to pul-

monary angiography (48). In this prospective study of 47 patients, readers in two institutions interpreted spiral CT images using films. Spiral CT technical factors included 5-mm collimation, pitch 1.0, and images reconstructed at 3-mm spacing. The spiral CT interpretations from the two institutions showed sensitivity values of 53% and 60%, and specificity values of 81% and 97%. The low-sensitivity values found in this study have not been replicated in previous or subsequent published series (Box 4-1). The authors noted that the scan acquisition parameters of 5-mm collimation, pitch 1.0, and the interpretation of images on film probably contributed to the low-sensitivity value. This study emphasizes that technical issues in scan acquisition and display may critically affect the results obtained with spiral CT in acute PE.

The first published study of multislice spiral CT in acute PE compared CT to pulmonary angiography in a prospective trial of 204 consecutive patients (50). In this study, there was no significant difference in the rate of suboptimal studies between dual-slice spiral CT (7%) and selective pulmonary angiography (6%). Compared to selective pulmonary angiography, dual-slice CTA demonstrated 94% specificity and 90% sensitivity.

Comparison With Ventilation–Perfusion Scintigraphy

A prospective comparison of spiral CT and ventilation–perfusion scintigraphy was performed in 142 patients (47). In both centers, two experienced observers independently assessed the results of both spiral CT and ventilation–perfusion scintigraphy. Spiral CT scans were obtained using 3-mm collimation and pitch values from 1.8 to 2.0. Images were interpreted on a workstation. The combination of a high-probability ventilation–perfusion scan and a spiral CT showing acute PE was considered diagnostic and no further imaging studies were required. The combination of normal, very low, or low-probability ventilation–perfusion scans and a negative spiral CT in a patient with a low clinical suspicion of PE was considered to be sufficient to exclude the disease. Patients who had intermediate ventilation–perfusion scans, discordance between the interpretation of ventilation–perfusion and spiral CT scans, and those with a high clinical index of suspicion underwent pulmonary angiography. Overall, spiral CT had a sensitivity of 87% and a specificity of 98% in the diagnosis of acute PE compared with a sensitivity of 41% and a specificity of 52% for a high-probability ventilation–perfusion scan. Twelve patients had discordant spiral CT and ventilation–perfusion results; using angiographic results as the gold standard, the spiral CT interpretation was correct in 11 and the ventilation–perfusion scan was correct in one. Analysis of the repeated interpretation of spiral CT and ventilation–perfusion scintigraphy images showed better interobserver agreement for CT, with values of 0.85 and 0.61, respectively (Kappa statistic). Comparable results were obtained in a subsequent similar trial of 149 patients (51). These authors reported 88% sensitivity, 95% specificity (averaged over two observers), and a Kappa value of 0.774.

A multicenter trial comparing spiral CT to ventilation–perfusion scintigraphy was performed in 10 European academic medical centers (52). Between January 1996 and April 1997, 758 patients were enrolled and 391 completed the study protocol. Similar to previous studies, all patients received spiral CT and ventilation–perfusion examinations. These two examinations served as a gold standard when they were in agreement and either normal or abnormal. In all other cases pulmonary angiography was performed. Initially, the images were interpreted locally, using a combination of film and cine viewing on a workstation. Films were then sent to two expert readers for interpretation. When the two expert readers disagreed, a third expert reader was used. In the local readings, spiral CT had a sensitivity of 95% and a specificity of 97%. In the pulmonary angiography subgroup, the local readers showed a sensitivity of 88% and specificity of 92%. The expert readers showed lower sensitivity of 87% and specificity of 90%. The improved performance of the local readers was ascribed to the interpretation of spiral CT images on the workstation using cine mode.

Clinical Utility Trials

Cross and coworkers compared spiral CT to ventilation–perfusion scintigraphy as the initial investigation in acute PE (53). This study was a randomized prospective trial performed in 78 patients. The authors

reported that a confident diagnosis was made in a significantly larger proportion of patients when spiral CT was used as the initial investigation (35/39, 90%) compared to using ventilation–perfusion scintigraphy (21/39, 54%, *p* less than 0.001). They found that the main difference between the two groups was that spiral CT demonstrated lesions other than pulmonary embolism, which accounted for the patient's symptoms. In the crossover segment of the study, spiral CT detected PE in two patients with nondiagnostic ventilation–perfusion scintigraphy. They recommended that where logistically feasible, spiral CT should replace ventilation–perfusion scintigraphy as the initial investigation for PE in patients with an underlying cardiorespiratory disorder.

Kim and associates prospectively determined the utility of spiral CT in 110 patients with clinically suspected acute PE (54). They compared spiral CT with at least one other imaging modality: ventilation–perfusion scintigraphy, ultrasonography of deep leg veins, or pulmonary angiography. Concordant findings between spiral CT and either ventilation–perfusion scintigraphy or ultrasonography of deep leg veins was considered sufficient to establish or refute the diagnosis of PE. In all cases where spiral CT disagreed with either ventilation–perfusion scintigraphy or ultrasonography of deep leg veins, pulmonary angiography was performed and regarded as the gold standard. Spiral CT allowed identification of 23 of 25 patients with acute PE (sensitivity 92%, specificity 96%). In 57 of 85 (67%) patients without PE, spiral CT provided additional information that suggested or confirmed the alternate clinical diagnosis, including pneumonia (Figure 4-12), cardiovascu-

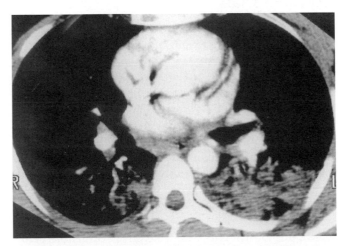

FIGURE 4-12. Bronchopneumonia clinically mimicking acute pulmonary embolism. Contrast-enhanced spiral CT at the level of the aortic root in a patient with pleuritic chest pain and shortness of breath. The scan demonstrates bilateral air-space consolidation in the lower lobes and slightly enlarged lymph nodes abutting the descending pulmonary arteries. There was no evidence of pulmonary embolism. The alternate diagnosis of community-acquired bronchopneumonia was confirmed by a prompt response to antibiotic therapy.

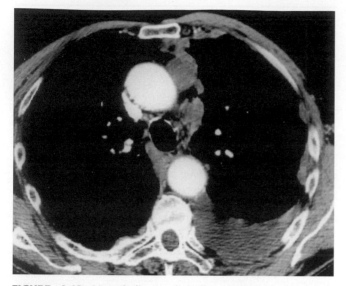

FIGURE 4-13. Mesothelioma clinically mimicking acute pulmonary embolism. This patient presented with pleuritic chest pain and left-sided pleural effusion and was suspected clinically of having acute PE. Spiral CT angiogram showed no evidence of pulmonary embolism but demonstrated nodular left pleural thickening, mediastinal lymphadenopathy, and left pleural effusion. Malignant mesothelioma was diagnosed at thoracoscopic biopsy of the left pleura.

lar disease, pulmonary fibrosis, trauma, postoperative change, malignancy (Figure 4-13), and pleural disease. Therefore, overall spiral CT provided useful information in 80 (73%) of the 110 patients studied.

Outcome Trials

Finally, the utility of a negative spiral CT study in the setting of suspected acute PE has been assessed in two prospective clinical outcome studies. The first included 164 consecutive patients suspected of having acute PE who were found to have intermediate probability ventilation–perfusion scans and negative leg ultrasound studies (55). Forty of the 164 patients (24%) were found to have PE by spiral CT (39/40) or pulmonary angiography (1/40). Three-month follow-up was obtained in 99% (163/164) of the study subjects. Recurrent PE occurred in 6 of 112 patients who had negative spiral CT findings and who did not receive anticoagulation therapy (5%). A second clinical outcome study was performed comparing 198 patients with a negative spiral CT to 350 patients with a negative ventilation–perfusion scan (normal, low probability) (56). In the 3-month follow-up period, subsequent PE occurred in 1% (2/198) of the CT cohort compared to 1.5% (5/162) of the ventilation–perfusion group (not statistically significant). However, differences in the patient dropout rate between the two cohorts has been raised as a potential confounding variable in this study (57).

Metaanalysis Studies

A recent systematic review of the literature has been performed to assess the safety of withholding anticoagulant therapy in patients who have clinically suspected PE and negative results at spiral CT. The authors reviewed all prospective English language studies, accepting 15 of 20 articles identified (58). Two authors used a priori, predefined criteria to independently assess each study. A third author resolved any disagreements by adjudication. Studies were assessed using predefined criteria including: inclusion of a consecutive series of all patients with suspect PE; inclusion of patients with and those without PE; a broad-spectrum of patient characteristics; performance of spiral CT and pulmonary angiography or other reference test in all patients; and independent interpretation of imaging tests. It was concluded that none of the 15 selected studies met all of these criteria to allow adequate evaluation of sensitivity and specificity. On the basis of their study, the authors concluded that the use of spiral CT in acute PE had not been adequately evaluated and therefore the safety of withholding anticoagulant treatment in patients with negative results on helical CT was uncertain. A second independent analysis of a published series on spiral CT for acute PE reached almost identical conclusions (59). It is noted that the studies reviewed in both of these analyses were performed on single-slice spiral CT scanners, using a mixture of film and workstation-based reading techniques.

Experimental Animal Trials

A limitation of human studies is the reliance on pulmonary angiography as the gold standard examination. Since the sensitivity and specificity of spiral CT in some trials has approached that of the pulmonary angiogram, inaccuracy could be introduced by the imperfect interpretation of the pulmonary angiogram. Baile and colleagues performed an experimental study in 16 ventilated anesthetized pigs to address this issue (32). In this repeated measures experimental design study, a methacrylate cast of the pulmonary vasculature was used as an independent gold standard against which both spiral CT and pulmonary angiography were compared. Colored methacrylate beads the diameter size of a human subsegmental pulmonary artery (4 mm) were embolized through a central venous catheter. Spiral CT angiography and three-view digital subtraction pulmonary angiography were performed in random order following embolization of the beads. At the completion of the imaging studies, the pig was euthanized and a clear methacrylate cast of the pulmonary arteries was made. The lungs were removed and the lung tissue was chemically removed, revealing the cast of the pulmonary arteries. Using this technique, the embolized colored methacrylate beads bonded to the clear methacrylate cast, demonstrating the exact location of the embolized beads in the live animal.

Ninety-eight percent of the embolized beads were recovered in the methacrylate casts. Using the methacrylate cast as the true gold standard, no significant difference ($p < 0.05$) was found between 3-mm collimation spiral CT or pulmonary angiography for either sensitivity (82% versus 87%) or positive predictive value (94% versus 88%). However, when the data were reinterpreted assuming pulmonary angiography as the gold standard (100% sensitivity and positive predictive value by definition), spiral CT sensitivity declined to 76% and positive predictive value declined to 86%. This change of spiral CT sensitivity and positive predictive value is secondary to the false-positive and false-negative results at pulmonary angiography. This same effect may affect the reported sensitivity and specificity values obtained in human trials when pulmonary angiography is assumed to be the gold standard.

SUMMARY

There is consensus that the published data support the use of single-slice spiral CT as a confirmatory study for acute PE. The data supporting single-slice spiral CT as a screening study for this condition are compelling at this time, but not yet felt to be conclusive by some authors. There are limited data evaluating multislice spiral CT for the evaluation of acute PE, but these are very encouraging. To convince all members of the medical community of their value, it would appear that a trial of spiral CT similar to that performed for ventilation–perfusion scintigraphy in the late 1980s would be required. This trial will need to be sufficiently large to provide adequate statistical power and employ multislice spiral CT technology. The reliability of the interpretation of all modalities will need to be assessed using blinded independent interpretations. Finally, clinical follow-up of negative patients must be performed to establish the safety of a negative spiral CT examination. It is anticipated that the results of such a trial will confirm the central role of spiral CT in the diagnostic algorithm for acute PE.

Based on the current literature (Table 4-1), we believe that spiral CT has a sensitivity of approximately 90% and a specificity of 90% to 95% in the diagnosis of acute PE. Therefore, we believe that spiral CT is clinically useful in patients with clinically suspected acute PE. Similar to what has been published recently in the clinical literature (60), we believe that patients who have symptoms or signs of deep vein thrombosis should first undergo Doppler ultrasound of the legs. Patients who have no signs or symptoms of deep venous thrombosis (DVT) and symptomatic patients with negative Doppler ultrasound examination and who have no COPD or parenchymal lung disease should undergo ventilation–perfusion scintigraphy. Patients with intermediate probability V/Q scans and patients with low probability scans but a high clinical index of suspicion for acute PE should undergo CT angiography. We believe that CT angiography should replace scintigraphy as the initial imaging modality for patients with COPD or parenchymal lung disease.

REFERENCES

1. Moser KM. State of the art: venous thromboembolism. *Am Rev Respir Dis* 1990;414:235–249.
2. Caranasos G, Stewart R, Cluff L. Drug-induced illness leading to hospitalization. *JAMA* 1974;228:713–717.
3. Henschke C, Mateescu I, Yankelevitz D. Changing practice patterns in the work up of pulmonary embolism. *Chest* 1995;107:940–945.
4. Remy-Jardin M, Remy J, Wattinne L, et al. Central pulmonary thromboembolism: diagnosis with spiral volumetric CT with the single-breath-hold technique. Comparison with pulmonary angiography. *Radiology* 1992;185:381–387.
5. Investigators P. Value of the ventilation–perfusion scans in acute pulmonary embolism: result of the prospective investigation of pulmonary embolism. *JAMA* 1990;263:2753–2759.
6. Sostman HD, Coleman RE, DeLong DM, et al. Evaluation of revised criteria for ventilation–perfusion scintigraphy in patients with suspected pulmonary embolism. *Radiology* 1994;193:103–107.
7. Freitas FE, Sarosi MG, Nagle CC, et al. Modified PIOPED criteria used in clinical practice. *J Nucl Med* 1995;36:1573–1578.
8. Worsley DF, Palevsky H, Alavi A. A detailed evaluation of patients with acute pulmonary embolism and low- or very-low-probability lung scan interpretations. *Arch Intern Med* 1994;154:2737–2741.
9. Hull RD, Raskob GE, Coates G, et al. A new noninvasive management strategy for patients with suspected pulmonary embolism. *Arch Intern Med* 1989;149:2549–2556.
10. Kelley MA, Carson JL, Palevsky HI, et al. Diagnosing pulmonary embolism: new facts and strategies. *Ann Intern Med* 1991;114:30.
11. Stein PD, Hull RD, Saltzman HA, et al. Strategy for diagnosis of patients with suspected acute pulmonary embolism. *Chest* 1993;103:1553–1559.
12. Oudkerk M, van Beek EJR, van Putten WLJ, et al. Cost-effectiveness analysis of various strategies in the diagnostic management of pulmonary embolism. *Arch Intern Med* 1993;153:947–954.
13. Stein PD, Athanasoulis C, Alavi A, et al. Complications and validity of pulmonary angiography in acute pulmonary embolism. *Circulation* 1992;85:462–468.
14. Grollman JH, Renner JW. Transfemoral pulmonary angiography: update on technique. *AJR* 1981;136:624–626.
15. Hudson ER, Smith TP, McDermott VG, et al. Pulmonary angiography performed with iopamidol: complications in 1,434 patients. *Radiology* 1996;198:61–65.
16. Musset D, Rosso J, Petipretz P, et al. Acute pulmonary embolism diagnostic value of digital subtraction angiography. *Radiology* 1988;166:455–459.
17. van Rooej WJ, den Heeten GJ, Sluzewski M. Pulmonary embolism: diagnosis in 211 patients with use of selective pulmonary digital subtraction angiography with a flow-directed catheter. *Radiology* 1995;195:793–797.
18. Johnson MS, Stine SB, Shah H, et al. Possible pulmonary embolus: evaluation with digital subtraction versus cut-film angiography—prospective study in 80 patients. *Radiology* 1998;207:131–138.
19. Ormond RS, Gale HH, Drake EH, et al. Pulmonary angiography and pulmonary embolism. *Radiology* 1966;86:658.
20. Weidner W, Swanson L, Wilson G. Roentgen techniques in the diagnosis of pulmonary thromboembolism. *AJR* 1967;100:397.
21. Weiner SN, Edelstein J, Charms BL. Observations on pulmonary embolism and the pulmonary angiogram. *AJR* 1966;98:859.
22. Quinn MF, Lundell CJ, Klotz TA, et al. Reliability of selective

pulmonary arteriography in the diagnosis of pulmonary embolism. *AJR* 1987;149:469–471.

23. Pond GD, Ovitt TW, Capp MP. Comparison of conventional pulmonary angiography with intravenous digital subtraction angiography for pulmonary embolic disease. *Radiology* 1983;147:345–350.

24. Schluger N, Henschke CI, King T, et al. Diagnosis of pulmonary embolism at a large teaching hospital. *J Thorac Imag* 1994;9:180–184.

25. Cooper TJ, Hayward MWJ, Hartog M. Survey on the use of pulmonary scintigraphy and angiography for suspected pulmonary thromboembolism in the UK. *Clin Radiol* 1991;43:243–245.

26. Mills SR, Jackson DV, Older RA, et al. The incidence, etiologies, and avoidance of complications of pulmonary angiography in a large series. *Radiology* 1980;136:295–299.

27. Perlmutt LM, Braun SD, Newman GE, et al. Pulmonary arteriography in the high-risk patient. *Radiology* 1987;162:187–189.

28. Godwin JD, Webb WR, Gamsu G, et al. Computed tomography of pulmonary embolism. *AJR* 1980;135(4):691–695.

29. Sinner WN. Computed tomography of pulmonary thromboembolism. *Eur J Radiol* 1982;2(1):8–13.

30. Breatnach E, Stanley RJ. CT diagnosis of segmental pulmonary artery embolus. *J Comput Assist Tomogr* 1984;8:762–764.

31. Kolebo P, Wallin J. Computed tomography in massive pulmonary embolism. *Acta Radiol* 1989;30:105–107.

32. Baile EM, King GG, Müller N, et al. Spiral computed tomography is comparable to angiography for the diagnosis of pulmonary embolism. *Am J Respir Crit Care Med* 2000;161:1010–1015.

33. Ghaye B, Szapiro D, Delannoy V, et al. How far does multidetector CT allow the analysis of peripheral pulmonary arteries? A comparative study with thin collimation single detector CT. *Radiology* 2000;217(P):508.

34. Remy-Jardin M, Remy J, Artaud D, et al. Peripheral pulmonary arteries: optimization of the spiral CT acquisition protocol. *Radiology* 1997;204:157–163.

35. Remy-Jardin M, Remy J, Artaud D, et al. Spiral CT of pulmonary embolism: technical considerations and interpretive pitfalls. *J Thorac Imag* 1997;12:103–117.

36. Remy-Jardin M, Remy J, Cauvain O, et al. Diagnosis of central pulmonary embolism with helical CT: role of two dimensional multiplanar reformations. *AJR* 1995;165:1131–1138.

37. Remy-Jardin M, Mastora I, Masson P, et al. Multislice CT of the thorax with reduced volume of contrast material: a comparative study with single slice CT. *Eur Radiol* 2001;11(P):167.

38. Brink JA, Woodard PK, Horesh L, et al. Depiction of pulmonary emboli with spiral CT: optimization of display window settings in a porcine model. *Radiology* 1997;204:703–708.

39. Remy-Jardin M, Duyck P, Remy J, et al. Hilar lymph nodes: identification with spiral CT and histologic correlation. *Radiology* 1995;196(2):387–394.

40. Bookstein JJ, Silver TM. The angiographic differential diagnosis of acute pulmonary embolism. *Radiology* 1974;110:25–33.

41. Sagel SS, Greenspan RH. Non-uniform pulmonary arterial perfusion: pulmonary embolism. *Radiology* 1970;99:541–548.

42. Coche EE, Müller NL, Kim W, et al. Acute pulmonary embolism: ancillary findings at spiral CT. *Radiology* 1998;207:753–758.

43. Shah AA, Davis SD, Gamsu G, et al. Parenchymal and pleural findings in patients with and patients without acute pulmonary embolism detected at spiral CT. *Radiology* 1999;211:147–153.

44. Schoepf UJ, Bruening R, Konschitzky H, et al. Pulmonary embolism: comprehensive diagnosis by using electron-beam CT for detection of emboli and assessment of pulmonary blood flow. *Radiology* 2000;217:693–700.

45. Remy-Jardin M, Remy J. Spiral CT angiography of the pulmonary circulation. *Radiology* 1999;212:615–636.

46. Remy-Jardin M, Remy J, Petyt L, et al. Diagnosis of acute pulmonary embolism with spiral CT: comparison with pulmonary angiography and scintigraphy. *Radiology* 1996;200:699–706.

47. Mayo JR, Remy-Jardin M, Müller NL, et al. Pulmonary embolism: prospective comparison of spiral CT with ventilation–perfusion scintigraphy. *Radiology* 1997;205(2):447–452.

48. Drucker EA, Rivitz SM, Shepard JO, et al. Acute pulmonary embolism: assessment of helical CT for diagnosis. *Radiology* 1998;209(1):235–241.

49. van Erkel AR, van Rossum AB, Bloem JL, et al. Spiral CT angiography for suspected pulmonary embolism: a cost effectiveness analysis. *Radiology* 1996;201:29–36.

50. Qanadli SD, Hajjam ME, Mesurolle B, et al. Pulmonary embolism detection: prospective evaluation of dual section helical CT versus selective pulmonary arteriography in 157 patients. *Radiology* 2000;217:447–455.

51. van Rossum AB, Pattynama PM, Ton ER, et al. Pulmonary embolism: validation of spiral CT angiography in 149 patients. *Radiology* 1996;201:467–470.

52. Herold C, Remy-Jardin M, Grenier PH, et al. Prospective evaluation of pulmonary embolism: initial results of the European Multicenter Trial (ESTIPEP). *Radiology* 1998;209(P):299 (abst).

53. Cross JJL, Kemp PM, Walsh CG, et al. A randomized trial of spiral CT and ventilation perfusion scintigraphy for the diagnosis of pulmonary embolism. *Clin Radiol* 1998;53:177–182.

54. Kim K-I, Müller NL, Mayo JR. Clinically suspected pulmonary embolism: utility of spiral CT. *Radiology* 1999;210:693–697.

55. Ferretti GR, Bosson J-L, Buffaz P-D, et al. Acute pulmonary embolism: role of helical CT in 164 patients with intermediate probability at ventilation–perfusion scintigraphy and normal results at duplex US of the legs. *Radiology* 1997;205:453–458.

56. Goodman LR, Lipchik RJ, Kuzo RS, et al. Subsequent pulmonary embolism: risk after a negative helical CT pulmonary angiogram— prospective comparison with scintigraphy. *Radiology* 2000;215:535–542.

57. Pattynama PMT. Meaning of a helical CT angiogram negative for pulmonary embolism [Letter to the Editor]. *Radiology* 2001;218:913–915.

58. Rathbun SW, Raskob GE, Whitsett TL. Sensitivity and specificity of helical computed tomography in the diagnosis of pulmonary embolism: A systematic review. *Ann Intern Med* 2000;132:27–232.

59. Mullins MD, Becker DM, Hagspiel KD, et al. The role of spiral volumetric computed tomography in the diagnosis of pulmonary embolism. *Arch Intern Med* 2000;160:293–298.

60. Fraser RS, Müller NL, Colman N, eds. *Diagnosis of diseases of the chest.* Philadelphia: WB Saunders, 1999:1773–1843.

61. Goodman LR, Curtin JJ, Mewissen MW, et al. Detection of pulmonary embolism in patients with unresolved clinical and scintigraphic diagnosis: helical CT versus angiography. *AJR* 1995;164:1369–1374.

62. Senac JP, Verhnet H, Bousquet C, et al. Embolie pulmonaire: apport de la tomodensitometrie helicoïdale. *J Radiologie* 1995;76:339–345.

63. van Rossum AB, Pattynama PM, Mallens WM, et al. Can helical CT replace scintigraphy in the diagnostic process in suspected pulmonary embolism? A retrolective-prolective cohort study focusing on total diagnostic yield. *Eur Radiol* 1998;8:90–96.

64. Garg K, Welsh CH, Feyerabend AJ, et al. Pulmonary embolism: diagnosis with spiral CT and ventilation–perfusion scanning: correlation with pulmonary angiographic results or clinical outcome. *Radiology* 1998;208:201–208.

65. Baghaie F, Remy-Jardin M, Remy J, et al. Diagnosis of peripheral acute pulmonary emboli: optimization of the spiral CT acquisition protocol. *Radiology* 1998;209(P):299(abst).

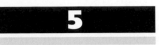

PULMONARY HYPERTENSION

Pulmonary hypertension is defined as a mean pulmonary artery pressure greater than 25 mm Hg at rest or greater than 30 mm Hg during exercise with increased pulmonary vascular resistance (1). In the great majority of cases, the hypertension is secondary to a recognizable cardiac or pulmonary apparent cause; in a small minority, no cause is apparent (2).

Pulmonary hypertension is often not recognized until it is advanced because the clinical findings are nonspecific. According to the diagnostic approach proposed in 1997 by Reaside and Peacock (3), there are two main categories of noninvasive methods of assessment. The first category includes tests that suggest the presence of pulmonary hypertension (clinical examination, electrocardiography, chest radiography, and conventional echocardiography). The second category includes tests that suggest a cause of pulmonary hypertension (pulmonary function tests, ventilation–perfusion scanning, and arterial blood gas tensions). There is an additional category of tests that estimate the severity of pulmonary hypertension, particularly Doppler echocardiography. Although in the 1997 study spiral CT was not even mentioned in the noninvasive approach of pulmonary hypertension, it currently plays an important role in the diagnosis and posttherapeutic management of pulmonary hypertension.

DEFINITION AND CAUSES OF PULMONARY HYPERTENSION

Pathologic Changes

Normal pulmonary arteries are composed of a monolayer of endothelial cells, a distinct medial layer of smooth muscle cells, and a collagenous adventitial layer (4). Pulmonary arteries with a diameter greater than 0.5 mm are defined as elastic pulmonary arteries. They course along the bronchi down to the subsegmental level and have a diameter similar to the adjacent airways (1). Beyond the subsegmental bronchi, these vessels transition to muscular arteries which accompany peripheral airways down to the level of the terminal bronchioles. As the smooth muscle layer progressively thins, these arteries become arterioles (0.15 to 0.015 mm in diameter) which proceed along the respiratory bronchioles and alveolar ducts to eventually form a capillary network in the alveolar walls (1).

The earlier vascular changes of pulmonary hypertension are not specific and are present irrespective of cause. In mild pulmonary hypertension, they consist of medial thickening, usually followed by subendothelial intimal fibrosis. In some conditions, further changes take place in the pulmonary arteries, described as plexogenic pulmonary arteriopathy. This entity has three main histologic features: localized foci of dilation of small muscular arteries (known as simple dilation lesions); wide thin-walled vessels which in turn feed into capillaries (known as plexiform lesions); and thin-walled cavernous spaces linking a muscular pulmonary artery to its capillary bed (known as angiomatoid lesions) (2). In severe obstruction of the pulmonary arterial bed, blood flow appears to be mainly, if not exclusively, via these newly formed collateral vessels (5). The plexiform lesions are unevenly distributed throughout the lungs. They occur mainly in small side branches (also known as supernumerary arteries), arising from larger parent arteries (0.2 to 0.4 mm in diameter) that are distally obliterated by intimal proliferation (2). The expansion of endothelial cells, together with the presence of a hypertrophied layer of smooth muscle cells in the media, form a sleeve along the compromised pulmonary arteries which results in an increase in the overall arterial diameter.

Classification of Pulmonary Hypertension

Several classifications have been proposed (6–8). The two most widely used are the classifications proposed by Wagenvoort (6) and by the World Health Organization (WHO) (7). Wagenvoort (6) classified pulmonary hypertension into four types according to the site and type of vascular obstruction (Box 5-1). The classification proposed at the WHO meeting in 1998 (7) divides pulmonary hypertension into five types: (a) primary pulmonary hypertension; (b) pulmonary venous hypertension; (c) pulmonary hypertension associated with disorders of the respiratory system and/or hypoxia; (d) pulmonary hypertension due to chronic thrombotic and/or embolic disease; and (e) pulmonary hypertension due to disorders directly affecting the pulmonary vasculature (Box 5-2).

BOX 5-1. CAUSES OF PULMONARY HYPERTENSION

- Precapillary: vasoconstrictive
   Hyperkinetic congenital heart disease
   Unknown (primary pulmonary hypertension)
   Chronic liver disease
   HIV infection
   Hypoxia (atmospheric or respiratory)
   Connective tissue disease
- Precapillary: embolic
   Thromboembolic
   Parasitic (schistosomial)
   Tumor emboli
- Capillary
   Widespread pulmonary fibrosis
   Capillary hemangiomatosis
   Diffuse smooth muscle proliferation
- Postcapillary
   Left-sided heart disease
   Venoocclusive disease

HIV, human immunodeficiency virus.
Source: Corrin B. Pathology of the lungs. New York: Churchill Livingstone, 2000 and Wagenvoort CA. Classifying pulmonary vascular disease. *Chest* 1973;64:503–504, with permission.

BOX 5-2. WORLD HEALTH ORGANIZATION CLASSIFICATION OF PULMONARY HYPERTENSION

1. Pulmonary arterial hypertension
   1.1. Primary pulmonary hypertension
      a. Sporadic
      b. Familial
   1.2. Related to:
      a. Collagen vascular disease
      b. Congenital systemic to pulmonary shunts
      c. Portal hypertension
      d. HIV infection
      e. Drugs/toxins
         (1) Appetite suppressing drugs
         (2) Other
      f. Persistent pulmonary hypertension of the newborn
      g. Other
2. Pulmonary venous hypertension
   2.1. Left-sided atrial or ventricular heart disease
   2.2. Left-sided valvular heart disease
   2.3. Extrinsic compression of central pulmonary veins
      a. Fibrosing mediastinitis
      b. Adenopathy/tumors
   2.4. Pulmonary venoocclusive disease
   2.5. Other
3. Pulmonary hypertension associated with disorders of the respiratory system and/or hypoxemia
   3.1. Chronic obstructive pulmonary disease
   3.2. Interstitial lung disease
   3.3. Sleep-disordered breathing
   3.4. Alveolar hypoventilation disorders
   3.5. Chronic exposure to high altitude
   3.6. Neonatal lung disease
   3.7. Alveolar–capillary dysplasia
   3.8. Other
4. Pulmonary hypertension due to chronic thrombolic and/or embolic disease
   4.1. Thromboembolic obstruction of proximal pulmonary arteries
   4.2. Obstruction of distal pulmonary arteries
      a. Pulmonary embolism (thrombus, tumor, ova and/or parasites, foreign material)
      b. *In situ* thrombosis
      c. Sickle cell disease
5. Pulmonary hypertension due to disorders directly affecting the pulmonary vasculature
   5.1. Inflammatory
      a. Schistosomiasis
      b. Sarcoidosis
      c. Other
   5.2. Pulmonary capillary haemangiomatosis

HIV, human immunodeficiency virus.
Source: Peacock AJ. Primary pulmonary hypertension. *Thorax* 1999;54:1107–1118, with permission.

CT FEATURES OF PULMONARY HYPERTENSION

Vascular Signs

Central Pulmonary Arteries

Several studies have shown that patients with pulmonary hypertension have central pulmonary arteries larger than patients with normal pulmonary arterial pressure. The possibility of pulmonary hypertension should be suspected on CT when the diameter of the main pulmonary artery is greater than 2.8 cm (9–14) or when the diameter of the pulmonary artery is greater than that of the aorta (14) (Figure 5-1). The diameter of the main pulmonary artery is measured in the scan plane of the bifurcation, at a right angle to its long axis and just lateral to the ascending aorta (10). Another finding is increased diameter of the right and left pulmonary arteries (upper normal limit: 1.6 cm). In severe forms of pulmonary hypertension, marked enlargement of proximal pulmonary arteries may be responsible for pseudodiaphragms on transverse CT scans which should not be mistaken for CT features of chronic pulmonary embolism (Figure 5-2).

The enlarged central pulmonary arteries may compress the surrounding anatomic structures. Rarely they may compress the phrenic nerve resulting in elevation of the hemidiaphragm (15) or compress the recurrent laryngeal nerve. In children, aneurysmal dilation of the pulmonary artery may lead to obstruction of the adjacent airway. Three-dimensional reconstructed images of the tracheobronchial tree and central pulmonary arteries are helpful in the assessment of these complications (16).

Peripheral Pulmonary Arteries

Enlargement of peripheral pulmonary arteries is a common CT finding in patients with pulmonary hypertension. This feature is visually assessed by comparing the arterial and bronchial diameters at the level of segmental and subsegmental divisions. The normal pulmonary artery to accompanying bronchus ratio usually ranges from 1.0 to 1.2 and is most accurately determined on bronchoarterial structures oriented perpendicular to the plane of section (apical segments of the upper lobes and basilar segments of the lower lobes) (Figure 5-3).

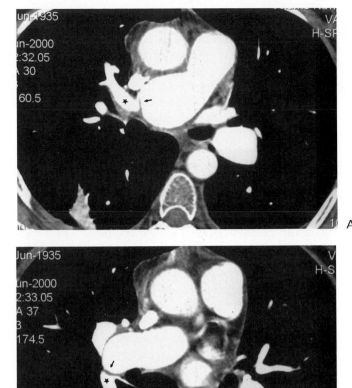

A

B

FIGURE 5-2. Cross-sectional CT angiogram images obtained at the level of the anterior segmental artery of the right upper lobe (**A**, *star*) and the apical segmental artery of the right lower lobe (**B**, *star*) in a patient with severe primary pulmonary hypertension. Marked dilation of proximal pulmonary arterial branches is responsible for pseudodiaphragms (**A** and **B**, *arrow*) on transverse CT scans, mimicking chronic pulmonary embolism.

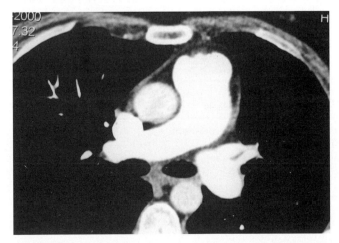

FIGURE 5-1. Cross-sectional CT angiogram obtained at the level of the main pulmonary artery in a patient with primary pulmonary hypertension. Note the abnormal diameter of the pulmonary artery trunk, greater than that of the aorta.

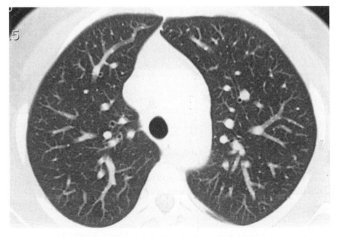

FIGURE 5-3. Noncontrast spiral CT scan of the lung parenchyma obtained at the level of the upper lung zones in a patient with primary pulmonary hypertension. Note the marked enlargement of the central and peripheral pulmonary arteries.

Pulmonary Veins

The analysis of pulmonary veins is an important morphologic clue in the investigation of the cause of pulmonary hypertension. The size of central and peripheral pulmonary veins can be easily assessed on CT. It is also important to systematically search for enlarged interlobular pulmonary veins, responsible for smooth dilation of interlobular septa in patients with elevated pulmonary venous pressure. Pulmonary veins are typically small-sized in patients with precapillary pulmonary hypertension and enlarged in patients with pulmonary hypertension secondary to left-sided heart disease.

Vascular Complications of Pulmonary Hypertension

Vascular complications include thrombosis of central pulmonary arteries, atherosclerotic calcifications of the pulmonary artery, dissecting aneurysm, and secondary effects on the right-sided heart structures.

Dissecting aneurysm of the pulmonary artery is a rare complication that may occur in patients with severe pulmonary hypertension. Atherosclerotic plaques and/or cystic necrosis of the media are often present. The dissection usually occurs at the level of the pulmonary artery trunk. The patients present with acute chest pain. Previously, the diagnosis was made by echocardiography and/or pulmonary angiography (17) but now can be made with spiral CT angiography (CTA). In the context of acute chest pain in a patient known for pulmonary hypertension, this CT examination should start by a noncontrast acquisition to search for pulmonary artery wall calcifications, followed by a spiral CT angiogram with retrospective electrocardiogram (ECG)-gated reconstructions (if available) for precise delineation of the dissection without motion artifacts. In addition, the use of automatic triggering of data acquisition when the predetermined level of vascular enhancement is reached is recommended to achieve optimal results in contrast studies. The CT features of a dissection of the pulmonary artery are similar to those of an aortic dissection (intimal flap, intraluminal thrombi, arterial wall calcifications) (18). Precise demonstration of the aneurysmal/dissection extent and the anatomic relationship with the adjacent structures is essential for determining the optimal surgical approach.

Pleuroparenchymal Signs

Mosaic Attenuation Pattern

A mosaic pattern of attenuation, with patchy areas of increased and decreased attenuation, is nonspecific and may be seen on thin-section CT scans of the lungs when vascular, infiltrative lung, or airway diseases are present (19). The differential diagnosis of these three causes of mosaic attenuation is based on recognizing differences in the relative size of vessels and secondary lobules between areas with increased and decreased attenuation, and the presence of air trapping on expiratory CT scans (Table 5-1). Patients with a mosaic pattern due to vascular diseases typically have enlarged vessels in the areas of increased (ground-glass) attenuation and decreased vascularity in the areas of decreased attenuation (a pattern also known as mosaic perfusion) (Figure 5-4). In patients with infiltrative parenchymal lung disease, the mosaic attenuation results from patchy areas of ground-glass attenuation and interposed normal lung parenchyma. The vessel and secondary lobule size is similar in the areas with increased and normal attenuation. In cases of airway disease, the mosaic pattern results from reflex vasoconstriction secondary to hypoventilation of alveoli distal to airway obstruction and blood flow redistribution to adjacent normal areas of lung. These patients typically show air trapping on expiratory CT, with associated distension of affected secondary lobules. It should be noted, however, that Worthy and coworkers have reported the presence of air trapping in 25% to 50% of patients with vascular disease (19), and suggested that the reduced arter-

TABLE 5-1. DISTINGUISHING FEATURES OF THE DISEASE THAT MAY CAUSE MOSAIC LUNG ATTENUATION ON CT SCANS

Type of Disease	Attenuation	CT Findings Vessels	Air Trapping (expiratory CT scans)
Infiltrative lung	Ground glass	Normal size and number throughout the lung	Not seen
Airway	■ Reduced (hypoxic vasoconstriction)	Decreased in size and number in areas of reduced attenuation	Present
	■ Increased (regional hyperperfusion)		
Vascular	■ Reduced (obstructed flow)	■ Decreased in size and number in areas of reduced attenuation	Uncommon
	■ Increased (regional hyperperfusion)	■ Increased in size and number in areas of increased attenuation	

Source: Worthy SA, Müller NL, Hartman TE, et al. Mosaic attenuation pattern on thin-section CT scans of the lung: differentiation among infiltrative lung, airway, and vascular diseases as a cause. *Radiology* 1997;205:465–470, with permission.

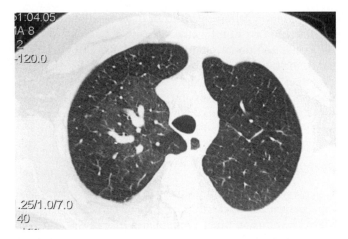

FIGURE 5-4. Mosaic perfusion. High-resolution CT scan obtained at the level of the upper lobes shows enlarged vessels within areas of ground-glass attenuation in the apical segment of the right upper lobe while decreased vascularity and lower attenuation are found in the periphery of the right upper lobe and throughout the entire left upper lobe.

ial carbon dioxide concentration in the areas of acute vascular occlusion could stimulate bronchoconstriction of small airways (20). Other helpful features in distinguishing mosaic attenuation of vascular from airway etiology are the presence of enlarged central pulmonary arteries in pulmonary hypertension and the presence of bronchial dilation in airway abnormalities.

A mosaic pattern of lung attenuation is seen commonly in patients with pulmonary hypertension due to vascular disease and seldom in patients with pulmonary hypertension due to cardiac or lung disease (21). Mosaic attenuation is seen much more commonly in patients with pulmonary hypertension secondary to chronic pulmonary thromboembolism than in patients with primary pulmonary hypertension (19).

Interlobular Septal Thickening

Interlobular septal thickening seen with pulmonary hypertension is characterized by the presence of smooth margins of secondary pulmonary lobules and is highly suggestive of postcapillary pulmonary hypertension. Associated CT findings often seen in cases of elevated pulmonary venous pressure include peribronchovascular interstitial thickening, thickening of the interlobar fissures, and pleural effusions.

Consolidation

Consolidation may be due to several different vascular or hemodynamic abnormalities. A common cause is hydrostatic pulmonary edema when pulmonary hypertension is complicated by left heart failure (22). A peripheral wedge-shaped area of consolidation is suggestive of pulmonary infarction and should suggest the possibility of acute or chronic thromboembolic disease.

Mediastinal and Cardiac Signs

Hilar and Mediastinal Lymph Node Enlargement

Mediastinal lymph node enlargement can be seen with chronic thromboembolic pulmonary hypertension (23). On histologic examination, these lymph nodes exhibit vascular transformation of the lymph node sinuses, often associated with variable degrees of sclerosis. Similar histologic features can be seen at the level of enlarged hilar lymph nodes in various causes of pulmonary hypertension (Figure 5-5). Patients with congestive heart failure and postcapillary pulmonary hypertension often have enlarged mediastinal lymph nodes and inhomogeneous or hazy attenuation of mediastinal fat. These findings have been related to edema within the mediastinal lymph nodes and fat (24).

Right Heart Abnormalities

Spiral CT, particularly with the use of multislice technology and cardiac gating, allows evaluation of right ventricular function in patients with pulmonary hypertension. It is therefore recommended to include the right ventricle in the surveyed volume and to obtain ECG-gated acquisitions to reconstruct images at predefined cardiac phases. A similar study design as that described for the estimation of the right ventricle volume with magnetic resonance (MR) can be applied, the main difference being the temporal resolution, which is between 125 and 250 milliseconds with CT compared to 60 to 80 milliseconds with MR (25). Right ventricular volume can be measured with no geometric assumptions by adding the volume of contiguous slices of the right ventricle, each obtained at the same phase of the cardiac cycle.

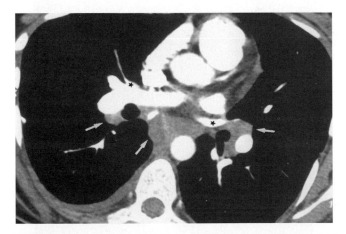

FIGURE 5-5. Cross-sectional CT angiogram image at the level of the interlobar pulmonary arteries shows enlarged hilar and subcarinal lymph nodes (*arrows*) in a patient with pulmonary hypertension secondary to venooclusive disease. Histologic examination of the subcarinal lymph node, surgically sampled, revealed hyperplasia of the lymph node sinuses. Note the small size of the right and left superior pulmonary veins (*stars*) suggestive of precapillary pulmonary hypertension.

Displacement of the interventricular septum on CT scans can be demonstrated by measuring the short axis of the right ventricle and left ventricle chambers in the axial planes at their widest points in diastole between the inner surface of the free wall and the surface of the interventricular septum (26,27) (Figure 5-6). The maximum diastolic dimensions of the right and left heart chambers may be at slightly different levels. Dilation of the right ventricle is considered present when the right ventricle/left ventricle ratio is greater than 1 and there is a posterior convexity of the interventricular septum.

With cardiac gating and subsecond scan times, it is now possible to study systolodiastolic changes in ventricular volume as well as cardiac motion artifact. It has been shown that the majority of patients with massive pulmonary embolism exhibit reduced cardiac motion artifact, presumably due to severe ventricular dyskinesis (26). Presence of cardiac motion artifacts and analysis of the shape of the interventricular septum are two findings easily depicted on unenhanced CT scans. Because there is a theoretical risk of right ventricular overload in patients showing a dilated right ventricle and leftward septal bowing, it would be prudent to

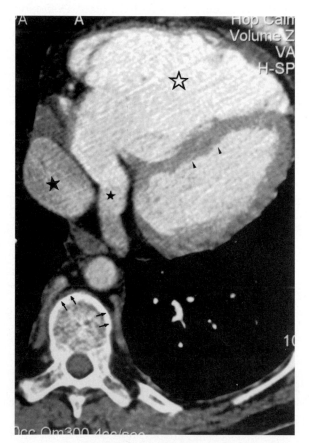

FIGURE 5-6. Right heart abnormalities secondary to pulmonary hypertension. Cross-sectional CT angiogram image shows marked dilation of the right ventricle (*open star*), coronary sinus (*small dark star*), inferior vena cava (*large dark star*), and intercostal veins (*arrows*) and the leftward septal bowing (*arrowheads*).

try to limit the volume of contrast material administered to a maximum of 140 mL (26).

Several additional parameters can be measured on CT scans, including the right ventricular myocardial thickness (less than 4 mm in normal subjects) and the degree of dilation of the coronary sinus and inferior vena cava. However, CT does not allow assessment of the presence of tricuspid or pulmonary valvular regurgitation.

Pericardial Changes

Patients with severe pulmonary hypertension often have mild pericardial thickening or a small pericardial effusion (28). The effusion often accumulates first in the anterosuperior pericardial recess (sagittal diameter greater than 15 mm measured between the ascending aorta and the pulmonary trunk). Because the clinical diagnosis of pulmonary hypertension may be difficult and delayed, this sign could be a useful indirect indicator of pulmonary hypertension, particularly when associated with dilation of the proximal pulmonary arteries. The pathogenesis of the pericardial effusion in these patients is unknown.

DIAGNOSTIC APPROACH OF PULMONARY HYPERTENSION

Chronic Thromboembolic Pulmonary Hypertension

It has been estimated that in the United States, approximately 500,000 episodes of pulmonary embolism occur each year, resulting in 500 to 2,500 cases of chronic thromboembolic pulmonary hypertension (29). Incomplete resolution of thrombi leads to complex restructuring processes, which include organization, recanalization, and retraction of emboli (30). The pulmonary arterial hypertension in patients with chronic thromboembolic disease can result from obstruction of either surgically accessible central arteries (main pulmonary artery to segmental arteries) or obstruction of surgically inaccessible distal arteries (subsegmental and distal vessels). The pulmonary hypertension results in small-vessel arteriopathy in the unobstructed vascular bed (31). Lung perfusion in obstructed areas can be maintained either by the recanalization process or via collateral systemic supply. The symptomatology is nonspecific and the average time from onset of symptoms to diagnosis usually exceeds 3 years (32). Approximately 80% of patients have normal pulmonary function tests and 20% of patients have mild to moderate restrictive lung function (15).

Vascular Signs

CT Signs of Pulmonary Hypertension

Pulmonary hypertension can be suspected based on the presence of dilation of the main pulmonary artery. Another finding in chronic pulmonary thromboembolism is marked variation in the diameter of segmental vessels presumably due to uneven distribution of emboli and subsequent sequelae within the lungs (31) (Figure 5-7). The arterial dilation and subsequent changes on lung attenuation on CT scans is unevenly distributed within the lung, an important criterion for the differential diagnosis between pulmonary hypertension secondary to chronic thromboembolism from that of other causes. The pulmonary veins are not dilated. Long-standing pulmonary artery hypertension results in right ventricular dysfunction, right-sided cardiomegaly, and dilation of the coronary sinus and azygos vein.

Chronic Thromboembolism

The CT features of chronic thromboembolism are similar to those described with conventional angiography (Box 5-3) (30–35). Occluded vessels may have a pouching amputation or an abrupt truncation convex to the periphery. This finding is easily related to chronic thromboembolism on CT due

BOX 5-3. VASCULAR CT FEATURES SUGGESTIVE OF CHRONIC THROMBOEMBOLISM

- Organized embolic material:
    Partial or complete filling defects
    Emboli eccentric and contiguous with the vessel wall
    Irregular contours of the intimal surface
- Retracted embolic material:
    Complete filling defects at the level of stenosed pulmonary arteries
    Abrupt cutoffs and narrowing
- Recanalized embolic material:
    Webs, bands, or stenoses with poststenotic dilation
- Calcified embolic material:
    Calcifications within filling defects

to the direct visualization and delineation of partial or complete filling defects within central pulmonary artery branches. A recanalized thrombus perpendicular to the artery wall generates webs or bands and focal stenoses with mild poststenotic dilation. Parallel to the arterial lumen, the incomplete recanalization thickens the artery walls (Figure 5-8), sometimes resulting in an irregular contour of the intimal surface (Figure 5-9). CTA allows identification of additional features not detectable on conventional angiography, such as peripheral clots lining the arterial wall and severely stenosed or occluded arteries, not recognized distal to the obstruction on angiography. The stenosed arterial diameter is considerably smaller than the diameter of the adjacent bronchus (Figures 5-7B and 5-10). Because partial or complete filling defects of normal-sized pulmonary arteries can be seen in acute and chronic pulmonary embolism (PE), these features alone should not lead to the assessment of chronic PE. The differential diagnoses of vascular features of chronic thromboembolism are listed in Box 5-4. It should be pointed out that, although most cases of chronic pulmonary embolism have multiple and bilateral arterial abnormalities, occlusion

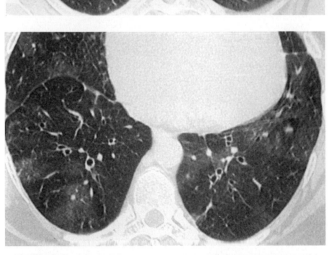

A

B

FIGURE 5-7. Chronic thromboembolic pulmonary hypertension. High-resolution CT scans at the level of the upper (**A**) and lower (**B**) lobes show mosaic perfusion, unevenly distributed within the lung. Note marked reduction in size of most pulmonary arterial sections in the lower lobes (**B**), suggestive of retracted embolic material, with mild dilation of their accompanying bronchi.

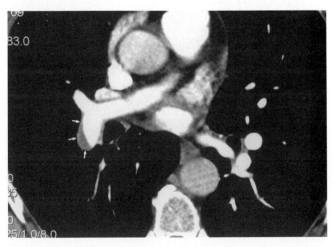

FIGURE 5-8. Chronic mural clot. Cross-sectional CT angiogram image shows a mural defect at the level of the outer wall of the right interlobar pulmonary artery (*arrows*).

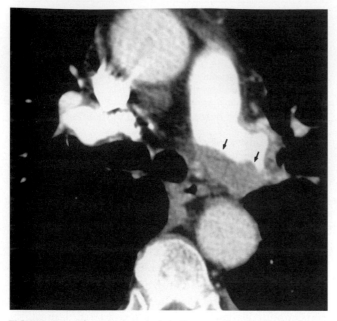

FIGURE 5-9. Chronic mural clot. Cross-sectional CT angiogram image at the level of the carina shows a large filling defect within the left pulmonary artery with irregular contours (*arrows*).

of one main pulmonary artery has been reported in approximately 3% of cases, mimicking proximal interruption (absence) of the pulmonary artery (36,37).

Calcifications within chronic thrombi are seen in a small number of patients. Visualization of calcified central thrombi may be difficult on spiral CT angiograms viewed at usual mediastinal window settings because they are obscured by the surrounding contrast material (Figure 5-11). Selection of wider window settings (greater than 450 HU) for the inter-

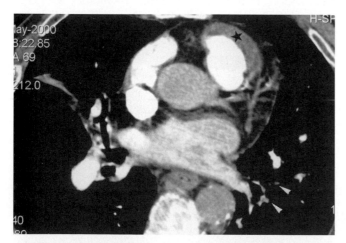

FIGURE 5-10. Retracted embolic material. Cross-section CT angiogram image at the level of the lower lung zones shows marked reduction in size of the left lower lobe pulmonary arterial sections (*arrowheads*), devoid of contrast material conversely to the right lower lobe pulmonary artery. In addition, note the marked myocardial hypertrophy at the level of the pulmonary artery infundibulum (*star*).

BOX 5-4. DIFFERENTIAL DIAGNOSES OF VASCULAR SIGNS OF CHRONIC THROMBOEMBOLIC DISEASE

- Congenital pulmonary artery stenosis:
    Usually diagnosed in children (vs. diagnosis of chronic thromboembolic disease in adult patients)
    Isolated proximal arterial stenoses (vs. proximal arterial stenoses associated with mural thrombi, mural and luminal calcifications without poststenotic dilation in chronic thromboembolic disease)
- Fibrosing mediastinitis:
    Enlarged and calcified hilar lymph nodes responsible for narrowing of proximal pulmonary arteries
    Presence of mediastinal lymph nodes
    Clinical context:
        History of tuberculosis, histoplasmosis, and other endemic granulomatous diseases
        Environmental exposure (silicosis)
- Takayasu's arteritis:
    High-attenuation wall thickening
    Delayed enhancement after contrast medium administration (after 1–2 min)
    Smooth tapering of the pulmonary artery without intraluminal thrombus
    Systemic arteritis (involvement of the aortic wall)
- Neurofibromatosis:
    Severe intimal fibrosis
    Responsible for multiple bilateral filling defects on CT scans
    Specific clinical context
- Pulmonary artery sarcoma:
    Isolated proximal filling defects, sometimes bilateral
    Delayed enhancement after contrast material administration (after 2–3 min)
- Unilateral pulmonary artery agenesis:
    Interpretive difficulty on angiograms (rather than on CT scans)
    Abrupt tapering of the pulmonary artery without endo- or periluminal changes
    Clinical context:
        Marked female predominance
        Young age of patients
- Acute thromboembolism:
    Partial and/or complete filling defects
    Smooth margins
    Absence of any other typical vascular features of chronic thromboembolism
- Anatomically and technically related pitfalls
    Partial volume effect on obliquely oriented vessels misinterpreted as abrupt narrowing
    Hilar lymph nodes misinterpreted as mural thrombi

pretation of cross-sectional images or creation of maximum intensity projections are helpful in the visualization of peripheral calcified thrombi. Calcified thrombi located within fifth- or sixth-order pulmonary arteries or smaller branches are often indistinguishable from calcified lung parenchymal micronodules on cross-sectional CT images. The distinction can be made on the basis of their microtubular shape and location at the site of arterial sections, two morphologic criteria readily identified by means of the sliding thin slab maximum intensity projection (STS-MIP) tech-

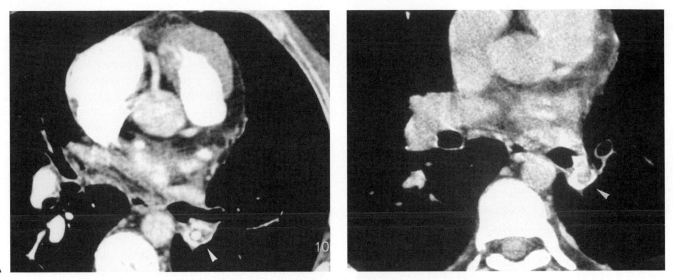

FIGURE 5-11. Chronic obstruction of the left lower lobe pulmonary artery by a partially calcified thrombus (**A**, and **B** *arrowheads*), difficult to detect on a cross-sectional CT angiogram image (**A**), often requiring a noncontrast CT scan (**B**) for adequate depiction.

nique (Figure 5-12). A summary of the reconstruction techniques useful in identifying the various vascular features of chronic thromboembolism is given in the Appendix.

The usefulness of spiral CT as an alternative to conventional angiography for diagnosis of chronic thromboembolic pulmonary hypertension was shown in two studies (30,31). The main advantage of CT over pulmonary angiography is the depiction of direct vascular signs of chronic thromboembolism, including peripheral residual thrombi, difficult to detect on angiograms if smoothly marginated (Figure 5-13), and completely occlusive clots depicted only as abrupt cutoffs on angiograms. However, difficulties in the recognition of peripheral morphologic changes on cross-sectional CT images performed using 4- to 5-mm collima-

tion scans have been reported by several groups of investigators (30,31,38). Causes of false-negative cross-sectional CT images included small thrombi concentric and adherent to the arterial wall or located tangentially at the bottom or the roof of a vessel, and mild arterial stenosis. These difficulties can be overcome by the availability of thin-collimation acquisition protocols on multislice CT scanners and by generating multiplanar reformations along the long axis of questionable arterial branches, if needed. In order to detect all the vascular changes reliably, it is also necessary to change the window settings. For example, small thrombi may be masked at the peak of vascular enhancement unless the window level is adjusted to optimize vascular contrast (33).

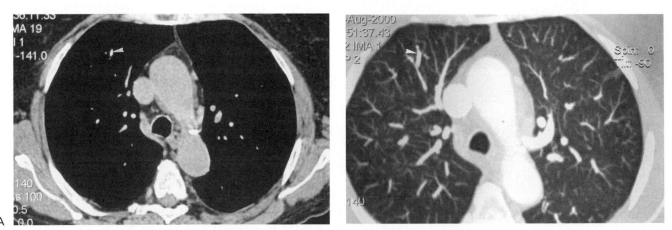

FIGURE 5-12. Calcified peripheral thrombus. Noncontrast thin-section CT scan at the level of the upper lobes shows a peripheral high-attenuating nodule (**A**, *arrowhead*), related to a calcified thrombus within a sixth-order pulmonary artery branch by means of the sliding thin slab maximum intensity projection image (**B**, *arrowhead*).

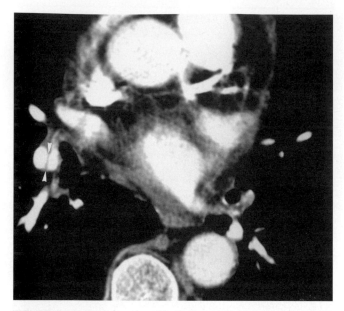

FIGURE 5-13. Peripheral residual thrombus. Cross-sectional CT angiogram image at the level of the right bronchus intermedius shows intraluminal web within the right interlobar pulmonary artery (*arrowheads*).

Systemic Collateral Supply

CT angiographic features of bilateral bronchial hypervascularization, similar to those seen with chronic bronchial disease, may also be found with chronic thromboembolism (39). The CT findings of bronchial artery hypervascularization consist of abnormal dilation of the proximal portions of bronchial arteries (i.e., a diameter greater than 1.5 mm) and arterial tortuosity (Figure 5-14). In chronic thromboembolic disease, the bronchial circulation is markedly increased due to the development of systemic-to-pulmonary arterial anastomoses. These anastomoses occur beyond the level of pul-

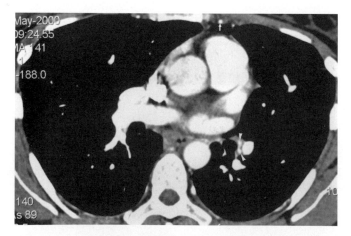

FIGURE 5-14. Systemic collateral supply. Cross-sectional CT angiogram image at the level of the lower lobe bronchus shows enlargement of left bronchial arteries (*arrowheads*) and left internal mammary artery (*arrow*) in a patient with unilateral chronic thromboembolic disease.

monary arterial obstruction and help to maintain pulmonary blood flow.

This systemic perfusion of the peripheral pulmonary arterial bed accounts for the presence of areas of ground-glass attenuation in patients with chronic pulmonary embolism (40). It is likely that subpleural septal lines sometimes identified in these patients reflect the presence of dilated bronchial arteries within interlobular septa. Development of bronchial hypervascularization may also be responsible for recurrent or massive bronchial bleeding (41). In this specific context, spiral CTA of bronchial arteries may help identify their ostia prior to an embolization procedure.

Surgery

Assessment of the proximal extent of chronic thromboembolism is critical in the preoperative evaluation of these patients. Current surgical techniques allow removal of chronic thrombi whose proximal location extends to the main, lobar, and segmental arteries. Those that begin more distally are not subject to endarterectomy. Perfusion scanning is incapable of determining the magnitude, location, or proximal extent of disease. Interpretive difficulties exist in the angiographic recognition of residual thromboembolic material incorporated concentrically in vessel walls with new epithelium smoothing the internal contour. As demonstrated by Bergin and colleagues (34), the sensitivity of MR imaging is limited by the spatial resolution needed to demonstrate mural thromboembolic material. Although pulmonary angioscopy has proven invaluable in determining whether chronic thromboembolic obstruction is amenable to surgical intervention, this technique is not widely available.

Only two studies have evaluated the role of CT in demonstrating surgical resectability of chronic thromboemboli (30,34). Schwickert and associates examined 74 patients with chronic thromboembolic pulmonary hypertension with both conventional and single-slice spiral CT and found that CT had 77% sensitivity and 80% accuracy in depicting central thromboembolism (30). These results led the authors to conclude that conventional angiography before surgery may not be necessary in all patients. Similar conclusions were drawn by Bergin and colleagues who evaluated 40 patients with single-slice CT, MR, and/or angiography and compared the imaging findings with the surgical findings in individual vessels (34). The sensitivity and overall accuracy for the demonstration of central disease was highest with spiral CT. Limitations of CT were due to misinterpretation of vessel curvature and to limited spatial resolution at the segmental level inherent to their selection of a 5-mm collimation. The marked increase in spatial resolution with current multislice CT makes it reasonable to postulate that this technique will become the gold standard in the assessment of patients for potential surgical resection. In a recent study, Bergin and coworkers have shown that CT angiographic evidence of extensive central vessel disease and limited small vessel involvement were good predictors of patient response to pulmonary thromboendarterectomy (42).

Parenchymal Signs

Mosaic Perfusion

Mosaic perfusion in chronic thromboembolic pulmonary hypertension can be recognized on CT as sharply demarcated regions of decreased and increased attenuation and vascularity that often conform to the boundaries of secondary pulmonary lobules, without evidence of destruction or displacement of pulmonary vessels (20,43). Correlations between CT and single photon emission CT (SPECT) images have shown that areas of low attenuation within the lung parenchyma CT are due to hypoperfusion (44). Regions of increased attenuation are due to the redistribution of blood flow to the patent arterial bed. A potential limitation in the sensitivity of CT scans for depicting areas of hypoperfusion may be collateral blood flow from the bronchial circulation, which can be abundant in chronic pulmonary thromboembolism (38,44).

Parenchymal Scarring

A common but nonspecific lung parenchymal finding in chronic pulmonary hypertension is wedge-shaped, pleural-based parenchymal areas of high attenuation. These are often multiple and predominantly affect the lower lobes (30). These areas do not enhance after administration of contrast medium and likely represent fibrotic residuals of pulmonary infarction. They have been reported to occur in 10% to 15% of thromboembolic events (33). According to Morris and associates (15), patients with chronic thromboembolic pulmonary hypertension who have restrictive lung function are more likely to have parenchymal scarring than those with normal lung function.

Cardiac Signs

Vascular obstruction in chronic thromboembolism results in pulmonary hypertension and right ventricular hypertrophy (45). Over time, right ventricular function deteriorates, even in the absence of recurrent embolism, presumably because of the development of hypertensive vascular lesions in the nonobstructed pulmonary artery bed. Right ventricular enlargement may be accompanied by dilation of the tricuspid valve annulus and resultant tricuspid valve regurgitation. The pressure and volume overload of the right heart lead to right ventricular enlargement and convex bulging of the interventricular septum toward the left ventricle. The presence of decreased right ventricular function should be suspected prior to administration of contrast medium. In such cases, it is recommended to increase the delay between the start of the contrast medium injection and the start of spiral CT data

acquisition, from 15 seconds to up to 25 seconds (33). Thrombi, sometimes calcified, may be identified within right heart cavities and coronary sinus.

Miscellaneous Signs

Patients with chronic thromboembolic pulmonary hypertension may have enlarged hilar lymph nodes. An accurate knowledge of the position of hilar lymph nodes in relation to major pulmonary arteries has become essential to differentiate enlarged hilar lymph nodes from mural thrombi (46).

Pleural effusions or, more often, sequelae of pleural effusions can be identified on CT scans of patients showing vascular features of chronic thromboembolic disease. Recurrent pleural effusions may result in pleural symphysis and the development of transpleural antegrade anastomoses between nonbronchial systemic and pulmonary arteries.

Remy-Jardin and coworkers, in a study of 33 patients with chronic pulmonary thromboembolic disease, have reported cylindric bronchial dilation in 64% of patients. The dilation was observed at the level of segmental and subsegmental bronchi and was associated with the presence of severely stenosed arterial branches (47) (Figure 5-15). The CT finding of bronchial dilation in patients without clinical and functional evidence of chronic obstructive lung disease raises the possibility that chronic pulmonary embolism can directly affect the adjacent airways.

Nonthromboembolic Pulmonary Hypertension

Venoocclusive Disease

Pulmonary venoocclusive disease is a rare disorder (approximately 150 reported cases), usually affecting children and young adults. The etiology of this disease is unknown but

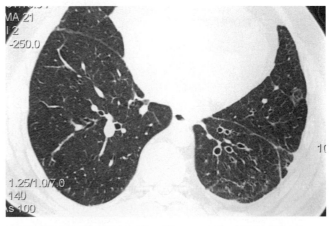

FIGURE 5-15. High-resolution CT scan at the level of the lower lobes shows marked stenosis of the left lower lobe pulmonary arteries and cylindric dilation of their accompanying bronchi. Note the additional presence of left lower lobe retraction.

has been observed in patients following bone marrow transplantation, using oral contraceptives, receiving treatment with chemotherapeutic agents, and recently, in a patient with human immunodeficiency virus (HIV) infection (48). It has also been associated with environmental toxins, autoimmune disease, intracardiac shunts, radiation injury, and genetic predisposition (49).

Histologically, the abnormalities characteristically involve pulmonary veins less than 0.1 mm in diameter and consist of occlusion and recanalization of the lumen, muscularization, and intimal fibrosis. Nonspecific findings secondary to venous hypertension are also present. These include venous medial hypertrophy, septal edema and fibrosis, paraseptal venous infarction, interstitial and pleural lymphatic dilation, intraalveolar hemosiderin-laden macrophages, and features of secondary pulmonary arterial hypertension (1).

The diagnosis is often missed initially because both the clinical presentation and radiographic findings are suggestive of interstitial lung disease. The standard clinical criteria for the disease include pulmonary hypertension, chronic airspace and interstitial edema, normal pulmonary capillary wedge pressure, and the absence of cardiac abnormalities. The most common CT findings consist of smooth interlobular septal thickening, multifocal ground-glass opacities, pleural effusions, enlarged central pulmonary arteries, and normal caliber (or small-sized) pulmonary veins (1,49,50) (Figure 5-16). Pathologic correlations have shown that the thickened interlobular septa correspond to the presence of fibrotic septa with associated venous sclerosis. Alveolar septal thickening is responsible for the ground-glass opacities but it may also result in diffuse, small, poorly defined nodular opacities with a bronchiolocentric (centrilobular) distribution. The absence of both left heart enlargement and the

features of mediastinal fibrosis are important negative findings to suggest the likelihood of pulmonary venoocclusive disease. Enlarged hilar and mediastinal lymph nodes can be seen, corresponding to reactive adenopathy or vascular transformation of the lymph node sinuses (51). In the latter situation, enhancement of these abnormally enlarged lymph nodes can be demonstrated on spiral CT angiograms (Figure 5-17). While *in situ* thrombus formation in the small muscular pulmonary arteries is common, the occurrence of proximal pulmonary arterial thrombus is unusual (51).

In one patient, there was complete resolution of the interstitial changes in the native lung following unilateral lung transplant (52). The preoperative CT findings, therefore, were due exclusively to pulmonary congestion and not to interstitial fibrosis (53) (Figure 5-18).

Pulmonary Capillary Hemangiomatosis

Pulmonary capillary hemangiomatosis is a rare cause of pulmonary hypertension that may occur in pediatric and young adult patients. This disease is characterized by the presence of precapillary pulmonary hypertension and subsequent right heart dysfunction, a reticulomicronodular pattern of lung infiltration, recurrent hemoptysis, and the absence of a cardiac abnormality. The presence of hemoptysis in a patient with pulmonary hypertension and without known pulmonary and cardiac disease should suggest two main diagnostic possibilities: pulmonary venoocclusive disease and pulmonary capillary hemangiomatosis.

Histologically, pulmonary capillary hemangiomatosis is a locally aggressive benign vascular neoplasm of the lung characterized by the presence of numerous cytologically benign, thin-walled, capillary-sized blood vessels proliferating diffusely through the pulmonary interstitium, in and around pulmonary vessels and airways, and pleura (53). The mechanism for development of pulmonary hypertension is multifactorial and consists of: (a) a secondary venoocclusive phenomenon resulting from invasion of the small pulmonary veins by the proliferating capillaries; (b) recurrent pulmonary hemorrhage with subsequent scar formation; and (c) progressive arterial obliteration secondary to *in situ* thrombosis and infarction, occasionally leading to occlusion of central pulmonary arteries (53).

Rare descriptions of CT findings in pulmonary capillary hemangiomatosis have been reported in the literature, based on thin-section CT images (50,53,54). They include: (a) enlargement of pulmonary arteries with atherosclerotic changes and *in situ* thrombosis; (b) a mosaic pattern of attenuation of pulmonary parenchyma; (c) thickening and nodularity of the central and peripheral compartments of lung interstitium, representing the proliferating capillary mass; (d) nonspecific infiltrates or areas of consolidation in relation with various stages of pulmonary hemorrhage and/or lung infarction; and (e) enlarged hilar lymph nodes. Focally enhanced perfusion to the hemangiomatous tissue

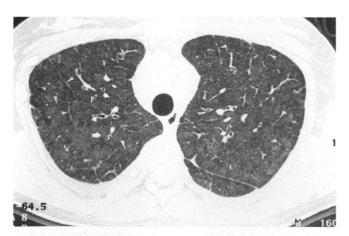

FIGURE 5-16. Venoocclusive disease (same patient as shown in Figure 5-5). High-resolution CT scan at the level of the upper lobes shows multifocal ground-glass opacities, smooth interlobular septal thickening (*arrowheads*), and mild dilation of peripheral pulmonary arterial sections despite marked pulmonary hypertension. The concurrent depiction of small-sized pulmonary veins are highly suggestive of precapillary pulmonary hypertension.

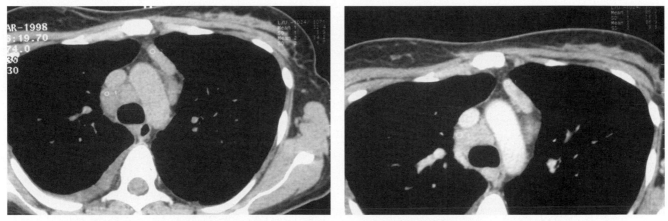

FIGURE 5-17. Venoocclusive disease (same patient as shown in Figure 5-5). Noncontrast CT scan at the level of the aortic arch (**A**) shows enlargement of mediastinal lymph nodes (mean attenuation values: 32 HU and 34 HU). Cross-sectional CT angiogram image obtained 2 minutes after injection of contrast material (**B**) shows enhancement of the enlarged lymph nodes (mean attenuation values: 87 HU and 96 HU) suggestive of hypervascularization. Autopsy findings revealed hyperplasia of mediastinal lymph node sinuses.

demonstrated with ventilation–perfusion scanning and angiography (55) could probably be detected on thin-section spiral CT angiograms. Because of the importance of subpleural capillary proliferation, and in the absence of malignant disease, the combination of diffuse interstitial lung disease and bloody pleural effusions in a child or a young adult is highly suggestive of pulmonary capillary hemangiomatosis (56).

Because of major similarities in the CT presentation of venoocclusive disease and pulmonary capillary hemangiomatosis, these two diagnostic possibilities should be suggested to the clinicians and clearly distinguished from other entities with precapillary pulmonary hypertension but normal lungs on CT. This distinction is of clinical importance because of the severe clinical deterioration that may occur in patients with pulmonary hypertension treated with pulmonary vasodilator therapy if the hypertension is secondary to venoocclusive disease and pulmonary capillary hemangiomatosis (57).

Tumor Embolism

In a patient with extrathoracic malignancy, the diagnosis of tumor emboli should be suspected in the presence of unexplained dyspnea, with or without signs of pulmonary hypertension. Tumor cells form emboli in the vena cava and subsequently occlude small muscular pulmonary arteries and arterioles (1). Numerous neoplasms can embolize and

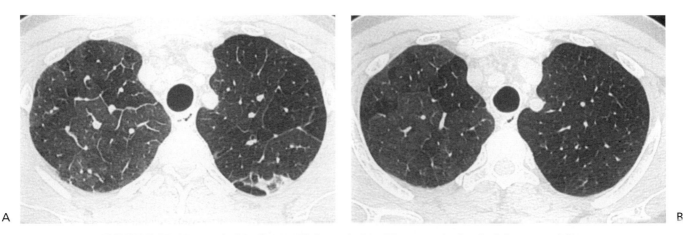

FIGURE 5-18. Venoocclusive disease. High-resolution CT scan at the level of the upper lobes (**A**) shows enlarged pulmonary arterial sections, a pattern of mosaic perfusion associated with thickened septal lines, more pronounced in the right lung. Note considerable reduction in size of pulmonary vascular sections and partial resolution of lung and interstitial infiltration after medical treatment of pulmonary edema (**B**), underlining the role of pulmonary congestion in this entity.

be responsible for pulmonary hypertension, including gastric, breast, prostate, lung, hepatocellular, renal, and ovarian carcinomas as well as osteosarcoma, lymphoma, choriocarcinoma, and right atrial myxoma. Unlike other malignancies, right atrial myxoma and renal cell carcinoma tend to embolize to the large central and segmental pulmonary arteries.

Findings of intravascular metastases include dilated and beaded peripheral pulmonary arteries (58), with or without companion radiologic manifestations of malignancy, including lymphadenopathy and CT features of lymphangitic carcinomatosis. CT may also be normal (59) or depict filling defects within proximal pulmonary arteries.

Pulmonary Hypertension in POEMS Syndrome and Neurofibromatosis

POEMS syndrome is a rare multisystem disorder, considered as a complication of plasma cell dyscrasia, mainly of osteosclerotic myeloma and solitary plasmocytoma. It is characterized by five main features: *P*olyneuropathy, *O*rganomegaly, *E*ndocrinopathy, *M*onoclonal gammopathy, and *S*kin changes (60). Pulmonary arteriopathy is similar to that observed in primary pulmonary hypertension, with a less severe clinical course and frequent improvement with corticosteroids. These lesions include fibrous thickening of arteriolar and capillary walls in affected organs. Other respiratory manifestations of POEMS syndrome include pleural effusion, phrenic neuropathy, and pulmonary tumorlets (61).

Neurofibromatosis has been known to involve blood vessels throughout the body. Pulmonary vascular involvement may be responsible for development of pulmonary hypertension which can mimic chronic thromboembolic pulmonary hypertension, with spiral CT features of multiple bilateral filling defects caused by extensive and irregular intimal fibrosis (62).

REFERENCES

1. Frazier AA, Galvin JR, Franks TJ, et al. From the archives of the AFIP. Pulmonary vasculature: hypertension and infarction. *Radiographics* 2000;20:491–524.
2. Corrin B. *Pathology of the lungs*. New York: Churchill Livingstone, 2000.
3. Reaside D, Peacock A. Making measurements in the pulmonary circulation: when and how? *Thorax* 1997;52:9–11.
4. Tuder RM, Lee SD, Cool CC. Histopathology of pulmonary hypertension. *Chest* 1998;114:1S–6S.
5. Yaginuma GY, Mohri H, Takahashi T. Distribution of arterial lesions and collateral pathways in the pulmonary hypertension of congenital heart disease: a computer aided reconstruction study. *Thorax* 1990;45:586–590.
6. Wagenvoort CA. Classifying pulmonary vascular disease. *Chest* 1973;64:503–504.
7. Peacock AJ. Primary pulmonary hypertension. *Thorax* 1999;54: 1107–1118.

8. Voelkel NF, Tuder RM. Severe pulmonary hypertensive diseases: a perspective. *Eur Respir J* 1999;14:1246–1250.
9. Kuriyama K, Gamsu G, Stern RG, et al. CT-determined pulmonary artery diameters in predicting pulmonary artery hypertension. *Invest Radiol* 1984;19:16–22.
10. Schmidt HC, Kauczor HU, Schild HH, et al. Pulmonary hypertension in patients with chronic pulmonary thrombo-embolism: chest radiography and CT evaluation before and after surgery. *Eur Radiol* 1996;6:817–825.
11. Murray Ti, Boxt LM, Katz J, et al. Estimation of pulmonary artery pressure in patients with primary pulmonary hypertension by quantitative analysis of magnetic resonance images. *J Thorac Imag* 1994;9:198–204.
12. Falashi F, Palla A, Formichi B, et al. CT evaluation of chronic thromboembolic pulmonary hypertension. *J Comput Assist Tomogr* 1992;16:897–903.
13. Tan RT, Kuzo R, Goodman LR, et al. Utility of CT scan evaluation for predicting pulmonary hypertension in patients with parenchymal lung disease. *Chest* 1998;113:1250–1256.
14. Ng CS, Wells AU, Padley SPG. A CT sign of chronic pulmonary arterial hypertension: the ratio of main pulmonary artery to aortic diameter. *J Thorac Imag* 1999;14:270–278.
15. Morris TA, Auger WR, Ysrael MZ, et al. Parenchymal scarring is associated with restrictive spirometric defects in patients with chronic thromboembolic pulmonary hypertension. *Chest* 1996; 110:399–403.
16. Sagy M, Poustchi-Amin M, Nimkoff L, et al. Spiral computed tomographic scanning of the chest with three dimensional imaging in the diagnosis and management of paediatric intrathoracic airway obstruction. *Thorax* 1996;51:1005–1009.
17. Steurer J, Jenni T, Medici C, et al. Dissecting aneurysm of the pulmonary artery with pulmonary hypertension. *Am Rev Respir Dis* 1990;142:1219–1221.
18. Wunderbaldinger P, Bernhard C, Uffman M, et al. Acute pulmonary trunk dissection in a patient with primary pulmonary hypertension. *J Comput Assist Tomogr* 2000;24:92–95.
19. Worthy SA, Muller NL, Hartman TE, et al. Mosaic attenuation pattern on thin-section CT scans of the lung: differentiation among infiltrative lung, airway, and vascular diseases as a cause. *Radiology* 1997;205:465–470.
20. Austin JHM, Sagel SS. Alterations of airway caliber after pulmonary embolization in the dog. *Invest Radiol* 1972;3:135–139.
21. Sherrick AD, Swensen SJ, Harman TE. Mosaic pattern of lung attenuation on CT scans: frequency among patients with pulmonary artery hypertension of different causes. *AJR* 1997;169: 79–82.
22. Primack SL, Muller NL, Mayo JR, et al. Pulmonary parenchymal abnormalities of vascular origin: high-resolution CT findings. *Radiographics* 1994;14:739–746.
23. Meysman M, Diltoer M, Raeve HD, et al. Chronic thromboembolic pulmonary hypertension and vascular transformation of the lymph node sinuses. *Eur Respir J* 1997;10:1191–1193.
24. Slanetz PJ, Truong M, Shepard JAO, et al. Mediastinal lymphadenopathy and hazy mediastinal fat: new CT findings of congestive heart failure. *AJR* 1998;171:1307–1309.
25. Boxt LM, Katz J. Magnetic resonance imaging for quantitation of right ventricular volume in patients with pulmonary hypertension. *J Thorac Imag* 1993;8:92–97.
26. Reid JH, Murchison JT. Acute right ventricular dilatation: a new helical CT sign of massive pulmonary embolism. *Clin Radiol* 1998;53:694–698.
27. Oliver TB, Reid JH, Murchison JT. Interventricular septal shift due to massive pulmonary embolism shown by CT pulmonary angiography: an old sign revisited. *Thorax* 1998;53:1092–1094.
28. Baque-Juston MC, Wells AU, Hansell DM. Pericardial thicken-

ing or effusion in patients with pulmonary artery hypertension. A CT study. *AJR* 1999;172:361–364.

29. Fedullo PF, Auger WR, Channinck RN, et al. Chronic thromboembolic pulmonary hypertension. *Clin Chest Med* 1995;16: 353–374.

30. Schwickert HC, Schweden F, Schild HH, et al. Pulmonary arteries and lung parenchyma in chronic pulmonary embolism: preoperative and postoperative CT findings. *Radiology* 1994;191: 351–357.

31. Bergin CJ, Hauschildt HP, Brown MA, et al. Identifying the cause of unilateral hypoperfusion in patients suspected to have chronic pulmonary thromboembolism: diagnostic accuracy of helical CT and conventional angiography. *Radiology* 1999;213:743–749.

32. Auger WR, Fedullo PF, Moser KM, et al. Chronic major-vessel thromboembolic pulmonary artery obstruction: appearance at angiography. *Radiology* 1992;182:393–398.

33. Roberts HC, Kauczor HU, Schweden F, et al. Spiral CT of pulmonary hypertension and chronic thromboembolism. *J Thorac Imag* 1997;12:118–127.

34. Bergin CJ, Sirlin CB, Hauschildt JP, et al. Chronic thromboembolism: diagnosis with helical CT and MR imaging with angiographic and surgical correlation. *Radiology* 1997;204:695–702.

35. Remy-Jardin M, Louvegny S, Remy J, et al. Acute central thromboembolic disease: posttherapeutic follow-up with spiral CT angiography. *Radiology* 1997;203:173–189.

36. Moser K, Olson L, Schlusselberg M, et al. Chronic thromboembolic occlusion in the adult can mimic pulmonary artery agenesis. *Chest* 1989;95:503–508.

37. Hirsch A, Moser K, Auger W, et al. Unilateral pulmonary artery thrombotic occlusion: is distal arteriopathy a consequence? *Am J Respir Crit Care Med* 1996;154:491–496.

38. Remy-Jardin M, Remy J, Deschildre F, et al. Diagnosis of pulmonary embolism with spiral CT: comparison with pulmonary angiography and scintigraphy. *Radiology* 1996;200:699–706.

39. Kauczor HU, Schwickert HC, Mayer E, et al. Spiral CT of bronchial arteries in chronic thromboembolism. *J Comput Assist Tomogr* 1994;18:855–861.

40. Tardivon AA, Musset D, Maitre S, et al. Role of CT in chronic pulmonary embolism: comparison with pulmonary angiography. *J Comput Assist Tomogr* 1993;17:345–351.

41. Thomas CS, Endrys J, Abul A, et al. Late massive haemoptysis from bronchopulmonary collaterals in infarcted segments following pulmonary embolism. *Eur Respir J* 1999;13:463–464.

42. Bergin CJ, Sirlin C, Deutsch R, et al. Predictors of patient response to pulmonary thromboendarterectomy. *AJR* 2000;174: 509–515.

43. Bergin CJ, Rios G, King MA, et al. Accuracy of high-resolution CT in identifying chronic pulmonary thromboembolic disease. *AJR* 1996;166:1371–1377.

44. King MA, Bergin CJ, Yeung DWC, et al. Chronic pulmonary thromboembolism: detection of regional hyperperfusion with CT. *Radiology* 1994;191:359–363.

45. King MA, Ysrael M, Bergin CJ. Chronic thromboembolic pulmonary hypertension: CT findings. *AJR* 1998;170:955–960.

46. Remy-Jardin M, Duyck P, Remy J, et al. Hilar lymph nodes: identification with spiral CT and histologic correlation. *Radiology* 1995;196:387–394.

47. Remy-Jardin M, Remy J, Louvegny S, et al. Airway changes in chronic pulmonary embolism: CT findings in 33 patients. *Radiology* 1997;203:355–360.

48. Chazova I, Robbins I, Loyd J, et al. Venous and arterial changes in pulmonary veno-occlusive disease, mitral stenosis and fibrosing mediastinitis. *Eur Respir J* 2000;15:116–122.

49. Swensen SJ, Tashjian JH, Myers JL, et al. Pulmonary venoocclusive disease: CT findings in eight patients. *AJR* 1996;167: 937–940.

50. Dufour B, Maître S, Humbert M, et al. High-resolution CT of the chest in four patients with pulmonary capillary hemangiomatosis or pulmonary venoocclusive disease. *AJR* 1998;171: 1321–1324.

51. Katz DS, Scalzetti EM, Katzenstein ALA, et al. Pulmonary venoocclusive disease presenting with thrombosis of pulmonary arteries. *Thorax* 1994;50:699–700.

52. Cassart M, Gevenois PA, Kramer M, et al. Pulmonary venoocclusive disease: CT findings before and after single-lung transplantation. *AJR* 1993;160:759–760.

53. Eltorky MA, Headley AS, Winer-Muram H, et al. Pulmonary capillary hemangiomatosis: a clinicopathologic review. *Ann Thorac Surg* 1994;57:7772–7776.

54. Lippert JL, White CS, Cameron EW, et al. Pulmonary capillary hemangiomatosis: radiographic appearance. *J Thorac Imag* 1998; 13:49–51.

55. Faber CN, Yousem SA, Dauber JH, et al. Pulmonary capillary hemangiomatosis. A report of three cases and a review of the literature. *Am Rev Respir Dis* 1989;140:808–813.

56. Canny GJ, Cutz E, MacLusky IB, et al. Diffuse pulmonary angiomatosis. *Thorax* 1991;46:851–853.

57. Humbert M, Maître S, Capron F, et al. Pulmonary edema complicating continuous intravenous prostacyclin in pulmonary capillary hemangiomatosis. *Am J Respir Crit Care Med* 1998;157: 1681–1685.

58. Shepard JA, Moore EH, Templeton PA, et al. Pulmonary intravascular tumor emboli: dilated and beaded peripheral pulmonary arteries at CT. *Radiology* 1993;187:797–801.

59. Hibbert M, Braude S. Tumour microembolism presenting as "primary pulmonary hypertension." *Thorax* 1997;52:1016–1017.

60. Lesprit PH, Godeau B, Authier FJ, et al. Pulmonary hypertension in POEMS syndrome. A new feature mediated by cytokines. *Am J Respir Crit Care Med* 1998;157:907–911.

61. Mokhlesi B, Jain M. Pulmonary manifestations of POEMS syndrome. *Chest* 1999;115:1740–1742.

62. Samuels N, Berkman N, Milgalter E, et al. Pulmonary hypertension secondary to neurofibromatosis: intimal fibrosis versus thromboembolism. *Thorax* 1999;54:858–589.

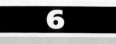

ACQUIRED VASCULAR DISEASES OF THE LUNG

PULMONARY ARTERITIS

This section includes the main inflammatory processes that involve medium and large pulmonary arteries, namely Behçet's disease, Hughes-Stovin's syndrome, and Takayasu's arteritis. Other conditions associated with pulmonary vasculitis, such as Wegener's granulomatosis and connective tissue diseases, involve small pulmonary vessels and capillaries. The vascular abnormalities in these entities are therefore below the resolution of CT angiography (CTA) and beyond the scope of this text.

Behçet's Disease

Behçet's disease was initially described as a syndrome characterized by the clinical triad of recurrent oral ulcers, genital ulcers, and uveitis (1,2). It is now recognized to be a systemic vasculitis that may involve arteries and veins of any size (3). The most common manifestations consist of aph-thous oral and genital ulcers, uveitis or retinal vasculitis, cutaneous vasculitis, gastrointestinal involvement, arthritis, and meningoencephalitis (3). The incidence is highest in the Middle East (Turkey, Israel, Lebanon) and the Far East (Japan, Korea, China) (3,4). The age of onset is usually between 20 and 30 years; men are affected more often than women (4). The cause is unknown.

The main intrathoracic manifestations of Behçet's disease consist of pulmonary artery aneurysm formation, pulmonary artery thrombosis, and thrombosis of the superior vena cava (SVC) (Figures 6-1 and 6-2) (3,4). Less common complications include aneurysm of the aorta or brachiocephalic artery and stenosis or occlusion of the brachiocephalic artery (4).

Pulmonary vascular involvement occurs in 5% to 10% of patients and usually first manifests several years after the onset of systemic disease (Box 6-1) (2,5). Pulmonary artery aneurysms are associated with poor prognosis. The most common and serious clinical symptom of pulmonary

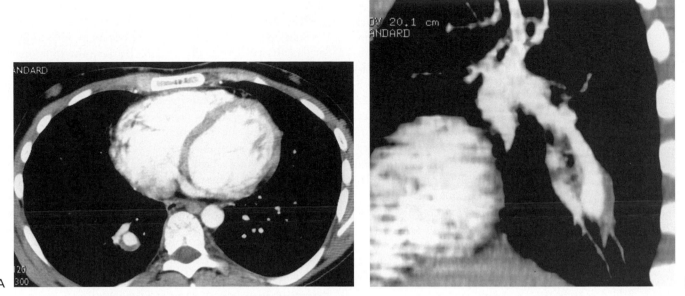

A   B

FIGURE 6-1. Behçet's disease with pulmonary artery aneurysm. Cross-sectional CT angiogram image (**A**) shows aneurysmal dilation of the right lower lobe posterior basal segmental artery. Note presence of intramural thrombus. Sagittal reconstruction (**B**) demonstrates the extent of the aneurysm. (Case courtesy of Dr. Jim Barrie, Department of Radiology, University of Alberta Medical Centre, Edmonton, Alberta, Canada.)

involvement is hemoptysis, which can be massive and lead to death (2,3).

The radiographic manifestations are nonspecific and include round perihilar opacities, lung nodule or mass, focal airspace consolidation, wedge-shaped opacities, rapid development of unilateral hilar enlargement, and mediasti-

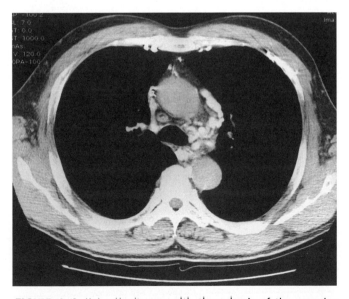

FIGURE 6-2. Behçet's disease with thrombosis of the superior vena cava. CT image shows extensive collateral venous circulation secondary to thrombosis of the innominate vein and superior vena cava in a 55-year-old male. (Case courtesy of Dr. Kyung Soo Lee, Department of Radiology, Samsung Medical Centre, Seoul, Korea.)

nal widening (4,6). The round perihilar opacities, lung nodules and masses, and hilar enlargement represent the pulmonary artery aneurysm. Focal areas of airspace consolidation and wedge-shaped opacities are due to pulmonary hemorrhage or infarction. The mediastinal widening may be secondary to SVC thrombosis or, less commonly, narrowing of the SVC or aortic aneurysm formation (3,4,6).

Contrast-enhanced CT allows assessment of the presence, size, and location of the pulmonary artery aneurysms, as well as other intrathoracic complications of Behçet's syndrome (Figure 6-1) (2,4,6). The aneurysms can be single or multiple and involve central or, less commonly, peripheral pulmonary arteries (2,7). The most commonly affected vessels are the descending branch of the right pulmonary artery, followed by the descending branch of the left pulmonary artery, and branches of the left upper lobe artery (7).

Erkan and colleague assessed the CT manifestations in nine patients with Behçet's disease who had lung involvement (2). Conventional CT (8-mm collimation) demonstrated aneurysms of the main, lobar, or segmental pulmonary arter-

BOX 6-1. BEHÇET'S DISEASE

- Oral ulcers, genital ulcers, and uveitis
- Pulmonary vascular involvement in 5%–10% cases
- Pulmonary artery aneurysms
- Single or multiple
- Central or, less commonly, peripheral
- Mural thrombosis common
- May lead to pulmonary artery occlusion

ies. One-mm thick sections allowed assessment of more peripheral branches, which showed irregularities of the vessel walls, focal enlargements, narrowings, and cutoffs (2). Ahn and associates reviewed the CT findings in nine patients with thoracic manifestations of Behçet's syndrome (6). Contrast-enhanced CT demonstrated airspace consolidation in five patients (56%), thrombosis of the SVC in four (44%), unilateral or bilateral pulmonary artery aneurysms in three (33%), and narrowing of the SVC in one patient (11%). Mural thrombosis was present in all pulmonary artery aneurysms. Numan and coworkers reviewed the findings in 15 patients with pulmonary arterial involvement (7). Twelve had multiple pulmonary aneurysms and three had single aneurysms. Fourteen aneurysms were located in the hilar or parahilar regions and one was subpleural. In six patients, the pulmonary artery aneurysm was accompanied by occlusion of the pulmonary artery. Occlusion occurred most commonly at the descending branch of the right pulmonary artery.

Recognition of occluded pulmonary artery aneurysms may be difficult because these aneurysms may not enhance following intravenous administration of contrast and cannot be visualized on conventional angiography (7). Conventional angiography should be avoided in these patients. Venous puncture and insertion of a venous catheter may initiate thrombosis or aggravate venous thrombosis (4). Arterial puncture can result in aneurysm formation at the puncture site (4). Magnetic resonance imaging (MRI) is recommended for further evaluation of suspected pulmonary artery aneurysms in patients with normal diagnostic CT findings (4,7).

Hughes-Stovin's Syndrome

Hughes-Stovin's syndrome is a rare idiopathic condition characterized by pulmonary artery aneurysm formation, pulmonary artery embolism or thrombosis, and systemic venous thrombosis (8,9). The radiographic and CT manifestations are identical to those of Behçet's disease. Because of the similarity of vascular manifestations, it has been suggested that Hughes-Stovin's syndrome may represent a manifestation of Behçet's disease (10).

Takayasu's Arteritis

Takayasu's arteritis, also known as nonspecific aortoarteritis, is an idiopathic arteritis that affects mainly the elastic arteries, including the aorta, its major branches, and, less commonly, the pulmonary arteries (11,12). It has a worldwide distribution but is seen most commonly in Southeast Asia, particularly Japan, Korea, China, and India (11–13). It characteristically affects young women, the average age of onset being approximately 30 years (14,15).

The most common manifestations of Takayasu's arteritis consist of short- or long-segment stenosis of the aorta and

are reviewed in Chapter 3. The discussion in this section is limited to the pulmonary vascular abnormalities.

Pulmonary vascular involvement occurs in 50% to 80% of patients (Box 6-2) (12,16,17). Because the pulmonary arteries have an elastic component down to the level of the lobular branches, Takayasu's arteritis may involve central and peripheral pulmonary vessels (18,19). The most characteristic manifestations consist of stenosis or occlusion of segmental and subsegmental arteries, or, less commonly, lobar or main pulmonary arteries (11,16). Pulmonary vascular involvement tends to be bilateral; upper lobe branches are affected more commonly than lower lobe, middle lobe, or lingular branches (11). In the vast majority of cases, pulmonary artery involvement is a late manifestation of the disease, but occasionally, pulmonary lesions may be present at the time of initial diagnosis (19,20).

The frequency of pulmonary artery involvement correlates with the severity of brachiocephalic artery disease but not with the extent or severity of aortic disease (16). The pathologic features of the pulmonary arteries are similar to the systemic artery lesions (16,17,21). The abnormalities consist of thinning of the media with disruption of the elastic fibers, fibrosis of the adventitia, and fibrosis and hyperplasia of the intima resulting in thickening of the arterial wall, luminal stenosis, and occlusion (22,23). There are usually no pulmonary symptoms; a small percentage of patients have hemoptysis or dyspnea (11,24). Occasionally, the clinical and radiologic features may mimic those of chronic thromboembolic disease (22). Because the pulmonary vascular lesions are usually asymptomatic but progressive, the pulmonary arteries should be assessed in all patients with suspected or proven Takayasu's arteritis (17).

The CT manifestations of pulmonary artery involvement include dilation of the pulmonary trunk, thickening and enhancement of the arterial wall, luminal stenosis and occlusion, aneurysm formation, and localized areas of decreased vascularity (Figure 6-3) (12,17,25). The presence of circumferential mural enhancement during the early arterial phase and/or mural enhancement on delayed scans are suggestive of active disease (Figure 6-4) (25).

Park and coworkers assessed the mural changes in the aorta and pulmonary arteries on conventional CT in 12 women with Takayasu's arteritis (25). Circumferential wall thickening of the aortic wall was present in all cases. In six of the eight patients with active disease, the aortic wall showed

BOX 6-2. TAKAYASU'S ARTERITIS

- Nonspecific aortoarteritis
- Pulmonary vascular involvement in 50–80% of cases
- Most commonly segmental and subsegmental arteries
- Stenosis or occlusion
- Thickening of the wall
- Wall enhancement with intravenous contrast
- Mosaic perfusion

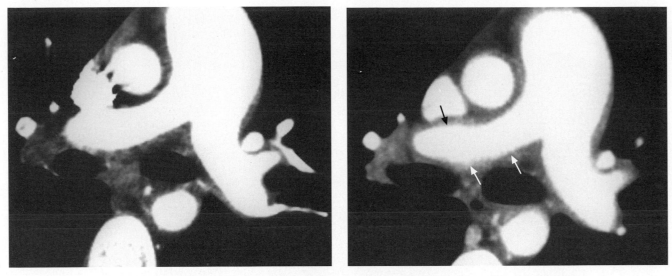

FIGURE 6-3. Takayasu's arteritis with pulmonary artery involvement. CT angiography (CTA) at the level of the pulmonary trunk (**A**) shows marked dilation of the central pulmonary arteries. CTA image performed 50 seconds later (**B**) shows thickening and enhancement of the wall of the right pulmonary artery (*arrows*). The patient was a 13-year-old girl with active Takayasu's disease affecting the aorta and pulmonary arteries. (Case courtesy of Dr. Mitsuhiro Koyama, Department of Radiology, Osaka University Medical School, Osaka, Japan.)

inhomogeneous enhancement following intravenous administration of contrast. Two patients showed thickening and enhancement of the wall of the pulmonary trunk and main pulmonary arteries. Paul and colleagues performed CTA using electron beam CT in 41 patients with Takayasu's arteritis (24). Pulmonary artery abnormalities were present in 22 patients (54%). These included dilation of the pulmonary artery trunk, right or left pulmonary arteries in 12 patients (29%), focal areas of hypoperfusion in 10 patients (24%), thickening of the arterial wall (thickness greater than 1.5 mm) in 6 patients (15%), and high attenuation of the arterial wall in 4 patients (10%). The focal areas of parenchymal hypoperfusion were patchy in distribution resulting in a mosaic pattern of attenuation and perfusion (Figure 6-5). Five patients had pulmonary arterial hypertension diagnosed by Doppler sonography and all of these five patients had

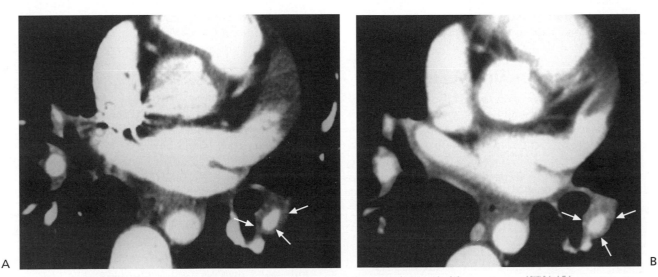

FIGURE 6-4. Takayasu's arteritis with pulmonary artery involvement. CT angiogram (CTA) (**A**) demonstrates increased soft tissue (*arrows*) surrounding the slightly narrowed lumen of the left interlobar pulmonary artery. CTA image performed 50 seconds (**B**) later shows enhancement of the arterial wall (*arrows*). The patient was a 13-year-old girl with active Takayasu's disease affecting the aorta and pulmonary arteries (same patient as shown in Figure 6-3 and Figure 3-1). (Case courtesy of Dr. Mitsuhiro Koyama, Department of Radiology, Osaka University Medical School, Osaka, Japan.)

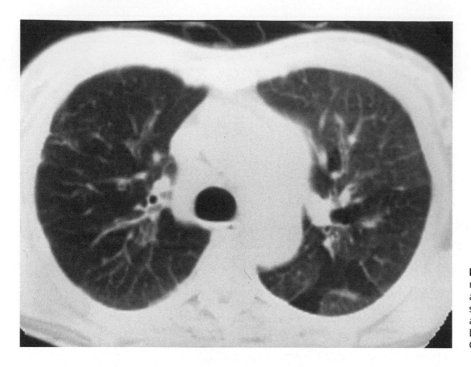

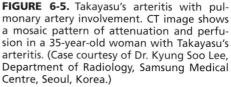

FIGURE 6-5. Takayasu's arteritis with pulmonary artery involvement. CT image shows a mosaic pattern of attenuation and perfusion in a 35-year-old woman with Takayasu's arteritis. (Case courtesy of Dr. Kyung Soo Lee, Department of Radiology, Samsung Medical Centre, Seoul, Korea.)

abnormalities of the pulmonary arteries on CTA. Two of these five patients had large right and left pulmonary arteries, one had bilateral pulmonary stenosis, one had unilateral pulmonary artery stenosis, and one had marked dilation of the pulmonary trunk (24).

Takahashi and coworkers assessed the CT findings of the pulmonary parenchyma in 25 patients with Takayasu's arteritis and compared these findings with those at angiography and perfusion scintigraphy (12). Eleven patients had a total of 33 localized areas of low attenuation and vascularity on CT. These areas corresponded to sites of staining voids on angiography and to perfusion defects at scintigraphy.

INFECTIOUS PULMONARY VASCULITIS

Infections can reach the pulmonary vessels by hematogenous spread or by direct extension from the adjacent parenchyma. Involvement of the pulmonary arteries may result in the development of aneurysms and pulmonary artery thrombosis (Box 6-3). Secondary manifestations include pulmonary hemorrhage, infarction, and septic embolism (Figure 6-6).

BOX 6-3. MYCOTIC PULMONARY ANEURYSMS

- Patients with left-to-right shunts
- Intravenous drug users
- Usually due to hematogenous seeding
- May be single or multiple
- Central or peripheral

Mycotic pulmonary aneurysms are rare (26). They are seen most commonly in patients with congenital heart disease who have left-to-right shunts complicated by endocarditis (26). They can also occur in intravenous drug users with endocarditis of the tricuspid or pulmonic valve, in patients with necrotizing pneumonia, and in patients with chronic tuberculosis (26–28). The vast majority of cases are due to *Staphylococcus aureus* or *Streptococcus* sp. (27,28). However, a number of other organisms have also been associated with mycotic pulmonary aneurysms including *Klebsiella* sp, *Aspergillus* sp, *Candida albicans*, *Mucor SP*, and *Micobacterium tuberculosis* (26,28).

The majority of mycotic aneurysms are secondary to endovascular seeding (28). The main exception are pulmonary artery aneurysms associated with *M. tuberculosis* (Rasmussen's aneurysms), which characteristically develop in vessels along the wall of tuberculous cavities (28).

Mycotic aneurysms may be single or multiple and involve the central or peripheral pulmonary arteries (26,28). Contrast-enhanced CT shows focal aneurysmal dilation with or without associated thrombus formation (26).

Invasion of pulmonary vessels is a characteristic manifestation of *A. fumigatus* infection in the immunocompromised host, particularly patients with severe neutropenia (neutrophil count less than 500) (29). Invasion of the pulmonary arteries by *Aspergillus* can lead to thrombus formation, tissue necrosis, and hemorrhage. The characteristic CT manifestations consist of nodules, often surrounded by a halo of ground-glass attenuation, and segmental areas of consolidation (Figure 6-7) (30,31). Correlation of the CT with histologic findings has shown that the nodules reflect the presence of nodular areas of lung infarction while the

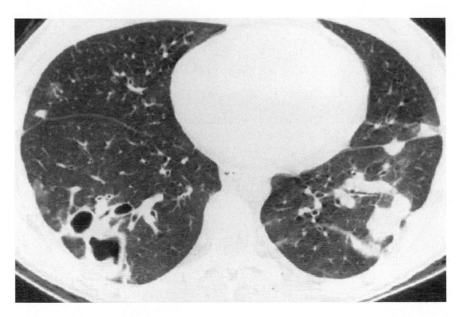

FIGURE 6-6. Septic embolism. High-resolution CT image demonstrates bilateral nodules and cavities involving mainly the subpleural lung regions of the lower lobes. The patient was a 23- year-old drug addict who developed bacterial endocarditis and septic embolism.

areas of ground-glass attenuation are due to surrounding hemorrhage (31–33). Cavitation of the nodules, often resulting with an air-crescent sign, is common but is usually a late manifestation of angioinvasive aspergillosis (29).

Rarely, pulmonary aspergillosis can invade the central pulmonary arteries and even the adjacent aorta and result in thrombus formation (34). Contrast-enhanced CT in these patients demonstrates low attenuation areas consistent with thrombi in the lumen of the pulmonary artery and adjacent descending aorta (34). These thrombi may progress and lead to complete occlusion of the pulmonary artery and aorta (34).

PULMONARY VASCULAR NEOPLASMS

Primary Vascular Tumors

Primary pulmonary vascular tumors are rare. The vast majority are sarcomas, most commonly leiomyosarcomas. Other subtypes include rhabdomyosarcomas, fibrosarcomas, chondromas, and undifferentiated sarcomas.

Almost all of the tumors occur in the mediastinum, hilar, or perihilar region (Box 6-4). In a review of 138 cases reported by 1997, 85% of the tumors involved the pulmonary trunk, 71% involved the right pulmonary artery, 65% the left pulmonary artery, 32% the pulmonary valve, and 10% involved the right ventricular outflow tract (35). Rarely, the sarcomas may originate from a central pulmonary vein (36). The tumors typically spread within the vascular lumen and often remain confined to the lumen. Complete vascular occlusion may occur due to the tumor itself or a combination of tumor and thrombus. Pulmonary vascular sarcomas can also extend across the vessel wall and invade the adjacent bronchial wall and lung parenchyma. Distal pulmonary metastases are common. Tumor emboli

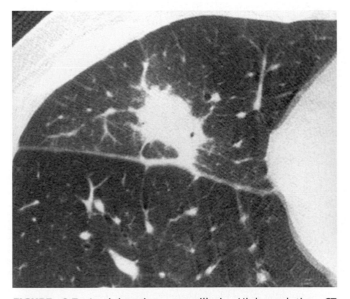

FIGURE 6-7. Angioinvasive aspergillosis. High-resolution CT images show right middle lower nodule surrounded by a halo of ground-glass attenuation. The patient was a 59-year-old man who had severe neutropenia following bone marrow transplantation for leukemia.

BOX 6-4. PULMONARY ARTERY SARCOMA

- Central pulmonary arteries
- Spread within vascular lumen
- Can invade adjacent structures
- Mimic pulmonary embolism
- Late enhancement on CT angiography

and tumor-related thromboemboli may result in pulmonary infarcts (37).

The clinical and radiologic features of the various pulmonary vascular sarcomas are similar. Clinical symptoms include chest pain, dyspnea, cough, and hemoptysis. The clinical presentation may mimic acute or chronic pulmonary thromboembolism (38,39). The radiographic manifestations include hilar enlargement, solitary or multiple lung nodules, and focal areas of consolidation (35,40).

Contrast-enhanced CT demonstrates the tumor as an intraluminal filling defect resembling acute or chronic pulmonary thromboembolism (41,42). The tumor may expand the involved vessel. Findings helpful in distinguishing a pulmonary artery sarcoma from thromboembolism include branching filling defects due to intraluminal tumor growth, extension into the mediastinum or lung, and peripheral pulmonary nodules (43). The tumor may also show delayed enhancement on CTA and enhancement on MRI following administration of gadopentetate dimeglumine (44).

Intravascular Metastases

Intravascular pulmonary metastases are commonly seen at autopsy, particularly in patients who have carcinoma of the breast, stomach, liver, kidney, or lung, or choriocarcinoma (45,46). The vast majority of these tumor emboli are microscopic and involve small arteries and arterioles. Grossly visible tumor emboli involving subsegmental and larger pulmonary arteries are uncommon.

The clinical symptoms of tumor embolism include dyspnea, cough, and hemoptysis (46). The radiographic manifestations are nonspecific and include dilation of the central pulmonary arteries due to pulmonary arterial hypertension, nodular opacities, and septal lines due to lymphangitic carcinomatosis (46).

Large tumor emboli can result in intraluminal filling defects in segmental or larger pulmonary arteries (Figure 6-8). These central tumor emboli resemble acute thromboembolic disease on CTA. Tumor emboli in subsegmental arteries result in a characteristic nodular or beaded thickening of these vessels, a finding that can be readily seen on CT without intravenous contrast (47). Smaller peripheral intravascular metastases cannot be identified on CT. Large and small tumor emboli may result in pulmonary infarction and pulmonary arterial hypertension (47,48). Rarely, pulmonary parenchymal metastases may grow into the lumen of a pulmonary vein and result in pulmonary venous tumor thrombosis and infarction (49).

PULMONARY VASCULAR INVOLVEMENT BY ADJACENT PROCESS

The discussion in this section is limited to the most common conditions associated with encasement and obstruction of the central pulmonary arteries and veins, namely, pulmonary carcinoma and fibrosing mediastinitis. The manifestations of involvement of parenchymal vessels by adjacent infectious processes were previously discussed under "Infectious Pulmonary Vasculitis."

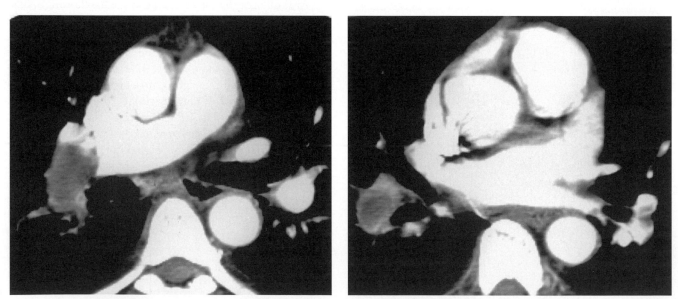

A   B

FIGURE 6-8. Intravascular pulmonary metastases. CT angiography (CTA) (**A**) shows large intraluminal filling defect in the right interlobar pulmonary artery. CTA at a lower level (**B**) demonstrates large embolus in the right lower lobe artery and smaller emboli in two of the segmental arteries of the left lower lobe. The patient was a 62-year-old man who had extensive pulmonary vascular metastases from renal cell carcinoma.

Pulmonary Arterial Involvement by Carcinoma

CT plays a major role in the preoperative diagnosis and staging of pulmonary carcinoma. It is helpful in determining the potential surgical resectability of the tumor and the type of surgery. Tumors encasing or surrounding the main pulmonary artery or proximal right or left pulmonary artery for more than 180 degrees are classified as T4 lesions and are unresectable (50,51). When the more distal portions of the right or left pulmonary artery are involved by tumor, complete resection may be possible but requires pneumonectomy. Involvement of the arch of the left pulmonary artery as it courses over left main bronchus requires pneumonectomy or left upper lobectomy with sleeve resection of the involved portion of the artery and anastomosis or interposition grafting (52,53). Involvement of the descending right pulmonary artery may necessitate bilobectomy.

It must be emphasized that for the tumor to be considered as definitely involving a central pulmonary artery it must encase the vessel or abut it for more than 180 degrees (54). Similar to the aorta, SVC, and central pulmonary veins, obliteration of the fat plane between the tumor and pulmonary artery, distortion of the artery by the tumor, and apparent intraluminal tumor extension are not reliable indicators of vascular involvement (54,55). Ninety-seven percent of pulmonary carcinomas that contact the mediastinum for 3 cm or less, abut the aorta for less than 90 degrees, or have a fat plane between the tumor and the mediastinum, are technically resectable (56). However, contact of greater than 3 cm with the mediastinum or contact of greater than 90 degrees but less than 180 degrees with the aorta or intrapericardial pulmonary artery are not reliable indicators of invasion or unresectability (54–56). The diagnostic accuracy of CT in the diagnosis of direct mediastinal invasion using the above described signs was assessed in an analysis of 785 mediastinal structures in 90 patients who underwent thoracotomy (54). All seven mediastinal structures or vessels with more than 180 degrees of contact with the tumor were involved (specificity 100%) but the sensitivity of this sign in detecting tumor involvement was only 28%. Greater than 90 degrees contact of tumor with a mediastinal structure or vessel had a sensitivity of 40% and a specificity of 99%. Only 11 of 17 mediastinal structures distorted by adjacent tumor (specificity 65%) and 5 of 7 structures with apparent intraluminal tumor on CT (specificity 71%) were shown to be involved by tumor (54).

Assessment of the relationship of pulmonary carcinoma to the pulmonary arteries in the mediastinal and hilar regions requires careful timing of the intravenous bolus of contrast, 3- to 5-mm collimation scans, and multiplanar reconstructions. In patients with extensive pulmonary artery encasement by carcinoma, the presence of encasement can be readily visualized on conventional cross-sectional images (Figure 6-9). These images also demonstrate secondary effects of the encasement such as decreased perfusion to the involved lung and blood flow redistribution to the remaining lung (Figure 6-10). Cross-sectional images, however, do not allow adequate assessment of vascular encasement when the interface between the vessel and the tumor is oriented horizontally. Therefore, multiplanar reconstructions (MPRs) are often required to determine the central extent of a tumor. The MPRs should be tailored to the site of suspected tumor involvement. Assessment of the proximal left pulmonary artery in the region of the aortopulmonary window is facilitated by the use of MPRs parallel to or perpendicular to the aortopulmonary (AP) window. The relationship of the central tumor to the superior and inferior margins of the proximal right pulmonary artery is best depicted on coronal reformations. Sagittal and oblique sagittal reformations provide optimal depiction of tumor extension along the right and left descending pulmonary arteries.

Pulmonary Venous Involvement by Carcinoma

Pulmonary carcinoma can encase and obstruct a pulmonary vein or grow into the lumen of the vein, extend along it,

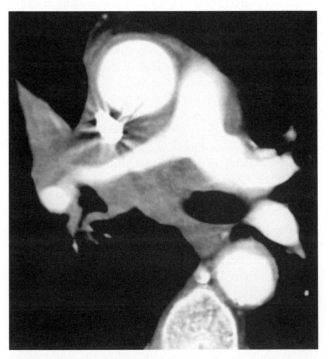

FIGURE 6-9. Pulmonary artery encasement by carcinoma. CT angiography demonstrates extensive tumor infiltration of the mediastinum with obliteration of fat planes and encasement of the right pulmonary artery in a 35-year-old woman with large cell carcinoma of the lung.

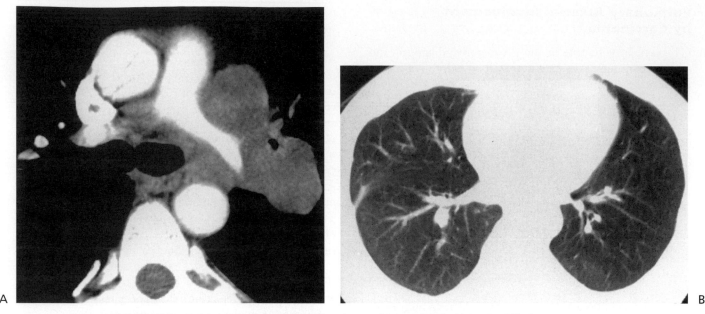

A   B

FIGURE 6-10. Pulmonary artery encasement by carcinoma. CT angiography (**A**) demonstrates increased soft tissue surrounding the left pulmonary artery with associated encasement of the vessel and narrowing of the lumen. Lung windows at the level of the inferior pulmonary veins (**B**) show decreased vascularity and attenuation of the left lung in a 64-year-old man with small cell carcinoma.

and invade the left atrium. A preoperative diagnosis of intraluminal venous extension is important, as surgical manipulation may result in multiple systemic tumor emboli (57). The CT manifestations of pulmonary venous invasion are those of venous obstruction. They include interlobular septal thickening, bronchial wall thickening, pulmonary edema, hemorrhage, and pleural effusion. On CTA, the invaded vein is typically nonopacified and increased in diameter. Tumor extension into the left atrium results in a filling defect at the venoatrial junction.

The value of obliteration of a pulmonary vein on CT in determining local extent of pulmonary carcinoma was assessed in a study of 325 patients who underwent thoracotomy (58). Obliteration of the pulmonary vein was considered present when the pulmonary vein was not visualized on contrast-enhanced CT and its place was occupied by tumor growth. Obliteration of the pulmonary vein up to its entrance into the left atrium, without associated filling defect in the left atrium, was present in 19 patients. Fourteen of these 19 patients (74%) had surgically proven tumor extension through the pulmonary vein beyond the pericardial reflection. Intrapericardial extension occurred in all 10 patients showing obliteration of either the right or left superior pulmonary vein, but in only 4 of 9 (44%) patients showing obliteration of either the right or left inferior pulmonary vein (58). Similar to the aorta or pulmonary artery, contact of greater than 90 degrees between tumor and pulmonary vein is not a reliable indicator of vascular involvement (55).

Fibrosing Mediastinitis

Fibrosing mediastinitis is a condition characterized by chronic inflammation and fibrosis of the mediastinal soft tissues. It can be focal or diffuse (Box 6-5). In North America, the vast majority of cases are secondary to histoplasmosis (59,60). In countries where histoplasmosis is not endemic, the most common cause is tuberculosis (61). A small percentage of cases occur in association with sarcoidosis, methysergide therapy, or following therapy for mediastinal nodal involvement by pulmonary carcinoma or Hodgkin's disease (60,62). Fibrosing mediastinitis may also be seen in association with autoimmune processes, retroperitoneal fibrosis, orbital pseudotumor, and Riedel's sclerosing thyroiditis (60). Occasionally, it may be idiopathic and not associated with other disease processes.

BOX 6-5. FIBROSING MEDIASTINITIS

- Focal: usually due to histoplasmosis or tuberculosis
- Foci of calcification: histoplasmosis or tuberculosis
- Diffuse: usually idiopathic
- Narrowing or obstruction of SVC
- Tracheobronchial narrowing
- Narrowing or occlusion of central pulmonary artery
- Most commonly right pulmonary artery

SVC, superior vena cava.

The clinical symptoms and signs are variable depending on which mediastinal structures are involved by the fibrotic process. The most common manifestations are cough, dyspnea, hemoptysis, and findings related to obstruction of the SVC (headache, cyanosis, and puffiness of the face, neck, and arms) (60,61). The radiographic findings include mediastinal widening, hilar enlargement, mediastinal calcification, and tracheobronchial narrowing (60,61).

Fibrosing mediastinitis is often progressive and can result in compression of the central airways, brachiocephalic veins, SVC, esophagus, pulmonary arteries, and veins (60). In one series of 33 patients with fibrosing mediastinitis, narrowing or obstruction of the SVC was present in 13 (39%), bronchial narrowing in 11 (33%), narrowing or obstruction of a central pulmonary artery in 6 (18%), and esophageal narrowing in 3 patients (9%) (60).

Involvement of the pulmonary arteries can be unilateral or bilateral but most commonly is limited to the right pulmonary artery (60,62). Fibrosing mediastinitis may result in complete obstruction of the main pulmonary artery, usually the right artery (60,63). Progressive narrowing of one or both pulmonary arteries can result in pulmonary arterial hypertension, cor pulmonale, and right-sided heart failure (64).

CT is performed almost routinely in the assessment of patients with suspected or proven fibrosing mediastinitis (60,61). It allows assessment of the extent of fibrosis, presence of calcification, and presence and severity of narrowing of the airways and vessels. CT is also helpful in the differential diagnosis and management. Patients with fibrosing mediastinitis secondary to histoplasmosis or tuberculosis typically have a localized pattern of fibrosis commonly associated with foci of calcification and do not respond to corticosteroid therapy (Figure 6-11) (60). Idiopathic fibrosing mediastinitis, on the other hand, is typically diffuse, not calcified, and often improves following corticosteroid therapy (60).

Although, CT without intravenous contrast is helpful in the detection of subtle foci of calcification, contrast enhancement is essential for the evaluation of presence and extent of involvement of the pulmonary arteries, pulmonary veins, and SVC.

POSTSURGICAL COMPLICATIONS

The most important postoperative pulmonary arterial complications in which CTA can play a key role are postoperative pulmonary embolism, clot in the pulmonary artery stump, anastomotic vascular stenosis following lung transplantation, and lobar torsion. The main pulmonary venous complication is obstruction.

A clot in the pulmonary artery stump is a relatively common finding following pneumonectomy but seldom leads to complications (65,66). Stump clots occur most commonly following right pneumonectomy because the right arterial stump is longer than the left. Occasionally, stump clots may result in recurrent embolism of the remaining lung (66). Stump clots may also enlarge over time and mimic tumor recurrence (65) (Figure 6-12).

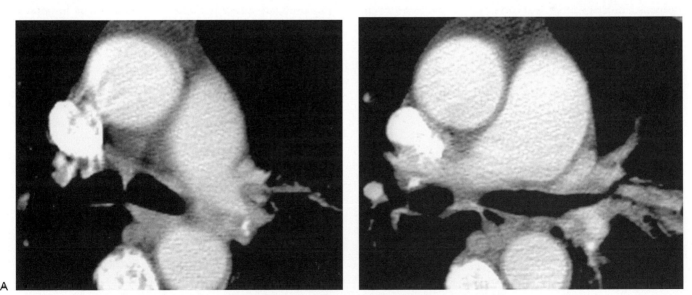

A   B

FIGURE 6-11. Fibrosing mediastinitis. Contrast-enhanced CT scan at the level of the tracheal carina (**A**) demonstrates increased soft tissue density and foci of calcification adjacent to the left pulmonary artery with associated encasement of the artery. CT image at the level of the left upper lobe bronchus (**B**) shows soft tissue density with poorly defined margins and foci of calcification in the left hilum. Also note parenchymal consolidation. The patient was a 60-year-old woman with surgically proven fibrosing mediastinitis secondary to tuberculosis.

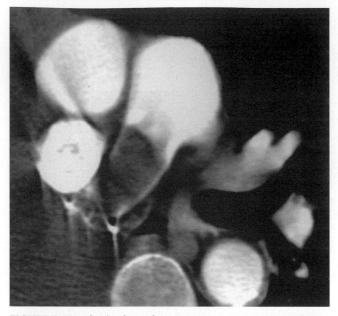

FIGURE 6-12. Clot in the pulmonary artery stump. CT angiography demonstrates large filling defect in the right pulmonary artery stump. The patient was a 79-year-old woman who had recurrent episodes of dyspnea following right pneumonectomy and had proven pulmonary embolism in the remaining left lung. (Case courtesy of Dr. Steve Kwong, Department of Radiology, Kelowna General Hospital, Kelowna, British Columbia, Canada.)

Anastomotic pulmonary vascular stenoses are an uncommon complication following lung transplantation (67,68). The diagnosis can be readily made using CTA. Pulmonary venous obstruction may occur secondary to reimplantation of pulmonary veins in the left atrium, as a consequence of traumatic injury at surgery, secondary to thrombosis, or in association with lobar torsion (69,70). Traumatic injury to the superior pulmonary vein is particularly common during middle lobectomy or middle and lower lobectomy in association with ligation of the lowermost branch or branches of this vein (70). CTA in these patients shows normal postoperative pulmonary arterial anatomy and absence of a venous phase.

Lobar torsion is a rare condition that occurs most commonly after lobectomy. Occasional cases have also been described following wedge resection, lung transplantation, severance of pleural adhesions, and pleurectomy (66,71,72). Early recognition of lobar torsion is important because a complete 180-degree torsion results in vascular obstruction and hemorrhagic pulmonary infarction (73). The radiographic findings include obstructive pneumonitis and atelectasis, abnormal position of the hilum in relation to the atelectatic lobe, abnormal position and orientation of the interlobar fissures, bronchi, and pulmonary vessels (66). The characteristic findings on CT consist of abnormal position and orientation of the interlobar fissures, twisting and narrowing or occlusion of the bronchus, and abnormal orientation and delayed opacification of the pulmonary vessels (66,72,74).

COMPLICATIONS OF DIAGNOSTIC AND MONITORING PROCEDURES

Several pulmonary vascular complications can occur in association with indwelling intravenous catheters, placement of balloon-tipped pulmonary arterial catheters, and during pulmonary angiography (66).

Indwelling Intravenous Catheters

The most important pulmonary vascular complications associated with indwelling intravenous catheters are pulmonary thromboembolism, septic embolism, and embolization of catheter fragments to the lungs (66,75,76).

Flow-Directed Balloon-Tipped Catheters

Pulmonary vascular complications secondary to flow-directed balloon-tipped (Swan-Ganz) catheters include pulmonary ischemia and infarction, perforation of the pulmonary artery, pseudoaneurysm formation, thrombus formation, and distal embolization (Box 6-6) (75,77,78). Pulmonary ischemia and infarction may be caused by occlusion of the pulmonary artery when the balloon is not deflated properly because of catheter malfunction or because the catheter is left too far out in a peripheral pulmonary artery (79,80). Pulmonary thromboembolism is relatively common, being demonstrated in 16 of 391 patients (4%) in one series (81). The main role of CTA is in the diagnosis of pulmonary embolism and of pulmonary artery pseudoaneurysm formation.

The most serious complication of Swan-Ganz catheters is pulmonary artery perforation, which occurs in approximately 3 cases for every 10,000 catheterizations and is often fatal (78). Perforation results in pulmonary hemorrhage, which is manifested radiographically as a focal area of consolidation. In patients who survive, the consolidation is gradually replaced over a period of 1 to 3 weeks by a nodular opacity or mass lesion ranging from 2 to 8 cm in diameter (82,83). However, the radiograph may be normal or show nonspecific findings (83). The diagnosis of pulmonary pseudoaneurysm can be readily be made on CTA. The characteristic findings on CT consist of a focal dilation of the pulmonary artery or an enhancing mass sometimes containing a partially thrombosed lumen (83,84). The adja-

BOX 6-6. COMPLICATIONS OF FLOW-DIRECTED, BALLOON-TIPPED CATHETERS

- Pulmonary artery occlusion
- Perforation of pulmonary artery
- Pseudoaneurysm formation
- Thromboembolism
- Pulmonary ischemia and infarction

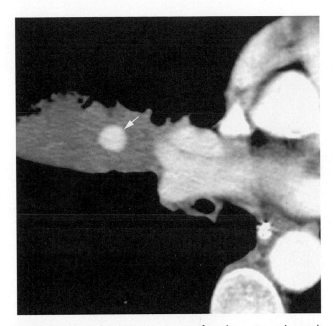

FIGURE 6-13. Pulmonary artery perforation at angiography. Contrast-enhanced CT shows increased diameter of the right middle lobe artery (*arrow*) and surrounding consolidation. The patient was a 56-year-old woman who developed a pseudoaneurysm of the middle lobe artery and severe pulmonary hemorrhage following pulmonary angiography. (Case courtesy of Dr. Cathy Staples, Department of Radiology, Kelowna General Hospital, Kelowna, British Columbia, Canada.)

cent lung parenchyma may show a halo of ground-glass attenuation surrounding the pseudoaneurysm (85).

Pulmonary Angiography

Pulmonary vascular complications of angiography are uncommon. They include pulmonary embolism from pelvic vein and inferior vena cava thrombus dislodgement during catheter placement, pulmonary artery dissection, perforation, contrast extravasation, and acute pulmonary arterial hypertension (86,87). In one series of 150 patients who had pulmonary angiography, three (2%) had vascular complications; one had pulmonary artery dissection, and two patients had contrast extravasation (86). All three patients had an uneventful recovery. Occasionally, however, pulmonary artery perforation may lead to severe hemorrhage and hypotension (Figure 6-13).

TRAUMATIC PULMONARY VASCULAR INJURIES

The majority of traumatic vascular injuries are iatrogenic. Pulmonary vascular injuries are relatively common during pulmonary and cardiac surgery and, as discussed in the previous section, as a complication of flow-directed balloon-tipped (Swan-Ganz) catheters. Pulmonary artery pseudo-

aneurysm secondary to blunt trauma is rare (28,88). Pseudoaneurysm formation and arteriovenous fistulas are more common following penetrating injuries (28,89).

Diagnosis of traumatic pulmonary pseudoaneurysms is important because they may result in fatal hemorrhage (90). The findings on chest radiography are nonspecific and consist of focal area of consolidation, ill-defined opacity, or lung nodule (90,91). The diagnosis can be readily made on CTA. CT demonstrates focal aneurysmal dilation of the pulmonary artery lumen (91).

MISCELLANEOUS PULMONARY VASCULAR ABNORMALITIES

Pulmonary Venoocclusive Disease

Pulmonary venoocclusive disease is a condition characterized by gradual fibrous obliteration of small pulmonary veins and venules leading to pulmonary arterial hypertension and pulmonary edema. It can occur at any age but is most common in children and young adults. The majority of cases are idiopathic (Box 6-7). Occasionally, it can occur following viral infection, use of contraceptives, inhaled toxins, or cytotoxic chemotherapy for malignant neoplasms or for bone marrow transplantation (92–94).

The patients present with progressive dyspnea, orthopnea, hemoptysis, and physical findings of cor pulmonale. The characteristic radiographic manifestations consist of a combination of findings of pulmonary arterial hypertension and interstitial pulmonary edema with septal (Kerley) lines. Because the edema is due to obstruction at the level of the pulmonary veins, the left atrium is not enlarged and there is no evidence of blood flow redistribution to the upper lobes. High-resolution CT demonstrates extensive thickening of the interlobular septa and ground-glass opacities due to interstitial edema (Figure 6-14) (95,96). The findings after transplantation have been reported in one patient who underwent unilateral lung transplantation because of severe hypoxemia and overt right ventricular failure (97). High-resolution CT prior to transplant demonstrated septal lines, ground-glass opacities, areas of consolidation, and small bilateral pleural effusions. After transplantation, all clinical signs of right-ventricular failure resolved within a few days. High-resolution CT 84 days after transplant showed almost complete resolution of the abnormalities in the native right lung and a normal transplanted left lung (97). The findings

BOX 6-7. PULMONARY VENOOCCLUSIVE DISEASE

- Usually idiopathic
- Signs of hydrostatic pulmonary edema
- Prominent septal lines
- Normal wedge pressure
- Signs of pulmonary arterial hypertension

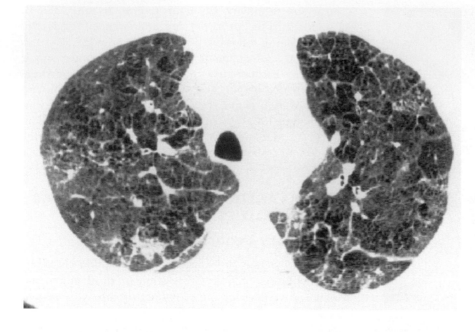

FIGURE 6-14. Pulmonary venoocclusive disease. High-resolution CT scan shows thickening of the interlobular septa and interlobar fissures consistent with interstitial pulmonary edema. Also noted is evidence of emphysema. The patient was a 51-year-old woman who presented with pulmonary arterial hypertension that was proven on surgical biopsy to be secondary to pulmonary venoocclusive disease.

on CTA have not been described. Definitive diagnosis requires surgical lung biopsy.

Pulmonary Capillary Hemangiomatosis

Pulmonary capillary hemangiomatosis is a locally aggressive benign neoplasm characterized by the proliferation of capillary-sized blood vessels through the pulmonary interstitium (98). It is a rare cause of pulmonary arterial hypertension and hemoptysis that occurs mainly in children and young adults. Pulmonary arterial hypertension results from progressive vascular obliteration due to *in situ* thrombosis and infarction, secondary venoocclusive disease, and recurrent pulmonary hemorrhage (98). Similar to primary venoocclusive disease, the pulmonary arterial hypertension in capillary hemangiomatosis is associated with a normal pulmonary wedge pressure (Box 6-8).

The clinical manifestations include slowly progressive dyspnea, recurrent hemoptysis, and signs of cor pulmonale (98). The chest radiograph demonstrates signs of pulmonary arterial hypertension and a diffuse reticulonodular pattern. The high-resolution CT findings resemble those of venoocclusive

disease and include thickening of the interlobular septa, focal ground-glass opacities, and small pleural effusions (96,98). Other high-resolution CT findings include poorly defined centrilobular nodular opacities and mediastinal lymphadenopathy (96). Contrast-enhanced CT in one patient demonstrated a focal thrombus in the left pulmonary artery and thrombosis and occlusion of the right interlobar artery (98). Definitive diagnosis requires surgical lung biopsy.

REFERENCES

1. Behçet H. Über rezidivierende, aphtöse, durch ein virus verursachte geschwüre am mund, am auge und an den genitalien. *Dermatologische Wochenschrift* 1937;105:1152–1157.
2. Erkan F, Çavdar T. Pulmonary vasculitis in Behçet's disease. *Am Rev Respir Dis* 1992;146:232–239.
3. Sullivan EJ, Hoffman GS. Pulmonary vasculitis. *Clin Chest Med* 1998;19:759–776.
4. Tunaci A, Berkmen YM, Gökmen E. Thoracic involvement in Behçet's disease: pathologic, clinical, and imaging features. *AJR* 1995;164:51–56.
5. Raz I, Okon E, Chajek-Shaul T. Pulmonary manifestations in Behçet's syndrome. *Chest* 1989;95:585–589.
6. Ahn JM, Im J-G, Ryoo JW, et al. Thoracic manifestations of Behçet syndrome: radiographic and CT findings in nine patients. *Radiology* 1995;194:199–203.
7. Numan F, Islak C, Berkmen T, et al. Behçet disease: pulmonary arterial involvement in 15 cases. *Radiology* 1994;192:465.
8. Teplick JG, Haskin ME, Nedwich A. The Hughes-Stovin syndrome. *Radiology* 1974;113:607–608.
9. Frater RWM, Beck W, Schrire V. The syndrome of pulmonary artery aneurysms, pulmonary artery thrombi, and peripheral venous thrombi. *J Thorac Cardiovasc Surg* 1975;49:330–338.
10. Durieux P, Bletry O, Huchon G, et al. Multiple pulmonary arterial aneurysms in Behçet's disease and Hughes-Stovin syndrome. *Am J Med* 1981;71:736–741.
11. Liu Y-Q, Jin B-L, Ling J. Pulmonary artery involvement in aor-

BOX 6-8. PULMONARY CAPILLARY HEMANGIOMATOSIS

- Benign neoplasm
- Proliferation of capillary-sized blood vessels
- Pulmonary arterial hypertension
- Hemoptysis
- Septal lines
- Normal wedge pressure
- Mimics venoocclusive disease

toarteritis: an angiographic study. *Cardiovasc Intervent Radiol* 1994;17:2–6.

12. Takahashi K, Honda M, Furuse M, et al. CT findings of pulmonary parenchyma in Takayasu arteritis. *J Comput Assist Tomogr* 1996;20:742–748.

13. Sharma S, Rajani M, Talwar KK. Angiographic morphology in nonspecific aortoarteritis (Takayasu's arteritis): a study of 126 patients from North India. *Cardiovasc Intervent Radiol* 1992;15:160–165.

14. Sekiguchi M, Suzuki J. An overview on Takayasu arteritis. *Heart Vessels Suppl* 1992;7:6–10.

15. Michet CJ. Epidemiology of vasculitis. *Rheum Dis Clin North Am* 1990;16:261–268.

16. Yamada I, Nakagawa T, Himeno Y, et al. Takayasu arteritis: evaluation of the thoracic aorta with CT angiography. *Radiology* 1998;209:103–109.

17. Matsunaga N, Hayashi K, Sakamoto I, et al. Takayasu arteritis: protean radiologic manifestations and diagnosis. *Radiographics* 1997;17:579–594.

18. Lie JT. Isolated pulmonary Takayasu arteritis: clinicopathologic characteristics. *Mod Pathol* 1996;9:469–474.

19. Hara M, Sobue R, Ohba S, et al. Diffuse pulmonary lesions in early phase Takayasu arteritis predominantly involving pulmonary artery. *J Comput Assist Tomogr* 1998;22:801–803.

20. Kerr KM, Anger WR, Fedrillo PF, et al. Large vessel pulmonary arteritis mimicking chronic thromboembolic disease. *Am J Respir Care Med* 1995;152:367–378.

21. Nasu T. Takayasu's truncoarteritis in Japan. A statistical observation of 76 autopsy cases. *Pathol Microbiol* 1975;43:140–146.

22. Kerr GS, Hallahan CW, Giordano J, et al. Takayasu arteritis. *Ann Intern Med* 1994;120:919–929.

23. Matsubara O, Yoshimura N, Tamura A, et al. Pathological features of the pulmonary artery in Takayasu arteritis. *Heart Vessels Suppl* 1992;7:18–25.

24. Paul J-F, Hernigou A, Lefebvre C, et al. Electron beam CT features of the pulmonary artery in Takayasu's arteritis. *AJR* 1999;173:89–93.

25. Park JH, Chung JW, Im J-G, et al. Takayasu arteritis: evaluation of mural changes in the aorta and pulmonary artery with CT angiography. *Radiology* 1995;196:89–93.

26. Loevner LA, Andrews JC, Francis IR. Multiple mycotic pulmonary artery aneurysms: a complication of invasive mucormycosis. *AJR* 1992;158:761–762.

27. Navarro C, Dickinson T, Kondlapoodi P, et al. Mycotic aneurysms of the pulmonary arteries in intravenous drug addicts: report of three cases and review of the literature. *Am J Med* 1984;76:1124–1131.

28. Bartter T, Irwin RS, Nash G. Aneurysms of the pulmonary arteries. *Chest* 1988;94:1065–1075.

29. McAdams HP, Rosado-de-Christenson ML, Templeton PA, et al. Thoracic mycoses from opportunistic fungi: radiologic–pathologic correlation. *Radiographics* 1995;15:271–286.

30. Kuhlman JE, Fishman EK, Burch PA, et al. CT of invasive pulmonary aspergillosis. *AJR* 1988;150:1015–1020.

31. Worthy SA, Flint JD, Müller NL. Pulmonary complications after bone marrow transplantation: high-resolution CT and pathologic findings. *Radiographics* 1997;17:1359–1371.

32. Hruban RH, Meziane MA, Zerhouni EA, et al. Radiologic–pathologic correlation of the CT halo sign in invasive pulmonary aspergillosis. *J Comput Assist Tomogr* 1987;11:534–536.

33. Brown MJ, Miller RR, Müller NL. Acute lung disease in the immunocompromised host: CT and pathologic examination findings. *Radiology* 1994;190:247–254.

34. Hayashi H, Takagi R, Onda M, et al. Invasive pulmonary aspergillosis occluding the descending aorta and left pulmonary artery: CT features. *J Comput Assist Tomogr* 1994;18:492–494.

35. Cox JE, Chiles C, Aquino SL, et al. Pulmonary artery sarcomas: a review of clinical and radiologic features. *J Comput Assist Tomogr* 1997;21:750–755.

36. Gyhra AS, Santander CK, Alarcón EC, et al. Leiomyosarcoma of the pulmonary veins with extension to the left atrium. *Ann Thorac Surg* 1996;61:1840–1841.

37. Moffat RE, Chang CH, Slaven JE. Roentgen considerations in primary pulmonary artery sarcoma. *Radiology* 1972;104:283–288.

38. Delany SG, Doyle TCA, Bunton RW, et al. Pulmonary artery sarcoma mimicking pulmonary embolism. *Chest* 1993;103:1631–1633.

39. Anderson MB, Kriett JM, Kapelanski DP, et al. Primary pulmonary artery sarcoma: a report of six cases. *Ann Thorac Surg* 1995;59:1487–1490.

40. Britton PD. Primary pulmonary artery sarcoma: a report of two cases with special emphasis on the diagnostic problems. *Clin Radiol* 1990;41:92–94.

41. Lamers RJS, Hochstenbag MMH, van Belle AF, et al. Unilateral hilar mass. *Chest* 1995;108:1444–1446.

42. Kauczor H-U, Schwickert HC, Mayer E, et al. Pulmonary artery sarcoma. *Cardiovasc Intervent Radiol* 1994;17:185–189.

43. Smith WS, Lesar MS, Travis WD, et al. MR and CT findings in pulmonary artery sarcoma. *J Comput Assist Tomogr* 1989;13:906–909.

44. Bressler EL, Nelson JM. Primary pulmonary artery sarcoma: diagnosis with CT, MR imaging, and transthoracic needle biopsy. *AJR* 1992;159:702–704.

45. Winterbauer RH, Elfenbein IB, Ball WC Jr. Incidence and clinical significance of tumor embolization to the lungs. *Am J Med* 1968;45:271–290.

46. Ralston DR, St. John RC. Progressive shortness of breath in a 50-year-old man with ulcerative colitis. *Chest* 1996;110:1608–1610.

47. Shepard JO, Moore EH, Templeton PA, et al. Pulmonary intravascular tumor emboli: dilated and beaded peripheral pulmonary arteries at CT. *Radiology* 1993;187:797–801.

48. Kane RD, Hawkins KH, Miller JA, et al. Microscopic pulmonary tumor emboli associated with dyspnea. *Cancer* 1975;36:1473–1482.

49. Nelson E, Klein JS. Pulmonary infarction resulting from metastatic osteogenic sarcoma with pulmonary venous tumor thrombus. *AJR* 2000;174:531–533.

50. Gay SB, Armstrong P, Black WC, et al. Chest CT of unresectable lung cancer. *Radiographics* 1988;4:735–748.

51. Primack SL, Lee KS, Logan PM, et al. Bronchogenic carcinoma: utility of CT in the evaluation of patients with suspected lesions. *Radiology* 1994;193:795–800.

52. Read RC, Ziomek S, Ranval TJ, et al. Pulmonary artery sleeve resection for abutting left upper lobe lesions. *Ann Thorac Surg* 1993;55:850–854.

53. Maggi C, Casadio C, Pischedda F, et al. Bronchoplastic and angioplastic techniques in the treatment of bronchogenic carcinoma. *Ann Thorac Surg* 1993;55:1501–1507.

54. Herman SJ, Winton TL, Weisbrod GL, et al. Mediastinal invasion by bronchogenic carcinoma: CT signs. *Radiology* 1994;190:841–846.

55. Takahashi M, Shimoyama K, Murata K, et al. Hilar and mediastinal invasion of bronchogenic carcinoma: evaluation by thin-section electron-beam computed tomography. *J Thorac Imag* 1997;12:195–199.

56. Glazer HS, Kaiser LR, Anderson DJ, et al. Indeterminate mediastinal invasion in bronchogenic carcinoma: CT evaluation. *Radiology* 1989;173:37–42.

57. Spencer DD, Garza JL, Walker WA. Multiple tumor emboli after pneumonectomy. *Ann Thorac Surg* 1993;55:169–171.

58. Choe DH, Lee JH, Lee BH, et al. Obliteration of the pulmonary

vein in lung cancer: significance in assessing local extent with CT. *J Comput Assist Tomogr* 1998;22:587–591.

59. Lloyd JE, Tillman BF, Atkinson JB, et al. Mediastinal fibrosis complicating histoplasmosis. *Medicine (Baltimore)* 1988;67:295–310.

60. Sherrick AD, Brown LR, Harms GF, et al. The radiographic findings of fibrosing mediastinitis. *Chest* 1994;106:484–489.

61. Mole TM, Glover J, Sheppard MN. Sclerosing mediastinitis: a report of 18 cases. *Thorax* 1995;50:280–283.

62. Schowengerdt CG, Suyemoto R, Main FB. Granulomatous and fibrous mediastinitis: a review and analysis of 180 cases. *J Thorac Cardiovasc Surg* 1969;57:365–379.

63. Mallin WH, Silberstein EB, Shipley RT, et al. Fibrosing mediastinitis causing nonvisualization of one lung on pulmonary scintigraphy. *Clin Nucl Med* 1993;18:594–596.

64. Espinosa RE, Edwards WD, Rosenow EC, et al. Idiopathic pulmonary hilar fibrosis: an unusual cause of pulmonary hypertension. *Mayo Clin Proc* 1993;68:778–782.

65. Takahashi T, Yokio K, Mori K, et al. Clot in the pulmonary artery after pneumonectomy. *AJR* 1993;161:1110.

66. Fraser RS, Müller NL, Colman N, et al. Complications of therapeutic, biopsy, and monitoring procedures. In: RS Fraser, NL Müller, N Colman et al., eds. *Diagnosis of diseases of the chest.* Philadelphia: WB Saunders, 1999:2659–2695.

67. Gaubert J-Y, Moulin G, Thomas P, et al. Anastomotic stenosis of the left pulmonary artery after lung transplantation: treatment by percutaneous placement of an endoprosthesis. *AJR* 1993;161:947–949.

68. Murray JG, McAdams HP, Erasmus JJ, et al. Complications of lung transplantation: radiologic findings. *AJR* 1996;166:1405–1411.

69. Van Son JAM, Danielson GK, Puga FJ, et al. Repair of congenital and acquired pulmonary vein stenosis. *Ann Thorac Surg* 1995;60:144–150.

70. Hovaguimian H, Morris JF, Gately HL, et al. Pulmonary vein thrombosis following bilobectomy. *Chest* 1991;99:1515–1516.

71. Moser ES, Proto AV. Lung torsion: case report and literature review. *Radiology* 1987;162:639–643.

72. Collins J, Kuhlman JE, Love RB. Acute, life-threatening complications of lung transplantation. *Radiographics* 1998;18:21–43.

73. Kelly MV, Kyger ER, Miller WC. Postoperative lobar torsion and gangrene. *Thorax* 1977;32:501–504.

74. Munk PL, Vellet AD, Zwirewich C. Torsion of the upper lobe of the lung after surgery: findings on pulmonary angiography. *AJR* 1991;157:471–472.

75. Trigaux JP, Goncette L, Van Beers B, et al. Radiologic findings of normal and compromised venous catheters. *J Thorac Imag* 1994;9:246–254.

76. Fisher KL, Leung AN. Radiographic appearance of central venous catheters. *AJR* 1996;166:329–337.

77. Sise MJ, Hollingsworth P, Brimm JE, et al. Complications of the flow-directed pulmonary artery catheter. *Crit Care Med* 1981;9:315–318.

78. Kearney TJ, Shabot MM. Pulmonary artery rupture associated with the Swan-Ganz catheter. *Chest* 1995;108:1349–1352.

79. Foote GA, Schabel SI, Hodges M. Pulmonary complications by the flow-directed balloon-tipped catheter. *N Engl J Med* 1974;290:927–931.

80. Ovenfors C-O. Iatrogenic trauma to the thorax. *J Thorac Imag* 1987;2:18–31.

81. Katz JD, Cronau LH, Barash PG, et al. Pulmonary artery flow-guided catheters in the perioperative period: indications and complications. *JAMA* 1977;237:2832–2834.

82. Dieden JD, Friloux LA III, Renner JW. Pulmonary artery false aneurysms secondary to Swan-Ganz pulmonary artery catheters. *AJR* 1987;149:901–906.

83. Feretti GR, Thony F, Link KM, et al. False aneurysm of the pulmonary artery induced by a Swan-Ganz catheter: clinical presentation and radiologic management. *AJR* 1996;167:941–945.

84. Davis SD, Neithamer CD, Schreiber TS, et al. False pulmonary artery aneurysm induced by Swan-Ganz catheter: diagnosis and embolotherapy. *Radiology* 1987;164:741–742.

85. Guttentag AR, Shepard J-AO, McLoud TC. Catheter-induced pulmonary artery pseudoaneurysm: the halo sign on CT. *AJR* 1992;158:637–639.

86. van Beek EJR, Reekers JA, Batchelor DA, et al. Feasibility, safety and clinical utility of angiography in patients with suspected pulmonary embolism. *Eur Radiol* 1996;6:415–419.

87. Smith TP. Pulmonary angiography—safety and complications. In: Oudkerk M, van Beek EJR, ten Cate JW, eds. *Pulmonary embolism: epidemiology, diagnosis, and treatment.* Oxford: Blackwell Science, 1999;160–174.

88. Dillon WP, Taylor AT, Mineau DE, et al. Traumatic pulmonary artery pseudoaneurysm simulating pulmonary embolism. *AJR* 1982;139:818–819.

89. Symbas PN, Goldman M, Erbesfeld MH, et al. Pulmonary arteriovenous fistula, pulmonary artery aneurysm, and other vascular changes of the lung from penetrating trauma. *Ann Surg* 1980;191:336–340.

90. Gavant ML, Winer-Muram HT. Traumatic pulmonary artery pseudoaneurysm. *Can Assoc Radiol J* 1986;37:108–109.

91. Crivello MS, Hayes C, Thurer RL, et al. Traumatic pulmonary artery aneurysm: CT evaluation. *J Comput Assist Tomogr* 1986;10:503–505.

92. Lombardd CM, Churg A, Winokur S. Pulmonary veno-occlusive disease following therapy for malignant neoplasms. *Chest* 1987;92:871–876.

93. Troussard X, Bernaudin JF, Cordonnier C, et al. Pulmonary veno-occlusive disease after bone marrow transplantation. *Thorax* 1984;39:956–957.

94. Wagenvoort CA, Wagenvoort N, Takahashi T. Pulmonary veno-occlusive disease: involvement of pulmonary arteries and review of the literature. *Hum Pathol* 1985;16:1033–1041.

95. Swensen SJ, Tashjian JH, Myers JL, et al. Pulmonary venoocclusive disease: CT findings in eight patients. *AJR* 1996;167:937–940.

96. Dufour B, Maître S, Humbert M, et al. High-resolution CT of the chest in four patients with pulmonary capillary hemangiomatosis or pulmonary venoocclusive disease. *AJR* 1998;171:1321–1324.

97. Cassart M, Gevenois PA, Kramer M, et al. Pulmonary venoocclusive disease: CT findings before and after single-lung transplantation. *AJR* 1993;160:759–760.

98. Eltorky M, Headley AS, Winer-Muram HT, et al. Pulmonary capillary hemangiomatosis: a clinicopathologic review. *Ann Thorac Surg* 1994;57:772–776.

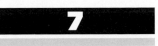

VASCULAR ANOMALIES OF THE LUNG

PULMONARY ARTERIOVENOUS MALFORMATIONS
Detection of Pulmonary Arteriovenous Malformations
Pretherapeutic Evaluation of Pulmonary Arteriovenous
  Malformations
Follow-up

PARTIAL ANOMALOUS PULMONARY VENOUS DRAINAGE
Scimitar Syndrome
Partial Anomalous Pulmonary Venous Return to
  the Superior Vena Cava
Partial Anomalous Pulmonary Venous Drainage of
  the Left Lung

PULMONARY SEQUESTRATION
Intralobar Sequestration
Extralobar Sequestration

Purely Vascular Sequestration
Atypical Pulmonary Sequestrations
  Ectopic sequestration
  Ectopic origin of the arterial blood supply
  Communicating bronchopulmonary foregut
   malformations
  Bilateral sequestrations

MISCELLANEOUS ANOMALIES
Anomalies of the Pulmonary Arteries
  Idiopathic dilation of pulmonary artery trunk
  Pulmonary artery sling
  Congenital pulmonary artery stenosis
  Proximal interruption (absence) of the pulmonary artery
Anomalies of the Pulmonary Veins
  Pulmonary varix
  Pulmonary vein stenosis and atresia

PULMONARY ARTERIOVENOUS MALFORMATIONS

Pulmonary arteriovenous malformations (PAVMs) are abnormal connections between pulmonary arteries and pulmonary veins. These are most commonly congenital (1,2), but also may represent acquired lesions. PAVMs are one of many causes of right-to-left shunt (Box 7-1). Spiral CT examinations are useful in the detection, characterization, and follow-up of PAVMs. The CT examination performed depends on the diagnostic question. Low-dose noncontrast spiral CT is used to screen patients suspected of harboring a PAVM. Once a suspicious lesion is identified, standard dose thin-section noncontrast spiral CT is used to precisely determine the angioarchitecture. This characterization CT scan utilizes thin-section transverse and surface-shaded display images. These allow the angioarchitecture of the PAVM to be noninvasively determined, including feeding arteries, draining veins, and the size of the aneurysm. These features determine the choice between surgical excision or interven-

tional radiologic embolotherapy. Finally, contrast-enhanced CT angiography is used to follow-up treated PAVMs to ensure that the aneurysm sac has been thrombosed.

Detection of Pulmonary Arteriovenous Malformations

Congenital Pulmonary Arteriovenous Malformations

Screening noncontrast spiral CT studies are indicated in several groups of patients who are suspected, or at high risk, of harboring PAVMs. Patients with extrathoracic manifestations of hereditary hemorrhagic telangiectasia (HHT, Rendu-Osler-Weber's syndrome) and their relatives require screening. Extrathoracic manifestations include cutaneous or neurologic arteriovenous malformations (AVMs). The screening of asymptomatic relatives is indicated as the condition is transmitted in an autosomal-dominant pattern. Patients with chest radiographs showing a prominent feeding pulmonary artery and draining

BOX 7-1. CAUSES OF RIGHT-TO-LEFT SHUNT

■ Cardiac:
  Congenital heart disease
  Pulmonary hypertension associated with a patent foramen
    ovale
  Diversion of blood flow from the inferior vena cava to the
    left atrium through a patent foramen ovale in the
    absence of pulmonary hypertension
■ Juxtacardiac:
  Left persistent superior vena cava or right superior vena
    cava draining to the left atrium
  Abnormal connection of the coronary sinus into the left
    atrium
  Levoatriocardinal vein
  Direct communication between the right pulmonary artery
    and left atrium (congenital or postsurgical)
■ Vascular:
  Pulmonary arteriovenous fistula (congenital and acquired)
  Portopulmonary venous derivations (spontaneous or
    postsurgical)
  Transpleural systemic: pulmonary venous collaterals
    (superior vena cava obstruction)
■ Parenchymal:
  Pneumonia: lung atelectasis without hypoxic vasoconstriction
  Bronchioloalveolar carcinoma
  Chronic tracheal or bronchial obstruction

vein require CT screening to exclude PAVM. Investigation of these asymptomatic patients is indicated due to the risk of stroke or cerebral abscess arising from the right-to-left shunt in an unrecognized PAVM. Finally, patients with conditions which may be related to PAVM complications (Box 7-2) should also be screened.

Since the potential screening population is large and the pulmonary vascular abnormalities are outlined by air, low-dose noncontrast spiral CT (see Appendix 7) can be used in addition to other noninvasive screening examinations (Fig-

BOX 7-2. COMPLICATIONS OF PULMONARY ARTERIOVENOUS MALFORMATIONS

■ Related to right-to-left shunting
  Hypoxemia/orthodeoxia
  Polycythemia
  Pulmonary hypertension
  Congestive heart failure
■ Related to rupture of the aneurysmal sac
  Hemothorax
  Life-threatening hemoptysis
  Anemia
■ Paradoxic cruoric or septic embolism
  Seizure
  Migraine headache
  Transient ischemic attack
  Cerebrovascular accident
  Brain abcess
  Infectious endocarditis

From Gossage JR, Kanj G. Pulmonary arteriovenous malformations. *Am J Respir Crit Care Med* 1998;158:643–661, with permission.

ure 7-1). The other screening studies include measurement of arterial blood gases (3), contrast echocardiography, and radioisotope measurement of a right-to-left shunt (4). Single-slice noncontrast spiral CT has been shown to have high sensitivity in detecting PAVMs (5,6). It is anticipated that the sensitivity will further increase using multislice spiral CT which can rapidly survey the lungs using narrower (1 to 2.5 mm) section collimation.

On screening noncontrast spiral CT, PAVMs present as soft tissue nodules connected to vascular pedicles. The soft tissue nodules represent the aneurysm of the malformation. At least one feeding artery and one draining vein must be identified. Small PAVMs may require 1-mm thick sections in order to allow adequate assessment of the angioarchitecture. The 1-mm thick transverse CT sections are optimally viewed using sliding thin slab maximum intensity projections (STS-MIPs) (7) (Figure 7-2). This volume-rendering technique enhances the visualization of the microfistula which may be oriented perpendicular or obliquely to the transverse CT sections. Feeding arteries and draining veins can be identified on STS-MIP images on the basis of their course from the hilar region. An alternate noninvasive screening technique, contrast-enhanced pulmonary magnetic resonance angiography (MRA) has recently been proposed for PAVMs with feeding arteries greater than 3 mm. However, the sensitivity of MRA is low for malformations with feeding arteries smaller than 3 mm in diameter (8).

Acquired Congenital Pulmonary Arteriovenous Malformations

Acquired PAVMs are found in patients with chronic liver disease and surgically treated congenital heart disease. The common feature of these two patient groups is the absence of normal hepatic venous blood flow into the pulmonary circulation (9). These acquired PAVMs can regress following liver transplantation or the channeling of hepatic venous blood into the pulmonary vasculature at corrective cardiac surgery (10). Histologic examination of lung tissue in these patients has shown dilation of both respiratory bronchiolar and terminal bronchiolar arteries (9). The pathogenesis of acquired PAVMs is unknown. It has been speculated that the liver secretes a factor that inhibits the growth of arteriovenous fistulas in the lung. Therefore, the exclusion of normal hepatic blood flow to the lung allows the development of PAVMs.

Hepatopulmonary syndrome (HPS), seen in approximately 15% of patients with end-stage liver disease, is a triad of hepatic dysfunction, intrapulmonary vascular dilation, and hypoxemia. The diagnosis of HPS requires demonstration of intrapulmonary shunting through subpleural vascular plexuses. These arteriovenous fistulae measure up to 12 mm in size and have many tortuous feeding vessels 0.2 to 1 mm in diameter. Some of these fistulae can be detected using spiral CT, which shows dilated peripheral

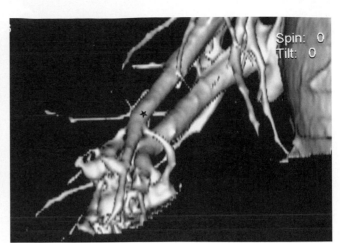

FIGURE 7-1. Low-dose noncontrast spiral CT evaluation of a right lower lobe pulmonary arteriovenous malformation in an asymptomatic young female (120 kVp; 20 mAs/slice; collimation: 4 × 1 mm). The feeding artery (**A** and **B**, *small star*) and draining vein (**B**, *large star*) are identified as enlarged vascular pedicles on these transverse CT scans, obtained 20 mm apart (reconstructed slice thickness: 5 mm). Determination of the optimal site for coil deposition, above the ramifications of the feeding artery (**C**, *star*) on the three-dimensional shaded-surface display of the malformation.

lung vessels that may extend to the pleura (11) in the lower lobes (12,13). Thick sections depict these vascular abnormalities better than thin-section (CT) scans (13). Volume-rendering using the maximum intensity projection algorithm on thick slabs can also demonstrate these fistulas. If the fistulas are not directly visualized, the diagnosis can be inferred by the detection of enlarged segmental pulmonary arteries in patients with HPS. Segmental artery enlargement can be quantified by comparing the ratio of segmental arterial diameter to bronchial diameter. This ratio is approximately one in nonhypoxic cirrhosis patients (1.2 ± 0.2) compared to two in patients with HPS (2.0 ± 0.2) (13). Alternately, the diagnosis can be inferred by demonstrating intrapulmonary arteriovenous shunting using microbubble enhanced echocardiography, technetium-99m (^{99m}Tc)-macroaggregated albumin (MAA) perfusion studies, right heart catheterization, or selective pulmonary arteriography (14).

PAVMs may develop in up to 25% of patients with congenital heart disease treated with the classic Glenn anastomosis, in which the superior vena cava is connected to the right pulmonary artery. The PAVMs develop in the right lung, which receives venous return only from the upper body with this shunt. The reported incidence of PAVMs is lower after other types of cavopulmonary anastomoses where there is the addition of hepatic blood flow to the lungs (e.g., Fontan or modified Fontan operation).

Other causes of acquired PAVMs are listed in Box 7-3 (15–17). Highly vascular neoplasms such as metastatic thyroid carcinoma, choriocarcinoma, and carcinoid tumors may be mistaken for PAVMs and represent potential pitfalls (18–20). Rarely, extensive hypervascular granuloma formation, which may occur with an intrapulmonary wooden foreign body, may simulate a pulmonary arteriovenous malformation (21).

Pretherapeutic Evaluation of Pulmonary Arteriovenous Malformations

Spiral CT has been shown to be useful in the pretherapeutic evaluation of the angioarchitecture of PAVMs. Accurate assessment of the number and orientation of the feeding arteries is critical to establish the approach and technical difficulty of an attempted embolization procedure. Eighty percent of PAVMs are simple, with a single feeding artery connected to the aneurysmal sac (22). The remaining 20% have

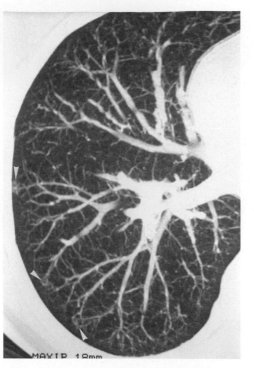

FIGURE 7-2. Sliding thin slab maximum intensity projection (STS-MIP) image obtained at the level of the right lower lobe (18-mm thick slab of lung parenchyma) showing numerous tiny pulmonary arteriovenous malformations (*arrowheads*).

a complex angioarchitecture with two or more feeding pulmonary artery branches. To fully characterize the angioarchitecture, a volumetric thin-section scan using a small field of view targeted to the lesion is required. Intravenous contrast material is not required in all cases, but it can exclude thrombosis within the malformation. It has been shown that recognition of tortuous feeding arteries and draining veins is facilitated using surface-shaded displays (5,23,24). In complex cases, two threshold values for the surface-shaded display may have to be used. The initial threshold value of −500 to −700 HU will outline the large vessels. Smaller arterial branches can then be searched for using a lower threshold value of −850 HU. The lower threshold value cannot be initially applied since the profusion of vessels identified may prevent identification of the aneurysmal sac.

It has been shown that the combined interpretation of three-dimensional, shaded-surface display images and transverse sections allows accurate evaluation of PAVM angioarchitecture in 95% of cases (23). Spiral CT assessment of the angioarchitecture can be superior to unilateral selective pulmonary angiography since the surface-shaded display allows an unlimited number of viewing angles. Additionally, selective pulmonary angiography can fail to opacify significant feeding arteries if the injection is performed too selectively. For these reasons, thin-section spiral CT with surface-shaded display is recommended prior to therapeutic pulmonary angiography for PAVM. In the future, volume rendering of thin-section spiral CT image sets may become the preferred technique (25). However, in a recent study comparing volume-rendered images and three-dimensional, surface-shaded displays of 52 PAVMs (unpublished data), we observed that volume-rendered images were less informative than shaded-surface displays due to inferior depth cues. This temporary limitation may be overcome through stereoscopic presentation of volume-rendered images.

Some patients with PAVMs have major arteriovenous malformations in the liver. Intrahepatic AVMs result in left-to-right shunts that worsen the intrapulmonary right-to-left shunt due to PAVMs. Embolization of hepatic AVMs results in considerable reduction in the diameter of the pulmonary malformations, which influences the technical conditions of PAVM embolotherapy. Because of these considerations, assessment of the liver is indicated in patients with PAVMs who have clinical findings suggestive of dominant liver involvement, including abdominal angina, portal hypertension, or high-output heart failure (26).

BOX 7-3. ACQUIRED PULMONARY ARTERIOVENOUS FISTULAE

- Chronic liver disease
- Pulmonary hypertension
- Atrio- and cavopulmonary anastomoses
- Rasmussen's aneurysm
- Uncommon:
    Metastatic (thyroid–choriocarcinoma) or primitive pulmonary tumors
    Schistosomiasis
    Chronic obstructive lung disease
    Mitral stenosis
    Penetrating trauma of the thorax
    Actinomycosis, coccidioidomycosis
    Fanconi's syndrome
    Mycotic aneurysms complicating right-sided valvular endocarditis

Follow-Up

PAVMs with feeding arteries greater than 3 mm are usually treated by embolotherapy (27). The long-term follow-up results of transcatheter embolotherapy indicate substantial decrease in the size of the aneurysmal diameter in the majority of PAVMs (5,28). Failure of reduction in the diameter of the aneurysmal sac has been reported in less than 10% of cases. This finding suggests persistent pulmonary perfusion, either because of recanalization of the originally occluded arterial pedicle(s), or because of the presence of an accessory feeding artery, undetected at the time of the initial evaluation. Rarely, the malformation has a systemic arterial supply that may arise from abnormal pleural vessels following pleural effusion or previous surgery. A systemic supply should be suspected when, after embolotherapy, the occluded feeding artery is no longer detectable but there is persistence of a large draining vein and no retraction of the aneurysmal sac (23).

Postembolotherapy follow-up of PAVMs can be easily made using unenhanced spiral CT examinations of the thorax (Figure 7-3). These noncontrast scans allow assessment of persistent PAVMs and recognition of the rare situation of a calcified thrombus of the aneurysmal sac, which could resemble persistent flow through of the aneurysm on spiral CT angiograms (28). However, the absence of resolution on unenhanced CT scans after successful embolotherapy requires confirmation of persistent aneurysmal perfusion with contrast-enhanced CT angiography (CTA) before definitive occlusion in a second embolotherapy session. This examination must include the analysis of the malformation during both pulmonic and systemic arterial phases.

When performed early after uneventful embolotherapy, CT enables the recognition of asymptomatic abnormalities within the lung parenchyma, such as transient ground-glass attenuation in the area of vascular occlusion, infiltrates, or pleural-based nodules. These changes usually spontaneously regress in the year following embolotherapy (5). Uncommonly, parenchymal infarction may occur and be associated with pleuritic chest pain in the days or weeks following uneventful and successful PAVM occlusion (5). In these cases CT may show a peripheral cavitating nodule.

CT follow-up of untreated PAVMs was reported over a mean follow-up period of 4 years (5). In 62 cases, characterization CT showed the PAVMs to be less than 3 mm in diameter. Embolotherapy is not indicated for these small PAVMs because it is impossible to occlude the feeding artery without loss of adjacent normal pulmonary artery branches. No significant change in the diameter of the aneurysms was detected, but precise follow-up of micronodules could not be confidently obtained because of limitations of the single-slice CT technique used in the study. In a study based on arterial blood gases measurement yearly after embolotherapy, White and colleagues reported persistent relief of hypoxemia after 5 years of follow-up (27). In the earlier patients who returned for occlusion of PAVMs not occluded on the first admission, these authors reported only minimal growth of the malformations. These studies suggest that the development of new PAVMs is low, but this hypothesis requires further confirmation with long-term follow-up which could help determine the optimal timing for follow-up with CT.

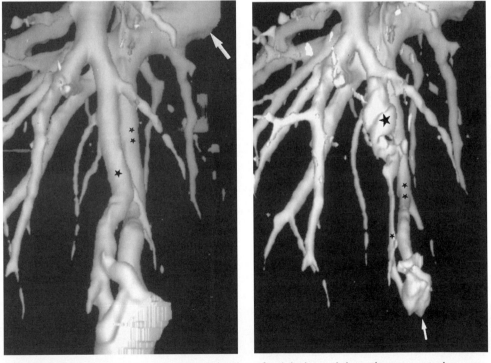

FIGURE 7-3. Pre- and posttherapeutic evaluation of a right lower lobe pulmonary arteriovenous malformation (PAVMs) using noncontrast spiral CT examination. Pretherapeutic three-dimensional shaded-surface display (SSD) of the malformation (**A**, posteroanterior view) shows one feeding artery (*single star*) and a single draining vein (*double stars*) joining the right inferior pulmonary vein (*arrow*), thus demonstrating a simple PAVM angioarchitecture. Postembolotherapy three-dimensional SSD of the malformation (**B**, posteroanterior view), obtained with similar acquisition and reconstruction parameters to those selected in **A**, demonstrates substantial decrease in size of the feeding artery (*single small star*), aneurysmal sac (*arrow*), and draining vein (*double small stars*). The large star (**B**) points to coils deposited within the feeding artery.

PARTIAL ANOMALOUS PULMONARY VENOUS DRAINAGE

Partial anomalous pulmonary venous drainage of one or more lobes occurs in 0.4% to 0.7% of individuals who have no other abnormalities (29). These congenital venous anomalies are easily identified by the abnormal course of the intraparenchymal pulmonary veins. In addition, these aberrant veins are usually larger in diameter than the adjacent normal pulmonary veins. Right-sided partial anomalous pulmonary venous connections occur twice as often as left-sided ones. Hemodynamically, partial anomalous pulmonary venous drainage of either lung results in a left-to-right shunt. Since these shunts only involve part of the venous blood flow to a lung, they are usually well tolerated and asymptomatic when seen as an isolated anomaly in an otherwise normal subject. In adults, a previously asymptomatic form of this malformation may become symptomatic following surgery to the opposite lung with normal pulmonary venous connections. The surgery unmasks the previously well-tolerated and clinically silent left-to-right shunt. In addition, these patients can develop asymmetric pulmonary edema with cardiac failure because the abnormal pulmonary vein drains into the right atrium and is protected from the effect of left atrial hypertension.

Embryologically, anomalous pulmonary veins connect to the nearest adjacent systemic vein (30). An anomalous right pulmonary vein can connect to the right superior vena cava, the azygos vein, the right atrium, the inferior vena cava, and a hepatic or portal vein. An anomalous vein from the left lung usually forms a left vertical vein which can connect to a persistent left superior vena cava, a hemiazygous vein or the coronary sinus. In clinical practice, three of these potential connections are commonly identified: scimitar vein, anomalous right superior pulmonary venous drainage to the superior vena cava, and anomalous left superior pulmonary venous drainage into a persistent left superior vena cava. Box 7-4 summarizes the regional consequences of partial anomalous pulmonary venous drainage to a systemic vein.

Scimitar Syndrome

The characteristic abnormality of scimitar syndrome (hypogenetic lung syndrome) is the abnormal vein draining a variable amount of the right lung to the inferior vena cava or, less commonly, the hepatic vein, or portal vein. Because the scimitar syndrome is usually associated with lobar agenesis, aplasia, or hypoplasia, it is also commonly known as the hypogenetic lung syndrome or the venolobar syndrome (31). The three main elements of this syndrome are the right-sided bronchopulmonary malformations, the partial anomalous pulmonary venous drainage (scimitar vein), and the systemic arterial supply to the right lung. This syndrome may also include variants and associated malformations (Box 7-5) (32). Females are affected more often than males and there are several reports of familial occurrences (31).

BOX 7-4. REGIONAL CONSEQUENCES OF PARTIAL ANOMALOUS PULMONARY VENOUS DRAINAGE TO A SYSTEMIC VEIN

- *Moderate enlargement of abnormally connected pulmonary veins.* This finding is related to lower pulmonary venous pressure in the area of left-to-right shunt.
- *Dilation of the systemic vein.* Detectability depends on the importance of the left-to-right shunt and the original diameter of this systemic vein. For example, partial anomalous pulmonary venous return of the right upper lobe into the azygos vein will dilate this vessel whereas the same malformation will not dramatically modify the diameter of the superior vena cava.
- *Area of partial anomalous pulmonary venous drainage:*
    is protected from the effect of left heart failure
    may show features of pulmonary edema in cases of right heart failure and superior vena cava obstruction
- *Degree of left-to-right shunting associated with partial anomalous pulmonary venous return* (96):
    ≤25% of cardiac output when seen as an isolated anomaly
    33% of cardiac output after lobectomy
    50% of cardiac output after controlateral pneumonectomy

Right Hemithoracic Malformations

Right upper lobe agenesis, aplasia, or hypoplasia represents the most constant component of the hypogenetic right lung. The right upper lobe bronchus is absent, replaced by a rudimentary bronchus that ends in a blind pouch or gives rise to a single segmental bronchus. The right upper lobe is small or absent, causing a shift of the heart and mediastinum to the right. Additional errors of segmentation and lobation are common. When one fissure is absent (usually the minor fissure), only two lobes are present and the bronchopulmonary pattern may mimic that of the left lung, also called levoisomerism. In this situation, the right bronchus is hyparterial and abnormally long, and a lingular bronchus distribution of bronchi is present. If both fissures are absent, the lung is unilobar. Even when three distinct lobes are present, the lung is still small, and there are no reported cases in which the bronchogram was completely normal (31).

The other right hemithoracic malformations are summarized in Box 7-6. Among them, special mention should be made of horseshoe lung, an associated malformation

---

BOX 7-5. MALFORMATIONS ASSOCIATED WITH A SCIMITAR SYNDROME

- Anomalies of the vena cava:
    Intraparenchymal course of the right superior vena cava (40)
    Persistent left superior vena
    Azygos continuation of an interrupted inferior vena cava
- Cardiac anomalies (97):
    Atrial septal defect
    Patent ductus arteriosus
    Tetralogy of Fallot
- Pulmonary arteriovenous malformations (98)
- Congenital pericardial defects
- Anomalies of the genitourinary tract and peripheral skeleton

BOX 7-6. RIGHT HEMITHORACIC MALFORMATIONS IN A SCIMITAR SYNDROME

- Hypogenetic right lung:
  Most frequent: right upper lobe agenesis, aplasia, or hypoplasia
  Various anomalies of lobation and segmentation
- Tracheobronchial abnormalities:
  Diverticula, bronchiectases
- Pulmonary artery abnormalities:
  Hypoplasia of the right pulmonary artery
  Absence of the right pulmonary artery
  Exclusion of the right pulmonary artery due to the development of sytemic collateral supply to the right lung and systemic-to-pulmonary artery retrograde shunting
- Pleural abnormalities:
  Accessory fissures, incomplete fissures, absence of pleural cavity
- Diaphragmatic abnormalities:
  Defects, cysts, partial duplication (also known as accessory hemidiaphragm)
- Pulmonary abnormalities:
  Horseshoe lung

more often described since the introduction of CT, and more commonly seen in pediatric than in adult forms of the scimitar syndrome (33). In horseshoe lung, the right and left lungs are fused posteriorly behind the cardiac apex by an isthmus of pulmonary parenchyma arising from the right lung base (32). The isthmus may be fused to the left lung without intervening pleura or with intervening pleura that resembles an accessory fissure. When this intervening pleura is present, the frontal chest radiograph shows a char-

acteristic linear or curvilinear fissure at the left lung base behind the heart. Because there is a single pleural cavity in horseshoe lung, also called "crossover lung segment," this malformation must be systematically searched for in the preoperative management of scimitar syndrome owing to the risk of postoperative bilateral pneumothorax.

Partial Anomalous Pulmonary Venous Return (Scimitar Vein)

The scimitar vein (Figure 7-4) drains a variable amount of the right lung to the inferior vena cava, and less often to the hepatic vein, or portal vein. This drainage constitutes a left-to-right shunt, which is usually small. However, it is important to note the presence of a second left-to-right shunt in many patients with scimitar syndrome because part of their right lung receives systemic arterial blood supply (discussed later in this Chapter). Rarely, stenosis of the anomalous pulmonary vein may be found at the level of its connection with the inferior vena cava.

Systemic Arterial Supply of the Lung

In scimitar syndrome, part or all of the hypogenetic lung may receive arterial blood supply from the thoracic or abdominal aorta and their branches. The absence of pulmonary arterial sections around segmental and subsegmental bronchi on CT scans suggests an exclusive systemic arterial supply (Figure 7-5). Once within the lung, these branches of variable size adopt the course and distribution of pulmonary arteries, resembling a pure vascular sequestration with a pulmonary venous return.

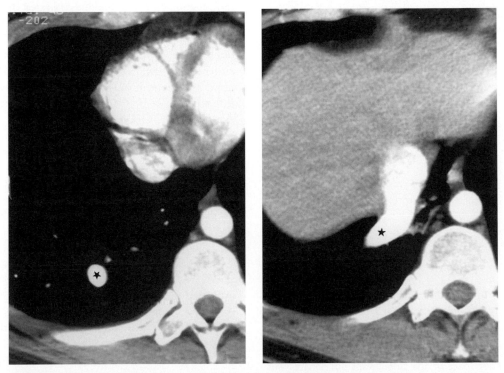

A   B

FIGURE 7-4. Cross-sectional CT angiogram images of a scimitar vein, coursing vertically in the right lung base (**A**, *star*), then draining into the right inferior vena cava (**B**, *star*).

Rarely, the systemic arteries supplying the right lower lobe arise from an ectopic artery, such as the internal mammary artery, the celiac trunk, or a renal artery. CTA has replaced conventional angiography in the determination of the number and diameter of these systemic arteries. This information is of importance for the surgeon or the radiologist in charge of occluding these vessels, which may be responsible for the clinical symptoms of hemoptysis or pulmonary hypertension.

Diagnosis and Treatment

Scimitar syndrome may be clinically silent when the degree of the left-to-right shunt secondary to the partial anomalous pulmonary venous return and systemic arterialization of the lung is moderate and when the associated anomalies are mild. It may be symptomatic because of the association with severe right hemithoracic malformations or important associated cardiac and noncardiac abnormalities. Two distinct types of scimitar syndrome have been described: the infantile form and the adult form (34,35). The infantile form is severe and associated with major cardiac lesions, including pulmonary vascular disease (35). The adult form is better tolerated, sometimes being asymptomatic (34). Pulmonary hypertension may develop in a previously asymptomatic adult due to stenosis of the anomalous pulmonary vein, intense systemic arterialization of the right lung, reduction of the pulmonary vascular bed on the right side, or increased blood flow resulting from the presence of an associated intracardiac defect (36).

Spiral CT, augmented with volume-rendered images, allows the complete noninvasive assessment of the main components of the scimitar syndrome. Using mediastinal window settings and segmenting out the vascular structures on three-dimensional display, the abnormal course and connection of the right pulmonary vein and the systemic arterial supply to the right lung can be clearly demonstrated. Lung window settings and three-dimensional reconstructions of the airways can demonstrate the abnormal lung lobation and anomalous

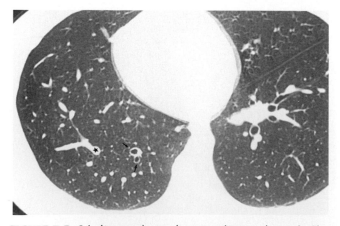

FIGURE 7-5. Scimitar syndrome (same patient as shown in Figure 7-4). High-resolution CT scan obtained at the level of the right lung base shows part of the anomalous pulmonary vein (*star*), two dilated peripheral bronchi (*arrows*) without accompanying pulmonary arterial sections, and dextrocardia.

bronchial branching pattern. Consequently, the pretherapeutic evaluation of a scimitar syndrome should no longer require angiography of the aorta, pulmonary arteries, and veins, nor bronchoscopy and bronchography (37).

Rarely is the presence of a scimitar vein on the chest radiograph not due to the aberrant draining vein of classic scimitar syndrome. Instead, the radiographic finding represents an aberrant scimitar-shaped anomalous vein draining normally into the left atrium (38,39) or a scimitar shadow produced by an anomalous superior vena cava that courses through the right lung before entering the right atrium (40).

Surgical repair of the venous abnormality in scimitar syndrome usually consists of reimplantation of the anomalous vein directly into the left atrium, or baffling the anomalous venous channel through the right atrium and into the left atrium through an atrial septal defect (36). Postoperative complications include thrombosis or stenosis of the reimplanted anomalous vein, which can give rise to acute unilateral pulmonary venous obstruction. CT may be useful to detect this postsurgical complication by demonstrating a localized region of pulmonary edema or hemorrhage with associated pleural effusion.

Partial Anomalous Pulmonary Venous Return to the Superior Vena Cava

This malformation consists of the drainage of part or all of the right upper lobe into the lower portion of the superior vena cava, just above the right atrium. This anomaly is easily missed on contrast-enhanced CT scans because there is no intraparenchymal aberrant vein and images of this portion of the superior vena cava may be degraded by streak artifacts.

The initial suspicion of this abnormality may arise from an anomalous, curved, vessel-like density seen on the chest radiograph. In this situation, we recommend obtaining either an unenhanced spiral CT (Figure 7-6) or scanning the upper lung zone at the time of pulmonary venous opacification when there is no contrast media remaining in the superior vena cava. Once this abnormal draining vein is identified, the patient should be evaluated for the presence of an atrial septal defect, which is seen in 90% of patients (41).

Therapeutic decision making depends on two factors: the hemodynamic status and the associated cardiac malformations. In the vast majority of patients, the abnormal drainage occurs at the superior vena cava–right atrial junction. Occasionally, the pulmonary venous drainage occurs into the high superior vena cava, which requires a different surgical approach (42). Therefore, whenever surgery is indicated, it is mandatory to provide the surgeon with precise information on the exact site of pulmonary-to-systemic vein junction and the length of the pulmonary vein able to be mobilized. These measurements will influence the surgical options for redirecting the pulmonary blood flow.

Other partial anomalous pulmonary venous drainage patterns can be seen on the right but are much less common. Partial pulmonary venous drainage to the right atrium is

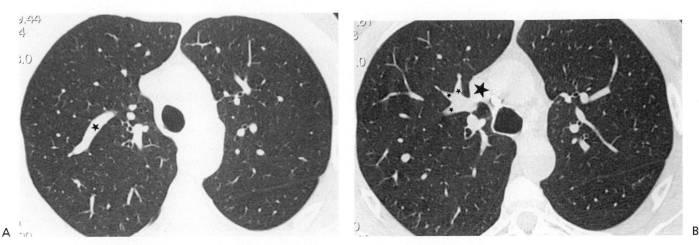

FIGURE 7-6. Partial anomalous pulmonary venous return to the superior vena cava. Noncontrast CT scans obtained at the level of the upper lung zones (**A, B**) show the enlarged anomalous veins (**A**, *star*) (**B**, *small stars*) joining the posterolateral wall of the superior vena cava (**B**, *large star*).

mainly seen in patients with visceral heterotaxia (43). Rarely, the partial anomalous venous return is to the azygos vein (44) or to the azygos arch (45). The azygos vein is often enlarged with these malformations. It may be difficult to make the distinction between an abnormal venous drainage to the distal portion of the azygos arch or to the posteroinferior portion of the superior vena cava. Thin-section imaging with multitrack scanners, visualized using three-dimensional rendering, may help in this unusual situation. Partial anomalous pulmonary venous drainage of the right lower lobe to the superior vena cava has also been described on CT (46).

Partial Anomalous Pulmonary Venous Drainage of the Left Lung

Partial anomalous venous drainage of the left lung usually is associated with a vertical vein that drains into the left bra-

chiocephalic vein (29,47). The vertical vein connecting the pulmonary and systemic circulations is believed to represent persistence of the embryonic left anterior cardinal vein. Diagnostically, this entity must be distinguished from a persistent left superior vena cava that drains into either the coronary sinus without associated shunt, or rarely, into the left atrium with an associated right-to-left shunt. Although all three of these venous anomalies may occur in isolation, they may also be associated with a wide variety of other vascular and cardiac defects (29).

CT of partial anomalous pulmonary venous drainage of the left upper lobe shows intraparenchymal pulmonary veins anomalously connecting to an aberrant vertical vein lateral to the aorticopulmonary window (Figure 7-7). The aberrant vertical vein abuts the lateral aspect of the aortic arch, and at that level is indistinguishable from a persistent left superior vena cava. The two are distinguished by their

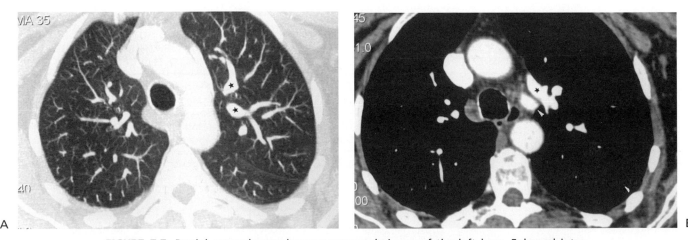

FIGURE 7-7. Partial anomalous pulmonary venous drainage of the left lung. Enlarged intra-parenchymal pulmonary veins (**A**, *stars*) anomalously connecting to an aberrant vertical vein (**B**, *star*) lateral to the aorticopulmonary window. Arrowhead points to the top of the pulmonary artery trunk.

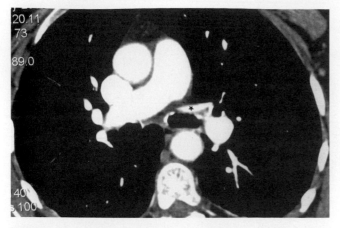

FIGURE 7-8. Cross-sectional CT angiogram image obtained at the level of the left main bronchus (same patient as shown Figure 7-7). A single, small-sized pulmonary vein (*star*), is seen anterior to the left main bronchus, corresponding to the lingular vein.

different hemodynamics and the appearance of the left hilum and coronary sinus. In contrast to a left-sided superior vena cava, the vertical vein is not densely opacified by administration of contrast material via a left-sided venous access. The enhancement pattern of the vertical vein follows that of other left-sided pulmonary veins. At the left hilum, the normal left superior pulmonary vein is not identified anterior to the left main bronchus. In its place is a single, small vessel, the lingular vein (Figure 7-8). Finally, in contrast to the findings with a left-sided superior vena cava with anomalous left pulmonary venous return via a vertical vein, the coronary sinus is of normal size and a normal sized left innominate vein is seen in the expected position. The CT findings enabling distinction between partial anomalous pulmonary venous drainage of the left upper lobe, persistent left superior vena cava draining into the coronary sinus, and persistent left superior vena cava draining into the left atrium are summarized in Table 7-1. The pre- and

postsurgical imaging management of left partial anomalous pulmonary venous return is identical to that for right-sided anomalous pulmonary venous return.

PULMONARY SEQUESTRATION

Pulmonary sequestration is defined as nonfunctioning lung tissue that is not in normal continuity with the tracheobronchial tree and that derives its blood supply from systemic vessels. The most common forms are intralobar and extralobar sequestrations. However, pulmonary sequestration encompasses a group of lesions with considerable diagnostic and therapeutic differences according to the presence or absence of bronchopulmonary malformations. If substantial parenchymal and bronchial anomalies are present, surgical resection is the only therapeutic option. Parenchymal anomalies in the sequestered lung can include: cysts containing air, mucus, or pus; hyperinflated or emphysematous lung surrounding cysts, nodules, or masses; or focal hypervascularity within part or all of the above-mentioned anomalies. Focal infiltration and calcifications have also been reported (48). If the malformation is limited to the systemic arterial supply of normal lung segments, simple ligation or embolization of the abnormal vascular pedicle is often sufficient treatment. Therefore, these therapeutic decisions are greatly influenced by vascular and airway findings on spiral CT.

Intralobar Sequestration

Intralobar sequestration accounts for 75% of all pulmonary sequestrations (49). It consists of an abnormal segment of lung tissue that shares the visceral pleural covering of an otherwise normal pulmonary lobe, but lacks a normal communication to the tracheobronchial tree. Variable amounts of air may be contained within the sequestered lung, delivered by collateral air flow through pores of Kohn. Ninety-eight

TABLE 7-1. CT FINDINGS ENABLING DISTINCTION BETWEEN PARTIAL ANOMALOUS PULMONARY VENOUS DRAINAGE OF THE LEFT UPPER LOBE, PERSISTENT LEFT SUPERIOR VENA CAVA DRAINING INTO THE CORONARY SINUS AND PERSISTENT LEFT SUPERIOR VENA CAVA DRAINING INTO THE LEFT ATRIUM

	Partial anomalous pulmonary venous drainage of the left upper lobe	Persistent left superior vena cava draining into the coronary sinus (i.e., duplication of the superior vena cava)	Persistent left superior vena cava draining into the left atrium
Parahilar intraparenchymal pulmonary veins of the left upper lobe	Enters the vertical vein	Enters the left superior pulmonary vein	Enters the left superior pulmonary vein
Blood flow direction in the vertical vein	Caudocranially	Craniocaudally	Craniocaudally
Left superior pulmonary vein	Small-sized or absent	Normal	Normal
Coronary sinus	Normal	Dilated	Normal
Left innominate vein	Normal or dilated	Normal in 20% of cases; absent or small-sized in 80% of cases	Normal, absent, or small-sized

percent of intralobar sequestrations occur within the lower lobes and are slightly more common on the left side. The anomalous systemic arterial supply arises from the lower thoracic or upper abdominal aorta. These vessels typically run in the inferior pulmonary ligament. The great majority of intralobar sequestrations are drained by normal pulmonary veins. Infection of the sequestered lung is the most frequently encountered complication. Rare complications include squamous cell carcinoma, adenocarcinoma, and tuberculous or fungal infection. Associated anomalies are relatively uncommon, occurring in 6% to 12% of cases (49).

Extralobar Sequestration

Extralobar sequestration represents approximately 15% to 25% of all pulmonary sequestrations (50). Most of them are diagnosed *in utero* or during the first 6 months of life, occurring more often in male than in female patients. Of all extralobar sequestrations, 60% to 90% are found on the left side. The typical presentation is as a mass within the pleural space in the posterior costodiaphragmatic sulcus between the diaphragm and the lower lobe. The blood supply is typically from systemic arteries and the venous drainage is usually systemic as well. Three features are specific to extralobar sequestrations: the ectopic location, the presence of communication to the gastrointestinal tract, and the frequency of associated anomalies. Ectopic locations include the mediastinum, the pericardial cavity, but mostly, the diaphragmatic and subdiaphragmatic regions. Because the lungs develop as a ventral diverticulum of the foregut, the sequestered tissue may communicate with the esophagus or stomach. Some 50% to 60% of extralobar sequestrations have associated congenital anomalies. The most common are congenital diaphragmatic hernia, diaphragmatic eventration, or paralysis. The differential diagnosis is extensive, but the main considerations are pulmonary or pleural mass, congenital cystic adenomatoid malformation, bronchial atresia, Swyer-James syndrome, and scar emphysema (48).

Purely Vascular Sequestration

Various combinations of the typical features of intra- and extralobar sequestrations account for the large number of anatomic, clinical, and radiologic presentations of pulmonary sequestration (51). Among this spectrum, one subset is commonly observed and warrants special description, the purely vascular sequestration, also known as Pryce type I sequestration (52), systemic arterial supply to normal lung, or systemic arterialization of lung without sequestration (53). In this variant of sequestration the only anomaly is systemic arterial supply to the lung. The anomalous artery supplies functional lung tissue that communicates with the tracheobronchial tree. There are no associated bronchial, parenchymal, or pleural malformations and no associated extrathoracic congenital anomalies. This variant is usually

found in the basal segments of the lung, and is most common on the left side. Although this anomaly may cause no symptoms, the recognition of purely vascular sequestration is important because massive hemoptysis may occur (54,55). The hemoptysis may be secondary to focal pulmonary hypertension in the involved lung as a consequence of long-term exposure to the systemic arterial pressure or to intrabronchial rupture of the abnormal systemic artery (54). This malformation may be suspected in patients with a continuous murmur, chest radiographic abnormalities at either lung base, high-output cardiac failure, hemothorax, or telengiectatic markings of the visceral pleura surface.

The systemic artery usually arises from the descending aorta and penetrates into the lung via the pulmonary ligament. The characteristic CT findings include a sigmoid-shaped anomalous systemic artery with a caudal course in its proximal segment, a cranial curve in its middle segment forming a hairpin loop, and a distal bulbous configuration before ramifying to peripheral branches (56). This artery substitutes for the normal pulmonary artery of the basal segments, associated with the absence of the lower lobe pulmonary artery distal to the origin of the superior segmental artery. Less commonly, the abnormal systemic artery may be just an accessory to the normal pulmonary artery supply. The proximal portion of the abnormal artery is often narrow while it appears enlarged when penetrating into the lung. This vessel may show atheromatous changes with mural calcifications evident during childhood. Intramural thrombus within distal ramifications of the anomalous artery have also been reported (53). Complete thrombosis of the proximal segment of the systemic artery with subsequent chest pain can also occur. In the absence of obstructive complications, the intralobar ramifications of the anomalous artery consist of dilated branches distributed along the normal bronchi in the basal segments of the lower lobes which are not supplied by normal pulmonary artery. This accounts for the early and massive filling of the inferior pulmonary vein identified on CT scans, corresponding to the left-to-left shunt which hemodynamically characterizes this malformation. Venous drainage occasionally occurs via systemic veins (azygos, hemiazygos, or portal vein), and results in a left-to-right shunt (57). When surgical treatment is considered, arterial ligation is followed by lower lobectomy. To prevent catastrophic bleeding during thoracotomy, it is important to provide precise description of the site of origin of the anomalous artery, which usually arises from the anterolateral border of descending aorta at the level of T9-T10 (56).

On CT, the search for the abnormal systemic supply to the lung must focus on the lower portion of the descending aorta and upper portion of the abdominal aorta. Thin collimation (1-mm) acquisition is recommended (58) to generate high-quality isotropic reconstructions. These images are reviewed to identify the anomalous systemic arteries, the bronchial arteries, intercostal arteries, and to attempt to visualize Adamkiewicz's artery (59). Coverage of approximately 20 cm and depiction of small-sized vessels require the administration of 140 mL of a 30% iodinated contrast agent. Because of the availability of thinner collimations to survey longer regions-of-interest, multislice CT is expected to provide a more accurate evaluation of purely vascular sequestrations than that obtained with single-slice spiral CT (60). Cross-sectional images are sufficient to make the diagnosis, but three-dimensional reconstructions may be helpful in demonstrating the course and the systemic relationship of the vessels (56,59,60–62) (Figure 7-9). Therefore, contrary to the recommendations on imaging of pulmonary sequestrations published in the early 1990s, we believe there is no requirement for angiography in these patients (63,64).

Apart from preoperative determination of the presence, number, and location of the abnormal systemic artery, the second objective of imaging study is analysis of the lung parenchyma, bronchial tree, and pleura to determine whether a conservative treatment can be reasonably considered. With regard to this second goal, spiral scanning also appears as the most appropriate imaging modality. In contradistinction to real-time sonography, color Doppler scanning, and MRA also suggested for the evaluation of this

entity (61), spiral CT is the only imaging study enabling the radiologist to provide precise information on the bronchopulmonary and pleural structures of the involved lobe (Figure 7-10).

The embryology of this entity has not been clearly established. Most authors favor the hypothesis of persistence of embryonic systemic arterialization of otherwise normally developing bronchial tree and lung parenchyma. It has also been postulated that the entity is acquired rather than congenital and that it represents hypertrophy of normal vessels within the inferior pulmonary ligament due to chronic inflammation (56).

Treatment is indicated for all patients with this anomaly, even if asymptomatic, because of the potential risks of hemoptysis, hemothorax, heart failure due to left-to-left shunt, and infection. In the absence of lung parenchyma and bronchial anomalies, surgical anastomosis of the anomalous artery with the lower lobe pulmonary artery can be performed. Alternatively, surgical ligation or embolization of the abnormal systemic artery may be sufficient to treat the malformation (65). If embolization is favored, spiral CT angiography should try to identify the ostium of the Adamkiewicz's artery to avoid iatrogenic occlusion (59). Coil embolization of pulmonary sequestration in infants is more frequently being considered as an alternative to surgery. Although short-term results are encouraging, there is a lack of information regarding the long-term efficacy of this therapeutic approach, justifying a CT follow-up of these patients (Figure 7-11). CT follow-up is facilitated by the absence of associated parenchymal lung disease (66).

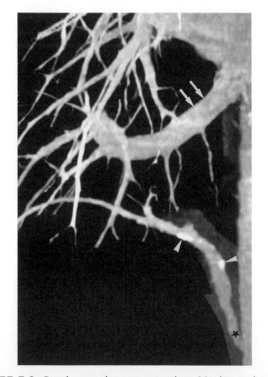

FIGURE 7-9. Purely vascular sequestration. Maximum intensity projection image of the right lower lung base (frontal view), obtained using spiral CT scanning (collimation: 4 × 1 mm), shows the abnormal systemic supply to the basal segments (*star*) originating from the upper portion of the abdominal aorta with venous drainage occurring via the right inferior pulmonary vein (*arrows*), normally connected to the left atrium. Note the presence of calcified atheromatous plaques at the level of the most dilated portion of the systemic artery (*arrowheads*).

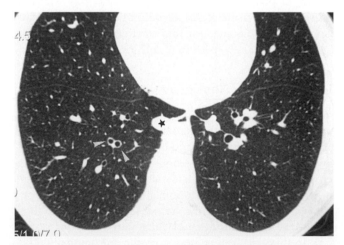

FIGURE 7-10. Purely vascular sequestration (same patient as shown in Figure 7-9). High-resolution CT scan at the level of the lower lung zones shows the abnormal course of the right inferior pulmonary vein (*star*), adjacent to the esophagus. Note the presence of two bronchi devoid of accompanying pulmonary arterial sections (*arrowheads*) in the right lower lobe, otherwise showing no parenchymal abnormality nor retraction.

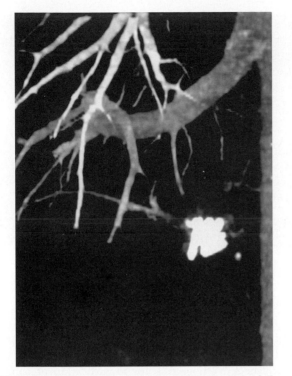

FIGURE 7-11. Posttherapeutic spiral CT angiography follow-up of a purely vascular sequestration (same patient as shown in Figure 7-9; similar acquisition and reconstruction protocols). Maximum intensity protocol image of the right lower lung base (frontal view), obtained several weeks after surgical ligation of the abnormal systemic artery, demonstrates the lack of opacification of the proximal portion of the systemic artery. Distal portion of this vessel is opacified by means of anastomoses with the pulmonary venous circulation.

Atypical Pulmonary Sequestrations

Ectopic Sequestrations

Approximately 10% to 15% of extralobar sequestrations are subdiaphragmatic. The diagnosis should be suspected in a patient of any age who is found to have a suprarenal, periadrenal mass, especially if there are no other retroperitoneal masses or adenopathy (67). This diagnosis can be strongly suspected if abnormal systemic supply can be identified on spiral CT angiograms. However, care should be taken to scan the patients with the thinnest available collimation as the malformation can be supplied by small-sized arteries (68).

Ectopic Origin of the Arterial Blood Supply

Seventy-five percent of pulmonary sequestrations derive their blood supply from the thoracic or abdominal aorta. The remaining 25% receive their blood flow from the subclavian, intercostal, pulmonary, pericardiophrenic, innominate, internal mammary, celiac axis, gastric, splenic, renal, or, rarely, coronary arteries (51,69,70). The arterial supply is usually a single vessel, with 15% to 20% of cases involving multiple aberrant arteries. Although rare, special note should be made of intralobar sequestrations with coronary artery supply (69,

70). This diagnosis should be suspected in infants or young adults with chronic left lower lobe consolidation and symptoms of myocardial ischemia, either related to vasospastic angina and stealing from the coronary circulation (70,71) or to severe arteriosclerotic changes (69). The most frequent source of ectopic coronary supply is the left circumflex artery whereas the existence of more than one aberrant vessel originating from the coronary vascular system has also been reported (70). In such cases, the use of electrocardiogram (ECG)-gated spiral CT acquisitions is recommended. Because an ectopic blood supply may also originate from renal arteries, suspicion of pulmonary sequestration should lead to scan a region-of-interest extending down to the level of these vessels. The anomalous artery can be found ascending through the diaphragm, then coursing through the leaves of the inferior pulmonary ligament (72).

Communicating Bronchopulmonary Foregut Malformations

This term underlines the embryologic relationships between the bronchopulmonary bud and the foregut. It also helps to emphasize that a pulmonary sequestration may communicate with the hollow viscus derived from the foregut (esophagus, stomach) or may include tissues derived from the foregut. Whenever the malformation is found in close contact with the gastrointestinal tract, its opacification should be obtained to search for communication. In cases of a cystic juxtadiaphragmatic thoracic mass lesion, the need for CT of the upper abdomen is justified because of a potential communication with the pancreatic ducts (73). Aberrant vascular supply of communicating bronchopulmonary foregut malformations is not systematically present.

Bilateral Sequestrations

Bilateral pulmonary sequestration is an exceedingly rare anomaly, either composed of similar or different types of sequestrations. Their blood supply may originate from the same vascular system or from different arteries (74).

MISCELLANEOUS ANOMALIES

Anomalies of the Pulmonary Arteries

Idiopathic Dilation of Pulmonary Artery Trunk

Idiopathic dilation of the pulmonary artery is a rare congenital abnormality which can be detected fortuitously on chest radiography or CT. This diagnosis refers to an abnormal enlargement of the pulmonary trunk without pulmonary valvular stenosis. Prior to the development of noninvasive imaging, definitive diagnosis was made by angiography. However, it is now supplanted by contrast-enhanced spiral CT (Figure 7-12) and magnetic resonance imaging in combination with echocardiography (75,76).

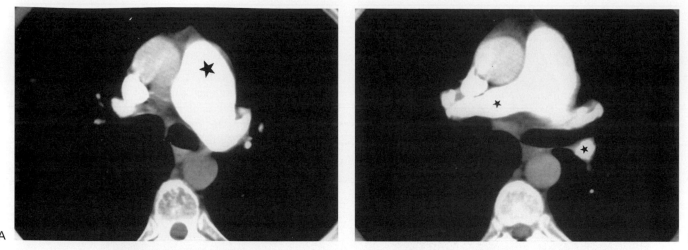

A   B

FIGURE 7-12. Idiopathic dilation of pulmonary artery trunk. Cross-sectional CT angiogram images illustrating the abnormal enlargement of the pulmonary trunk (**A**, *large star*) without abnormal dilation of the right and left pulmonary arteries (**B**, *small stars*).

Pulmonary Artery Sling

Pulmonary artery sling or anomalous left pulmonary artery is a developmental abnormality in which the left pulmonary artery arises from the right pulmonary artery and courses between the trachea and esophagus to reach the left hilum. It usually is diagnosed in neonates and young infants. It is often associated with tracheobronchial or cardiovascular anomalies, and is usually fatal if untreated. Rare cases have been reported in asymptomatic adults (77,78) (Figure 7-13).

The left pulmonary artery sling should be regarded as a multiplanar anomaly as it requires multiple planes of reformation for an optimal pretherapeutic approach. Until recently, multiple imaging techniques were required in the

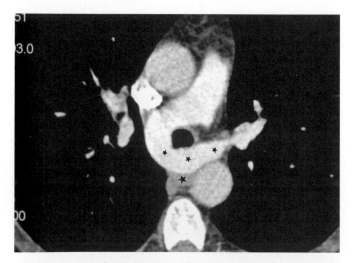

FIGURE 7-13. Pulmonary artery sling. Cross-sectional CT angiogram image obtained at the level of the pulmonary artery trunk shows the abnormal course of the left pulmonary artery (*small stars*), between the lower portion of the trachea and the esophagus (*large star*), originating from the right pulmonary artery.

preoperative assessment, including: (a) chest radiograph for the diagnosis of ventilatory disturbances; (b) bronchoscopy and tracheobronchography for identification of compression and associated abnormalities; (c) barium swallow for depiction of an anterior esophageal indentation by the aberrant left pulmonary artery; (d) echocardiography for demonstration of the anomalous origin of the left pulmonary artery; and (e) pulmonary angiography for the definitive preoperative diagnosis. Most of these modalities can now be replaced with spiral CT.

Spiral CT cross-sectional images are optimal to depict both the abnormal origin and abnormal course of the left pulmonary artery. It is superior to the frontal angiogram because on the angiogram, the abnormal origin of the left pulmonary artery can be hidden by the proximal right pulmonary artery (79). Moreover, spiral CT, particularly with the use of double-thresholding segmentation, allows evaluation of the tracheobronchial abnormalities that may be present in these patients (Figure 7-14). Park and colleagues have recently reported the use of spiral CT in the diagnosis of this entity (80). Contrast-enhanced CT with three-dimensional reformatted images allowed excellent evaluation of vascular and tracheobronchial anomalies, identifying the anomalous left pulmonary artery and diffuse and smooth tracheal narrowing. In addition, a respiratory dynamic CT scan showed no change in caliber and shape of the trachea during a forced vital capacity maneuver, leading to the suspicion of a complete cartilaginous ring, further confirmed by bronchoscopy.

Congenital Pulmonary Artery Stenosis

Stenosis of the pulmonary artery may be single or multiple, short or long, unilateral or bilateral, and may occur anywhere from the pulmonary valve to small peripheral pul-

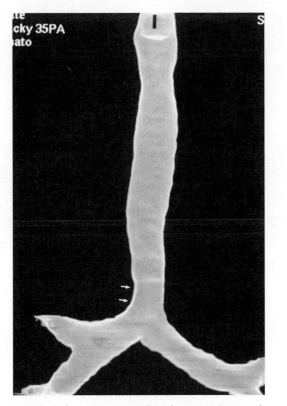

FIGURE 7-14. Pulmonary artery sling (same patient as shown in Figure 7-13; volume-rendered image obtained from the same data set). Bronchographiclike reconstruction showing mild tracheal stenosis above the carina (*arrows*) and symmetric angulation of the right and left main bronchi.

monary arteries (81). In children, this entity is often associated with congenital syndromes including Williams-Beuren's, Noonan's, Alagille's, Silver's, and congenital rubella. The hemodynamic consequences in childhood are often well tolerated and, in general, it is the noncardiac comorbid effects of these syndromes that determine the prognosis in these patients. In contrast, 12 adult patients with peripheral pulmonary artery stenosis have been described in a recent review (82). The patients presented with severe dyspnea, pulmonary hypertension, and unmatched radionuclide lung ventilation/perfusion studies, and were, therefore, all initially diagnosed as having chronic pulmonary thromboembolism. The second main differential diagnosis in adults is Takayasu's arteritis, which typically demonstrates stenosis of the pulmonary arteries (50% of cases) together with stenosis or aneurysms of the aorta and great vessels. Accurate diagnosis usually follows pulmonary angiography and hemodynamic studies, but could take advantage from spiral CT angiography, especially prior to treatment with balloon angioplasty (83). CT angiography can provide complementary information as to the precise shape, site, and length of proximal stenoses and can be appreciated with two-dimensional and three-dimensional reformations in various viewing angles.

Proximal Interruption (Absence) of the Pulmonary Artery

Proximal interruption is a rare congenital anomaly that can affect either the right or left pulmonary artery (Figure 7-15). Although rare examples of complete absence of both intrapulmonary and extrapulmonary artery branches have been described, this anomaly, described as "occult pulmonary artery," is better designated proximal interruption of the right or left pulmonary artery because the vessels in the lung are usually intact and patent (84). The affected lung is supplied by systemic collaterals, mainly bronchial arteries, while pulmonary venous return is usually normal. Proximal interruption of the left pulmonary artery is often associated with congenital cardiovascular anomalies, including tetralogy of Fallot, right aortic arch, septal defects, and patent ductus arteriosus, whereas right pulmonary artery agenesis is an isolated finding in most instances.

The majority of cases are diagnosed and treated during the patient's first year of life. Occasionally, however, in patients with a benign clinical course the diagnosis may not be made until adulthood. Symptomatic patients usually present with recurrent pulmonary infections but hemoptysis may appear as a consequence of systemic-to-pulmonary arterial shunting. The diagnosis of unilateral proximal interruption of a pulmonary artery is based on clinical and imaging examinations including CT. Bouros and coworkers described the CT findings in six adult patients (85). The main pulmonary artery and the arteries supplying the normal lung and its branches were always identified. The abnormal pulmonary artery was seen in all cases to terminate within 1 cm of its origin from the main pulmonary artery. Peripheral collateral arteries were identified in the affected lung in all patients examined. This finding may be

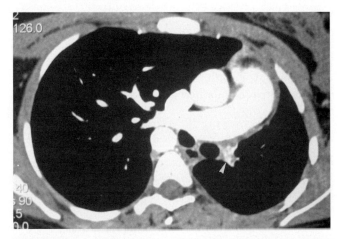

FIGURE 7-15. Proximal interruption (absence) of the left pulmonary artery. Cross-sectional CT angiogram image obtained at the level of the carina shows the absence of the proximal portion of the left pulmonary artery and numerous enlarged bronchial arteries (*arrowhead*) in the left hilum. Note presence of right aortic arch and marked mediastinal levorotation.

of great importance whenever selective embolization of systemic collaterals has to be considered in the context of massive hemoptysis (86). ECG-gated spiral CT could be particularly helpful in identifying abnormal collateral supply from coronary arteries, an exceptional situation incompletely depicted by nongated spiral CT acquisitions (87). In addition, acquired causes of pulmonary artery obstruction, such as vascular or lung tumor, and unilateral forms of chronic thromboembolic disease can be excluded. MR is also characteristic and has the advantage of aiding in the identification of accompanying congenital cardiac and great vessel abnormalities (88,89). These techniques are excellent depictions of the abnormal vascular anatomy, obviating the need for more invasive procedures. Additional advantages of CT over MR are the possibility to demonstrate bronchiectasis, sometimes present in the involved lung, but also the absence of air trapping, thus allowing distinction with the main differential diagnosis, namely Swyer-James syndrome.

Anomalies of the Pulmonary Veins

Pulmonary Varix

A varicosity of the pulmonary veins may be congenital or arise as a consequence of chronic pulmonary venous hypertension. Treatment is usually unnecessary once the vascular nature of the lesion has been established. However, surgical resection should be considered in patients with hemoptysis or symptoms suggestive of cerebral embolism.

This anomaly is an uncommon cause of a solitary pulmonary nodule in an asymptomatic patient but may also present as a mediastinal mass (90). The introduction of dynamic scanning allowed the noninvasive diagnosis of pulmonary varices (91–93). Contrast-enhanced dynamic CT allowed demonstration of the filling of the mass simultaneously with normal pulmonary vascular structures and continuity between the mass and the adjacent pulmonary vein. However, cross-sectional CT images are sometimes difficult to analyze because the malformation may be complex and depicted on several contiguous slices. In such cases, spiral CT with three-dimensional reconstructions provides better visualization of the vascular anatomy.

Pulmonary Vein Stenosis and Atresia

Congenital pulmonary vein stenosis and atresia usually are seen in association with other congenital abnormalities such as partial or total anomalous pulmonary venous connection, transposition of the great arteries, ventricular septal defect, and other anomalies (94,95). Occasionally, it may occur as an isolated finding. The stenosis or atresia is usually located at the pulmonary venous–left atrial junction (Figure 7-16), but additional stenosis may be present in the intraparenchymal segment. This entity induces progressive medial thickening and intimal fibrosis in pulmonary arteries and veins

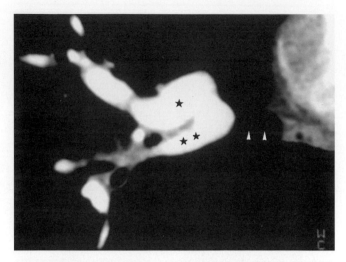

FIGURE 7-16. Right pulmonary vein atresia. Maximum intensity projection image of the right lung base showing confluence of the enlarged right middle lobe pulmonary venous return (RV4+5; *single star*) and the superior vein draining the apical segment of the right lower lobe (RV6; *double stars*). Note the discontinuity between the juxtaatrial part of the pulmonary veins and left atrium (*arrowheads*).

without plexiform lesions or more advanced stages of pulmonary vascular disease, which may explain the reversibility of pulmonary hypertension in these patients (95).

The diagnosis can be made with a combination of thin-section CT of the lung parenchyma and spiral CT angiography based on the presence of the following abnormalities: pleural thickening, absence of pulmonary venous reflux from the left atrium, discontinuity between the juxtaatrial part of the pulmonary veins and left atrium, and retrograde systemic-to-pulmonary artery shunt (24).

REFERENCES

1. Gossage JR, Kanj G. Pulmonary arteriovenous malformations. *Am J Respir Crit Care Med* 1998;158:643–661.
2. Shovlin C, Letarte M. Hereditary haemorrhagic telangiectasia and pulmonary arteriovenous malformations: issues in clinical management and review of pathogenic mechanisms. *Thorax* 1999; 54:714–729.
3. Kjeldsen AD, Oxhoj H, Andersen PE, et al. Pulmonary arteriovenous malformations. Screening procedures and pulmonary angiography in patients with hereditary hemorrhagic telangiectasia. *Chest* 1999;116:432–439.
4. Thompson RD, Jackson J, Peters M, et al. Sensitivity and specificity of radioisotope right–left shunt measurements and pulse oximetry for the early detection of pulmonary arteriovenous malformations. *Chest* 1999;115:109–113.
5. Remy J, Remy-Jardin M, Wattinne L, et al. Pulmonary arteriovenous malformations: evaluation with CT on the chest before and after treatment. *Radiology* 1992;182:809–816.
6. Remy-Jardin M, Remy J, Giraud F, et al. Pulmonary nodules: detection with thick-section spiral CT versus conventional CT. *Radiology* 1993;187:513–520.
7. Napel S, Rubin GD, Jeffrey RB. STS-MIP: a new reconstruction

technique for CT of the chest. *J Comput Assist Tomogr* 1993;17: 832–838.

8. Khalil A, Farres MT, Mangiapan G, et al. Pulmonary arteriovenous malformations. Diagnosis by contrast-enhanced magnetic resonance angiography. *Chest* 2000;117:1399–1403.

9. Srivastava D, Preminger T, Lock JE, et al. Hepatic venous blood and the development of pulmonary arteriovenous malformations in congenital heart disease. *Circulation* 1995;92:1217–1222.

10. Shah MJ, Rychik J, Fogel MA, et al. Pulmonary AV malformations after superior cavopulmonary connection: resolution after inclusion of hepatic veins in the pulmonary circulation. *Ann Thorac Surg* 1997;63:960–963.

11. Schraufnagel DE, Kay JM. Structural and pathologic changes in the lung vasculature in chronic liver disease. *Clin Chest Med* 1996;17:1–15.

12. Lee KN, Lee HJ, Shin WW, Webb WR. Hypoxemia and liver cirrhosis (hepatopulmonary syndrome) in eight patients: comparison of the central and peripheral pulmonary vasculature. *Radiology* 1999;211:549–553.

13. Oh YW, Kang EY, Lee NJ, et al. Thoracic manifestations associated with advanced liver disease. *J Comput Assist Tomogr* 2000;24: 699–705.

14. McAdams HP, Erasmus J, Crockett R, et al. The hepatopulmonary syndrome: radiologic findings in 10 patients. *AJR* 1996; 166:1379–1385.

15. Lundell C, Finck E. Arteriovenous fistulas originating from Rasmussen aneurysms. *AJR* 1983;140:687–688.

16. Braun RA, Buchmiller TL, Khankhanian N. Pulmonary arteriovenous malformation complicating coccidioidal pneumonia. *Ann Thorac Surg* 1995;60:454–457.

17. Stagaman DJ, Presti C, Rees C, et al. Septic pulmonary arteriovenous fistula. An unusual conduit for systemic embolization in right-sided valvular endocarditis. *Chest* 1990;97:1484–1486.

18. Cirimelli KM, Colletti PM, Beck S. Metastatic choriocarcinoma simulating an arteriovenous malformation on chest radiography and dynamic CT. *J Comput Assist Tomogr* 1988;12:317–319.

19. Aronchick JM, Wexler JA, Christen B, et al. Computed tomography of bronchial carcinoid. *J Comput Assist Tomogr* 1986;10:71–74.

20. Halsguth A, Schulze W, Ungeheuer E, et al. Pitfall in the CT diagnosis of pulmonary arteriovenous malformation. *J Comput Assist Tomogr* 1983;7:710–712.

21. Davis SW, Heitmiller RF, Davis F, et al. Intrapulmonary foreign body simulating pulmonary AVM: CT findings. *J Comput Assist Tomogr* 1997;21:769–770.

22. White RI, Pollak JS. Pulmonary arteriovenous malformations: diagnosis with three-dimensional helical CT—a breakthrough without contrast media. *Radiology* 1994;191:613–614.

23. Remy J, Remy-Jardin M, Giraud F, et al. Angioarchitecture of pulmonary arteriovenous malformations: clinical utility of three-dimensional helical CT. *Radiology* 1994;191:657–664.

24. Remy-Jardin M, Remy J. Spiral CT angiography of the pulmonary circulation. *Radiology* 1999;212:615–636.

25. Hofmann LV, Kuszyk BS, Mitchell SE, et al. Angioarchitecture of pulmonary arteriovenous malformations: characterization using volume-rendered 3-D CT angiography. *Cardiovasc Intervent Radiol* 2000;23:165–170.

26. Chavan A, Galanski M, Wagner S, et al. Hereditary hemorrhagic telangiectasia: effective protocol for embolization of hepatic vascular malformations—experience in five patients. *Radiology* 1998;209:735–739.

27. White RI, Lynch-Nyhan AL, Terry P, et al. Pulmonary arteriovenous malformations: techniques and long-term outcome of embolotherapy. *Radiology* 1988;169:663–669.

28. Lee DW, White RI, Egglin TK, et al. Embolotherapy of large pulmonary arteriovenous malformations: long-term results. *Ann Thorac Surg* 1997;64:930–940.

29. Dillon EH, Camputaro C. Partial anomalous pulmonary venous drainage of the left upper lobe vs duplication of the superior vena cava: distinction based on CT findings. *AJR* 1993;160:375–379.

30. Greene R, Miller SW. Cross-sectional imaging of silent pulmonary venous anomalies. *Radiology* 1986;159:279–281

31. Godwin JD, Tarver RD. Scimitar syndrome: four new cases examined with CT. *Radiology* 1986;159:15–20.

32. Woodring JH, Howard TA, Kanga JF. Congenital pulmonary venolobar syndrome revisited. *Radiographics* 1994;14:349–369.

33. Dupuis C, Remy J, Remy-Jardin M, et al. The "horseshoe" lung: six new cases. *Pediatr Pulmonol* 1994;17:124–130.

34. Dupuis C, Charaf LAC, Breviere GM, et al. The "adult" form of the scimitar syndrome. *Am J Cardiol* 1992;70:502–507.

35. Dupuis C, Charaf LAC, Breviere GM, et al. "Infantile" form of the scimitar syndrome. *Am J Cardiol* 1993;71:1326–1330.

36. Najm HK, William WG, Coles JG, et al. Scimitar syndrome: twenty years' experience and results of repair. *J Thorac Cardiovasc Surg* 1996;112:1161–1169.

37. Schramel FMNH, Westermann CJJ, Knaepen PJ, et al. The scimitar syndrome: clinical spectrum and surgical treatment. *Eur Respir J* 1995;8:196–201.

38. Cukier A, Kavakama J, Teixeira LR, et al. Scimitar sign with normal pulmonary venous drainage and systemic arterial supply. *Chest* 1994;105:294–295.

39. Takeda SI, Imachi T, Arimitsu K, et al. Two cases of scimitar variant. *Chest* 1994;105:292–293.

40. Heron CHW, Pozniak AL, Hunter GJS, et al. Case report: anomalous systemic venous drainage occurring in association with the hypogenetic lung syndrome. *Clin Radiol* 1988;39:446–449.

41. Zwetsch B, Wicky S, Meuli R, et al. Three-dimensional image reconstruction of partial anomalous pulmonary venous return to the superior vena cava. *Chest* 1995;108:1743–1745.

42. Black MD, Freedom RM. Azygos vein agenesis and PAPVR: a potential surgical hazard. *Ann Thorac Surg* 1997;64:1829–1831.

43. Van Praagh S, Carrera ME, Sanders S, et al. Partial or total direct pulmonary venous drainage to right atrium due to malposition of septum primum. *Chest* 1995;107:1488–1498.

44. Thorsen MK, Erickson SJ, Mewissen MW, et al. CT and MR imaging of partial anomalous pulmonary venous return to the azygos vein. *J Comput Assist Tomogr* 1990;14:1007–1009.

45. Posniak HV, Dudiak CM, Olson MC. Computed tomography diagnosis of partial anomalous pulmonary venous drainage. *Cardiovasc Intervent Radiol* 1993;16:319–320.

46. Schatz SL, Ryvicker MJ, Deutsch AM, et al. Partial anomalous pulmonary venous drainage of the right lower lobe shown by CT scans. *Radiology* 1986;159:21–22.

47. Pennes DR, Ellis JH. Anomalous pulmonary venous drainage of the left upper lobe shown by CT scans. *Radiology* 1986;159:23–24.

48. Ikezoe J, Murayama S, Godwin JD, et al. Bronchopulmonary sequestration: CT assessment. *Radiology* 1990;176:375–379.

49. Frazier AA, Rosado-de-Christenson ML, Stocker JT, Templeton PA. From the archives of the AFIP. Intralobar sequestration: radiologic–pathologic correlation. *Radiographics* 1997;17:725–745.

50. Rosado-de-Christenson ML, Frazier AA, Stocker JT, et al. From the archives of the AFIP. Extralobar sequestration: radiologic–pathologic correlation. *Radiographics* 1993;13:425–441.

51. Savic B, Birtel FJ, Tholen W, et al. Lung sequestration: report of seven cases and review of 540 published cases. *Thorax* 1979;34: 96–101.

52. Pryce DM. Lower accessory pulmonary artery with intralobar sequestration of lung: a report of seven cases. *J Pathol Bacteriol* 1946;58:457–467.

53. Miyake H, Hori Y, Takeoka H, et al. Systemic arterial supply to normal basal segments of the left lung: characteristic features on chest radiography and CT. *AJR* 1998;171:387–392.

54. Fabre OH, Porte HL, Godart FR, et al. Long-term cardiovascular

consequences of undiagnosed intralobar pulmonary sequestration. *Ann Thorac Surg* 1998;65:1144–1146.

55. Rubin EM, Garcia H, Horowitz MD, et al. Fatal massive hemoptysis secondary to intralobar sequestration. *Chest* 1994; 106:954–955.

56. Ko SF, Ng SH, Lee TY, et al. Anomalous systemic arterialization to normal basal segments of the left lower lobe: helical CT and CTA findings. *J Comput Assist Tomogr* 2000;24:971–976.

57. Tokel K, Boyvat F, Varan B. Coil embolization of pulmonary sequestration in two infants. *AJR* 2000;175:993–995.

58. Frush DP, Donnelly LF. Pulmonary sequestration spectrum: a new spin with helical CT. *AJR* 1997;169:679–682.

59. Kobayashi Y, Tanaka O, Adachi H, et al. Visualization of Adamkiewicz's artery using multislice helical CT for the preoperative assessment of thoraco-abdominal aortic disease. *Radiology* 2000;217(P):466.

60. Chung JW, Park JH, Im JG, et al. Spiral CT angiography of the thoracic aorta. *Radiographics* 1996;16:811–824.

61. Franco J, Aliaga R, Domingo ML, et al. Diagnosis of pulmonary sequestration by spiral CT angiography. *Thorax* 1998; 53:1089–1092.

62. Di Maggio EM, Dore R, Preda L, et al. Spiral CT findings in a case of pulmonary sequestration. *Eur Radiol* 1997;7:718–720.

63. Yamanaka A, Hirai T, Fujimoto T, et al. Anomalous systemic arterial supply to normal basal segments of the left lower lobe. *Ann Thorac Surg* 1999;68:332–338.

64. Felker R, Tonkin ILD. Imaging of pulmonary sequestration. *AJR* 1990;154:241–249.

65. Hirai T, Ohtake Y, Mutoh S, et al. Anomalous systemic arterial supply to normal basal segments of the left lower lobe. *Chest* 1996;109:286–289.

66. Mata JM, Caceres J, Lucaya X. CT diagnosis of isolated systemic supply to the lung: a congenital broncho-pulmonary vascular malformation. *Eur J Radiol* 1991;13:138–142.

67. Kopecky KK, Bodnar A, Morphis JG, Tao LC. Subdiaphragmatic pulmonary sequestrian simulating metastatic testicular cancer. *Clin Radiol* 2000;55:794–808.

68. Shaffrey JK, Brinker DA, Horton KM, et al. Atypical extralobar sequestration: CT–pathological correlation. *Clin Imag* 1999;23: 223–226.

69. Silverman ME, White CS, Ziskind AA. Pulmonary sequestration receiving arterial supply from the left circumflex coronary artery. *Chest* 1994;106:948–949.

70. Bertsch G, Markert T, Hahn D, et al. Intralobar lung sequestration with systemic coronary arterial supply. *Eur Radiol* 1999;9: 1324–1326.

71. Nakayama Y, Kido M, Minami K, et al. Pulmonary sequestration with myocardial ischemia caused by vasospasm and steal. *Ann Thorac Surg* 2000;70:304–305.

72. Pedersen ML, LeQuire MH, Spies JB, et al. Computed tomography of intralobar bronchopulmonary sequestration supplied from the renal artery. *J Comput Assist Tomogr* 1988;12:874–875.

73. Rahman GF, Bhardwaj N, Suster B, et al. Communicating bronchopulmonary pancreatic foregut malformation. *Ann Thorac Surg* 1999;68:2338–2339.

74. Wimbish KJ, Agha FP, Brady TM. Bilateral pulmonary sequestration: computed tomographic appearance. *AJR* 1983;140:689–690.

75. Silverman JM, Julien PJ, Herfkens RJ, et al. Magnetic resonance imaging evaluation of pulmonary vascular malformations. *Chest* 1994;106:1333–1338.

76. Ugolini P, Mousseaux E, Sadou Y, et al. Idiopathic dilatation of the pulmonary artery: report of four cases. *MRI* 1999;17:933–937.

77. Procacci C, Residori E, Bertocco M, et al. Left pulmonary artery sling in the adult: case report and review of literature. *Cardiovasc Intervent Radiol* 1993;16:388–391.

78. Stone DN, Bein ME, Garris JB. Anomalous left pulmonary artery: two new adult cases. *AJR* 1980;135:1259–1263.

79. Backer CL, Idriss FS, Holinger LD, et al. Pulmonary artery sling. Results of surgical repair in infancy. *J Thorac Cardiovasc Surg* 1992;103:683–691.

80. Park HS, Im JG, Jung JW, et al. Anomalous left pulmonary artery with complete cartilaginous ring. *J Comput Assist Tomogr* 1997;21:478–480.

81. Fraser RS, Muller NL, Colman N, et al. Developmental anomalies affecting the pulmonary vessels. In: *Diagnosis of diseases of the chest*, 4th ed. Philadelphia: WB Saunders, 1999:637–675.

82. Kreutzer J, Landsberg MJ, Tamar JP. Isolated peripheral pulmonary stenosis in the adult. *Circulation* 1996;93:1418–1423.

83. Fontaine AB, Wood DE, Borsa JJ, et al. Endovascular treatment of life-threatening peripheral pulmonary artery stenosis. *JVIR* 1998;9:965–967.

84. Anderson RC, Char F, Adams P Jr. Proximal interruption of a pulmonary arch (absence of one pulmonary artery): case report and new embryologic interpretation. *Dis Chest* 1958;34:73–76.

85. Bouros D, Pare P, Panagou P, et al. The varied manifestation of pulmonary artery agenesis in adulthood. *Chest* 1995;108: 670–676.

86. Rene M, Sans J, Dominguez J, et al. Unilateral pulmonary artery agenesis presenting with hemoptysis: treatment by embolization of systemic collaterals. *Cardiovasc Intervent Radiol* 1995;18: 251–254.

87. Mahnken AH, Wildberger JE, Spuntrup E, et al. Unilateral absence of the left pulmonary artery associated with coronary-to-bronchial artery anastomosis. *J Thorac Imaging* 2000;15:187–190.

88. Debatin JF, Moon RE, Spritzer CE, et al. MRI of absent left pulmonary artery. *J Comput Assist Tomogr* 1992;16:641–645.

89. Catala FJ, Marti-Bonmati L, Morales-Marin P. Proximal absence of the right pulmonary artery in the adult: computed tomography and magnetic resonance findings. *J Thorac Imag* 1995;8: 244–247.

90. Sirivella S, Gielchinski I. Pulmonary venous aneurysm presenting as a mediastinal mass in ischemic cardiomyopathy. *Ann Thorac Surg* 1999;68:241–243.

91. Chaise LS, Soulen R, Teplick S, et al. Computed tomographic diagnosis of pulmonary varix. *J Comput Tomogr* 1983;7:281–284.

92. Ferretti G, Arbib F, Bertrand B, et al. Haemoptysis associated with pulmonary varices: demonstration using computed tomography angiography. *Eur Respir J* 1998;12:989–992.

93. Vanherreweghe E, Rigauts H, Bogaerts Y, et al. Pulmonary vein varix: diagnosis with multislice helical CT. *Eur Radiol* 2000; 10:1315–1317.

94. Mortensson W, Lundstrom NR. Congenital obstruction of the pulmonary veins at their atrial junctions. Review of the literature and a case report. *Am Heart J* 1974;87:359–362.

95. Endo M, Yamaki S, Ohmi M, et al. Pulmonary vascular changes induced by congenital obstruction of pulmonary venous return. *Ann Thorac Surg* 2000;69:193–197.

96. Black MD, Shamji FM, Goldstein W, et al. Pulmonary resection and contralateral anomalous venous drainage: a lethal combination. *Ann Thorac Surg* 1992;53:689–691.

97. Olson MA, Becker GJ. The scimitar syndrome: CT findings in partial anomalous pulmonary venous return. *Radiology* 1986; 159:25–26.

98. Le Rochais JPH, Icard PH, Davani S, et al. Scimitar syndrome with pulmonary arteriovenous fistulas. *Ann Thorac Surg* 1999;68: 1416–1418.

HEMOPTYSIS

PATHOPHYSIOLOGY OF BRONCHIAL BLEEDING

ROLE OF CT IN DIAGNOSIS

SPIRAL CT ANGIOGRAPHY IN THE MANAGEMENT OF HEMOPTYSIS

Hemoptysis of Bronchial Artery Origin

Hemoptysis of Systemic Nonbronchial Artery Origin

Hemoptysis of Pulmonary Artery Origin

RARE VASCULAR CAUSES OF HEMOPTYSIS

Computed tomography (CT) has gained widespread acceptance in the evaluation of patients with hemoptysis. It allows noninvasive depiction of vascular abnormalities and identification of associated bronchopulmonary disorders, which may be unsuspected clinically and/or radiographically. The objective of this chapter is to provide the reader with a practical overview of the role and optimal technique for spiral CT angiography in the diagnostic and pretherapeutic evaluation of patients with hemoptysis. The discussion is limited to hemoptysis secondary to bronchial bleeding due to abnormalities of the systemic and pulmonary arteries.

PATHOPHYSIOLOGY OF BRONCHIAL BLEEDING

In the vast majority of cases, bronchial bleeding is secondary to hypervascularization of the lung, originating from bronchial, and less often from nonbronchial, systemic arteries. Systemic hypervascularization is a nonspecific response to several stimuli: reduced pulmonary arterial flow, hypoxemia, alveolar hypoxia, fibrosis, inflammation, and chronic suppuration. Whereas bronchial arteries are part of the normal systemic vascular supply of the lung, development of nonbronchial systemic hypervascularization requires preexisting pleural symphysis to allow perithoracic systemic arteries to penetrate into the lung parenchyma. Bleeding may also originate from the pulmonary arterial circulation, usually secondary to an underlying destructive lung process. CT angiography protocols have to be adapted to the expected source of bronchial bleeding. In approximately

90% of cases, the bleeding is related to bronchial arteries, in 5% to nonbronchial systemic arteries, and in 5% to pulmonary arteries (1).

The contribution of CT can be extended to the evaluation of other forms of endothoracic bleeding such as that occurring in the pleura, mediastinum, pericardium, lung, or esophagus (2,3). CT is also helpful in the diagnostic and pretherapeutic assessment of highly vascularized lesions that may require embolization prior to surgery, percutaneous biopsy, or drainage. These lesions may be located in the mediastinum, pleura, chest wall, or lung parenchyma and include a heterogenous group of entities such as paragangliomas, Castleman's disease, and hemangiopericytomas (4).

ROLE OF CT IN DIAGNOSIS

CT and fiberoptic bronchoscopy are the most useful diagnostic tests in the evaluation of patients presenting with hemoptysis of unknown origin (5). The role of fiberoptic bronchoscopy is twofold: the identification of the site of bleeding whenever an embolization procedure has to be planned, and the recognition of the cause of bronchial bleeding, especially when the diagnosis has to be confirmed histologically. CT has been shown to play a complementary role to fiberoptic bronchoscopy in the diagnostic approach of hemoptysis (5). When the source of bleeding is identified bronchoscopically, CT confirms the presence of bronchial disease and provides additional information on associated abnormalities, particularly helpful in the context of bronchial carcinoma requiring pretherapeutic staging. When fiberoptic bronchoscopy is not contributive, CT may help identify occult endobronchial lesions, detectable by means of bronchial wall abnormalities, or demonstrate bronchiectasis, a diagnosis often missed with bronchoscopy. Although CT and bronchoscopy are complementary, there are advantages of performing CT prior to bronchoscopy. CT may identify bronchiectasis as the cause of hemoptysis thus obviating bronchoscopy. It is also helpful as a guide to the optimal type and site of biopsy in patients with focal lung lesions. Furthermore, in the clinical context of active bronchial bleeding, it is recommended to perform CT examination before fiberoptic bronchoscopy in order to avoid iatrogenic complications such as fatal hemorrhage reported after taking a biopsy sample of a vascular or hypervascularized endobronchial lesion at bronchoscopy (6,7) (Figure 8-1).

When interpreting CT scans of patients with hemoptysis, it is important to realize that parenchymal and airway hemorrhage may mimic focal lung or airway lesions. Depending on the amount of blood, parenchymal bleeding may result in areas of ground-glass attenuation, airspace nodules, or consolidation. Whereas ground-glass opacities are easily recognized as being due to hemorrhage, it may be impossible to differentiate airspace nodules and focal parenchymal consolidation from lung infection or carcinoma, two potential causes of hemoptysis. The amount of bronchial bleeding also influences the extent of blood-related infiltration of the lung parenchyma, and thus the value of CT in localizing the site of bronchial bleeding. Identification of the site of bleeding is facilitated by the presence of a focal infiltrate. However, such a focal infiltrate usually hampers accurate detection of underlying mild bronchial or parenchymal abnormalities. Interpretive pitfalls also exist at the level of central and peripheral airways. Intrabronchial blood clots may thicken the bronchial wall or appear on CT scans as obstructive intraluminal masses, mimicking intrabronchial tumors especially when seen in association with lobar or segmental atelectasis (8). Additional interpretive pitfalls may be seen in patients with

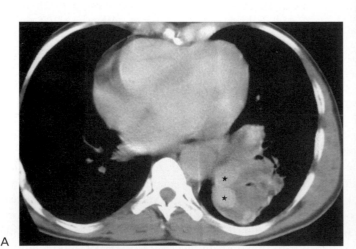
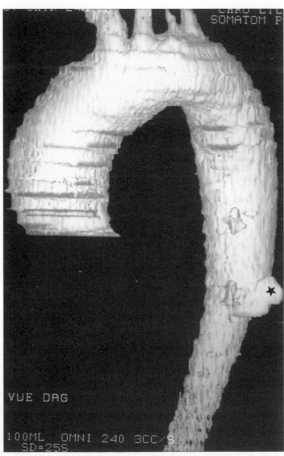

FIGURE 8-1. Sentinel hemoptysis, several hours before massive hemoptysis, in an 18-year-old patient with a purely vascular sequestration of the left lower lobe. Preoperative conventional CT scan at the level of the lower lung zones (**A**) shows suboptimal enhancement of the large systemic artery (*stars*), responsible for active bleeding in the left lower lobe bronchus. Postoperative three-dimensional shaded-surface display of the aorta (**B**) shows the stump of the abnormal systemic artery (*star*), surgically ligated. Note the marked dilation of descending aorta above the level of origin of the abnormal systemic artery.

preexisting bronchial and/or parenchymal lung disease. For example, a lung cyst or cavity filled by blood may resemble a nodule or mass. An intracavitary blood clot may mimic intracavitary aspergilloma, not only because of the overall shape of the lesion, but also because of its positional characteristics. Preexisting bronchiectasis may appear as bronchoceles. Because of these potential pitfalls, cautious interpretation of CT findings is recommended in the clinical context of recent hemoptysis, justifying a comparative analysis with prior or follow-up CT scans.

SPIRAL CT ANGIOGRAPHY IN THE MANAGEMENT OF HEMOPTYSIS

Hemoptysis of Bronchial Artery Origin

Bronchial arteries are the main source of systemic arterial supply to the lung. This blood supply normally constitutes 1% of the cardiac output. The bronchial arteries may enlarge greatly after birth to provide collateral flow to the pulmonary arteries when the pulmonary artery supply is obstructed or in the presence of inflammatory or neoplastic tissue in the lungs, particularly in patients with hypoxemia (9). In these various disease states, blood circulation in the bronchi can increase and represent as much as 30% of cardiac output (10).

Abnormal systemic arterial supply to the lung may be secondary to developmental or acquired abnormalities (Box 8-1) Developmental abnormalities occur in associa-

BOX 8-1. CAUSES OF ABNORMAL SYSTEMIC BLOOD SUPPLY TO THE LUNG

1. Developmental abnormalities in the systemic blood supply to the lungs (9):
   - Anomalous systemic arterial supply to the lungs in *congenital heart disease*:
     Congenital heart disease with pulmonary obstruction
     Unilateral pulmonary artery obstruction (stenosis, agenesis, atresia)
   - Anomalous systemic arterial supply to the lungs in *congenital lung disease*:
     Bronchopulmonary sequestration
     Scimitar syndrome
     Congenital cystic adenomatoid malformation
   - Anomalous systemic arterial supply to *apparently normal lung*:
     Pure vascular pulmonary sequestration
2. Acquired causes of abnormal systemic blood supply to the *lungs*:
   - Tuberculosis
   - Silicosis (coal worker's pneumoconiosis)
   - Bronchiectasis
   - Intracavitary aspergilloma
   - Tumor
   - Chronic obstructive bronchial disease
   - Cardiovascular causes
   - Lung abscess
   - Cystic fibrosis

tion with congenital heart disease, congenital lung disease, and rarely with apparently normal heart and lungs (9,11). The most frequent causes of acquired bronchial hypervascularization are tuberculosis, silicosis (and coal worker's pneumoconiosis), and bronchiectasis. The highest degree of bronchial hypervascularization is seen in congenital disorders, bronchiectasis, and intracavitary aspergilloma.

Enlarged bronchial arteries can be seen as abnormal tubular structures within the mediastinum or as nodular structures around the wall of the central airway that mimic focal thickening of the bronchial wall. The most common locations of the hypertrophied bronchial arteries are the retrotracheal area, the retroesophageal area, and the posterior wall of the main bronchus on the patient's right side and the aorticopulmonary window and the anterior and posterior walls of the main bronchus on the patient's left side (12,13). The presence of hypertrophied bronchial arteries that protrude into the lumen of the bronchi should alert the bronchoscopist to avoid accidental biopsy (13). Whereas bronchial bleeding is usually related to underlying bronchial hypervascularization, there is no strict correlation between the severity of hemoptysis and the degree of bronchial artery hypervascularization. Marked hypervascularization may be present in the absence of bronchial bleeding (Figure 8-2) and angiographically normal bronchial arteries have been shown to be responsible for massive hemoptysis (1).

Spiral CT is helpful in identifying the origin of bronchial arteries, thus providing a road map for the interventional radiologist prior to therapeutic embolization. Apart from the common origin at the level of proximal descending aorta, more than 20% of bronchial arteries have an anomalous origin from the great vessels (Figure 8-3) and another 10% originate from the aortic arch. To confirm that vessels originating from the thoracic aorta are bronchial arteries, demonstration of continuous vessels is important (Figure 8-4). This can be obtained by using curved reformation technique (14). Optimal evaluation of the bronchial artery requires the systematic search for the anterior spinal artery, a collateral of the right intercostobronchial trunk. The presence of this vessel is a contraindication to bronchial artery embolization. Moreover, spiral CT angiography represents the unique means of identifying mediastinal aneurysms of the bronchial arteries, an uncommon abnormality with potentially fatal hemorrhagic complications (15) (Figure 8-5). The parameters for adequate depiction of bronchial arteries on spiral CT are summarized in the Appendix.

Hemoptysis of Systemic Nonbronchial Artery Origin

In some patients, bronchial bleeding is secondary to nonbronchial systemic arteries. The most frequently involved arteries are the internal mammary, intercostal, esophageal,

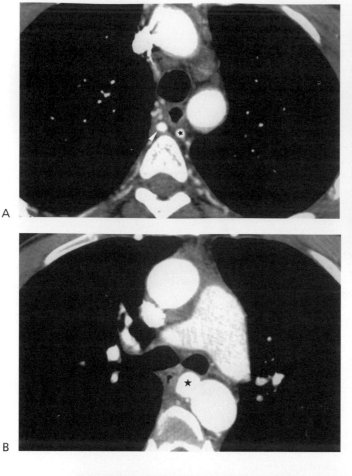

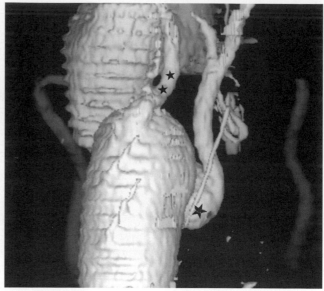

FIGURE 8-2. Spiral CT depiction of enlarged intercostal arteries in a patient with aortic coarctation. Cross-sectional CT angiogram images at the level of the aorticopulmonary window (**A**) and pulmonary artery trunk (**B**) show marked enlargement of the right (**A**, *arrowhead*) and left (**A**, *star*) intercostal arteries and saccular aneurysm of the origin of the right intercostobronchial artery (**B**, *star*). Three-dimensional shaded-surface display (posteroanterior view; **C**) shows the aneurysmal dilation of the origin (*single large star*) of the right intercostobronchial trunk and the enlarged left intercostal artery (*double small stars*).

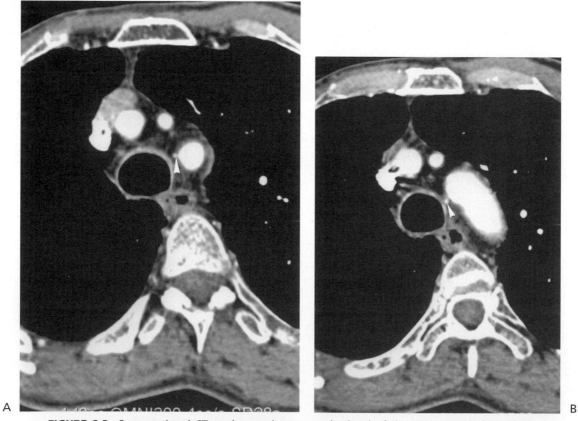

FIGURE 8-3. Cross-sectional CT angiogram images at the level of the great vessels (**A** and **B**) show the anomalous origin of the left bronchial artery from the medial border of the left subclavian artery (**A**, *arrowhead*), then seen between the trachea and aortic arch (**B**, *arrowhead*) in its downward course toward the left hilum.

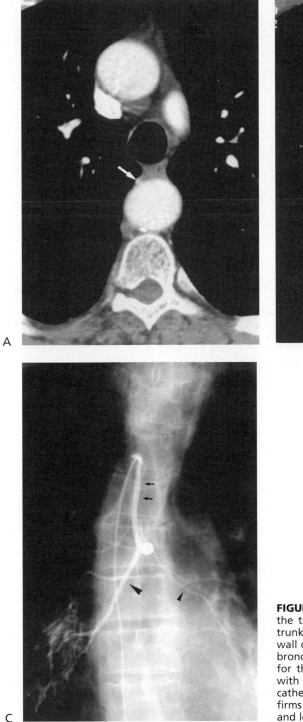

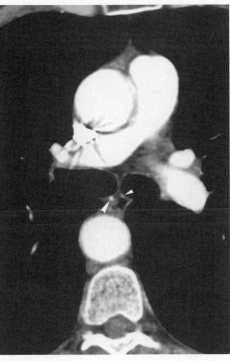

FIGURE 8-4. Cross-sectional CT angiogram images at the level of the trachea (**A**) and carina (**B**) show the origin of a common trunk for the right and left bronchial arteries from the anterior wall of the descending aorta (**A**, *arrow*), then giving rise to two bronchial arteries behind the carina (**B**) with a larger diameter for the right bronchial artery (**A**, *large arrowhead*) compared with the left bronchial artery (**B**, *small arrowhead*). Selective catheterization of the common arterial trunk (**C**, *arrows*) confirms the asymmetric diameter of the right (**C**, *large arrowhead*) and left (**C**, *small arrowhead*) bronchial arteries.

and coronary arteries and the systemic arteries coursing within the pulmonary ligament (16,17). Knowledge of this source of bronchial bleeding is important in the management of intracavitary aspergillomas in patients with poor lung function who cannot undergo surgery. These patients are often referred to the radiologist for percutaneous drainage of the cavity and subsequent instillation of antifungal treatment (18). Apart from the development of a rich blood supply from the bronchial arteries around the cavity, enlarged intercostal arteries are often seen in the vicinity of intracavitary aspergillomas. Their depiction on spiral CT angiograms is mandatory prior to the therapeutic decision as inadvertent puncture of enlarged intercostal arteries may lead to fatal massive hemorrhage.

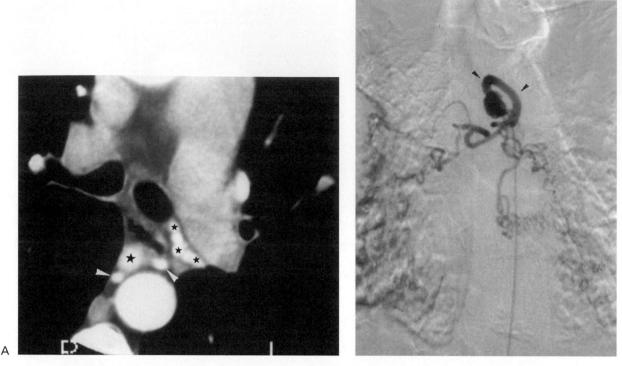

FIGURE 8-5. Bilateral cystic bronchiectasis responsible for recurrent episodes of hemoptysis in a 50-year-old woman. Cross-sectional CT angiogram image at the level of the carina (**A**) shows the aneurysmal dilation of the origin of a common trunk (**A**, *large star*) for the right and left bronchial arteries, posterior to the esophageal wall. The enhanced dots (**A**, *arrowheads*) surrounding the aneurysm correspond to the hairpin turn of the proximal portion of the common trunk around the aneurysm, clearly demonstrated on the anteroposterior view of the selective bronchial angiogram (**B**, *arrowheads*). On **A**, note the additional presence of small nodular enhancing areas (*small stars*), posterior to the left pulmonary artery, corresponding to an enlarged left upper bronchial artery.

Hemoptysis of Pulmonary Artery Origin

Several clinical situations should suggest the possibility of pulmonary artery origin of bronchial bleeding. One of these is persistence of bronchial bleeding after a technically adequate systemic embolization. Evaluation of pulmonary arteries is also justified in any patient presenting with hemoptysis and a destructive process of the lung as the latter can erode any vessel in its vicinity (19) (Figure 8-6). In this context, it is important to emphasize the possibility of "sentinel" bleeding, a clinical sequence of mild hemoptysis followed by massive and sometimes fatal bleeding after a free interval of a few hours or days. Lastly, several radiographic patterns should be underlined with the objective of preventive or curative treatment of massive bleeding from the pulmonary circulation: a cavity in close contact to a central pulmonary artery, and the replacement of a cavity by a nodule or a mass growing rapidly (19).

Among the destructive processes of the lung that can cause bronchial bleeding, of particular note is the Rasmussen's aneurysm (1,19,20). The aneurysm develops in tuberculous cavities as the granulation tissue destroys the elastic fibers of the arterial medial media. The vessel "wall," then only limited to the intima, herniates into the cavity. This intracavitary protrusion explains the episodic character of bleeding when the aneurysm ruptures. If the cavity is poorly drained, an intracavitary clot tamponades the bleeding. With retraction of the clot, bleeding may recur. Apart from tuberculous vascular erosion, the term "Rasmussen's aneurysm" has also been used for various infectious erosive processes, including pulmonary mycoses such as invasive aspergillosis and mucormycosis (Box 8-2) (Figure 8-7). An

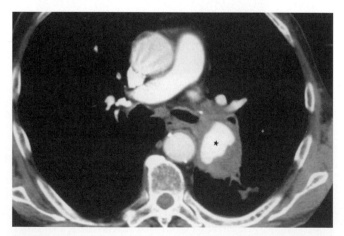

FIGURE 8-6. Cross-sectional CT angiogram at the level of the left hilum shows a pseudoaneurysm of the left lower lobe pulmonary artery (*star*), which developed into a cavitated lung carcinoma.

BOX 8-2. ANEURYSMS OF THE PULMONARY ARTERIES

Infection (mycotic aneurysm)
- Tuberculosis (Rasmussen's aneurysm)
- Syphilis
- Other bacteria and fungi

Cardiovascular diseases
- Congenital:
  Patent ductus arteriosus
  Atrial septal defect
- Acquired:
  Mitral stenosis, pulmonary stenosis
  Tricuspid incompetence, pulmonary incompetence

Vasculopathies
- Congenital
- Cystic medial necrosis:
  Acquired (atheroma)
  Marfan's syndrome
- Vasculitides:
  Behçet's disease
  Takayasu's disease
  Kawasaki's disease

Pulmonary hypertension
Hughes-Stovin syndrome
Traumatic
Miscellaneous

From Bartter T, Irwin RS, Nash G. Aneurysm of the pulmonary arteries. *Chest* 1988;94:1065–1075, with permission.

additional cause for pulmonary artery origin of bronchial bleeding is represented by pulmonary artery pseudoaneurysm, an uncommon sequela of pulmonary artery instrumentation and of blunt or penetrating thoracic trauma (21–24) (Figure 8-8). Rarely, hemoptysis may be due to endobronchial rupture of a pulmonary arteriovenous malformation.

The optimal technique for depiction of pulmonary artery aneurysms on CT scans depends on aneurysm size. The CT angiographic protocol for depiction of large-sized lesions is similar to that proposed for evaluation of acute pulmonary embolism. Identification of small-sized aneurysms requires use of the thinnest collimation available to cover the region-of-interest while administrating a highly concentrated contrast agent (300 mg I per mL).

Rare Vascular Causes of Hemoptysis

Focal or diffuse pulmonary venous stasis is partially derived toward bronchopulmonary venous anastomoses. These enlarged anastomoses are responsible for the presence of congestive submucosal bronchial veins, sometimes described as varices, which are prone to endobronchial rupture. Such a mechanism of hemoptysis can be seen in congenital left heart diseases and in various causes of pulmonary venous obstruction. Rarely, bronchial bleeding results from rupture of a proximal pulmonary varix (see Chapter 7).

Several mediastinal vessels can be involved in specific clinical situations. Most commonly seen in patients with aortic aneurysms, fistulas between the aorta and the tracheobronchial tree are highly lethal conditions (25). Aortobronchial fistula should be suspected in patients with a mediastinal mass and recurrent hemoptysis. Currently, atherosclerotic aneurysms and complications of cardiovascular and chest surgery have replaced infective aneurysms as the main causes of aortobronchial fistula (26). Traumatic fissuration of the brachiocephalic artery must be searched for after tracheostomy, long-standing tracheal intubation, or reconstructive surgery of the trachea. Such a lesion is usually located between the anterolateral border of the trachea and the posterior wall of the brachiocephalic artery. Fistulas

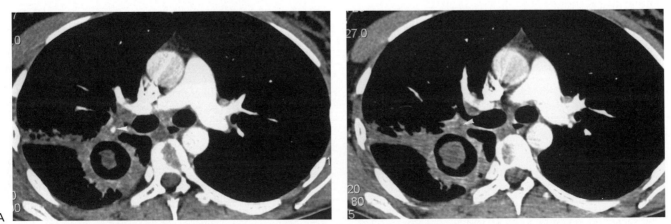

A   B

FIGURE 8-7. Mild hemoptysis in a patient with invasive aspergillosis. Cross-sectional CT angiogram images at the level of the upper lobes (**A** and **B**), spaced 10 mm apart, show the close contact between the lung cavity and RA3 (i.e., the posterior segmental artery of the right upper lobe; **A** and **B**, *arrowhead*). Note the absence of contrast enhancement of RA3 on **B**, suggestive of arterial thrombosis.

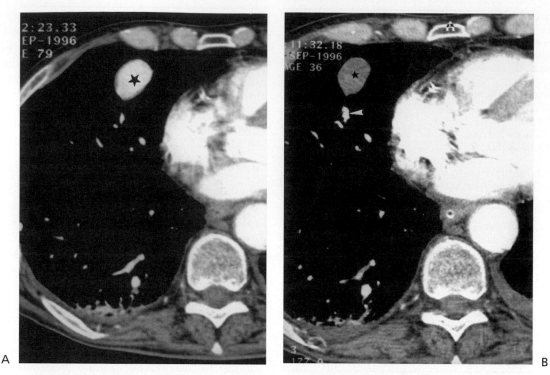

FIGURE 8-8. Cross-sectional image at the level of the right lung base (**A**) shows a pulmonary artery pseudoaneurysm (*star*) in the medial segment of the right middle lobe, a few days after cardiac surgery monitored with a Swan-Ganz catheter. Postembolotherapy CT angiogram image (**B**) demonstrating the thrombosed aneurysmal sac (*star*), below the level of deposited coils (*arrowhead*).

between the trachea and common carotid artery may be seen as a consequence of various laryngotracheal disorders or regional surgery. Any traumatic or mycotic aneurysm of the subclavian artery may rupture into the adjacent upper lobe. A tumoral process invading the superior vena cava may lead to the fissuration or rupture of this vessel into the trachea or right upper lobe. Lastly, rupture of congenital or postischemic aneurysms of the left ventricle into the airways may be exceptionally seen.

REFERENCES

1. Remy J, Remy-Jardin M, Voisin C. Endovascular management of bronchial bleeding. In: Butler J, ed. *Bronchial circulation.* New York: Marcel Dekker Inc, 1992:667–723.
2. Jones BV, Vu D. Diagnosis of posttraumatic pericardial tamponade by plain film and computed tomography and control of bleeding by embolotherapy of the left inferior phrenic artery. *Cardiovasc Intervent Radiol* 1993;16:183–185.
3. Hubler B, Earls JP, Stevens K. Trauma cases from Harborview Medical Center: traumatic pulmonary arterial and venous pseudoaneurysms. *AJR* 1997;169:1354.
4. Morandi U, Stefani A, De Santis M, et al. Preoperative embolization in surgical treatment of mediastinal hemangiopericytoma. *Ann Thorac Surg* 2000;69:937–939.
5. Naidich DP, Funt S, Ettenger NA, et al. Hemoptysis: CT–bronchoscopic correlations in 58 cases. *Radiology* 1990;177:357–362.
6. Gibbs PM, Hami A. Pulmonary arterial aneurysm presenting as an endobronchial mass. *Thorax* 1995;50:1013–1014.
7. Van Der Werf TS, Timmer A, Zijlstra. Fatal haemorrhage from Dieulafoy's disease of the bronchus. *Thorax* 1999;54:184–185.
8. Eisenhuber E, Brunner C, Bankier AA. Blood clots mimicking peripheral intrabronchial tumors in patients with hemoptysis: CT and bronchoscopic findings. *J Comput Assist Tomogr* 2000; 24:47–51.
9. Ellis K. Developmental abnormalities in the systemic blood supply to the lungs. *AJR* 1991;156:669–679.
10. Defabach ME, Charan NB, Lakshiminaryan S, et al. The bronchial circulation: small but vital attribute to the lung. *Am Rev Respir Dis* 1987;135:463–481.
11. Sharma S, Kothari SS, Krishnakumar R, et al. Systemic-to-pulmonary artery collateral vessels and surgical shunts in patients with cyanotic congenital heart disease: perioperative treatment by transcatheter embolization. *AJR* 1995;164:1505–1510.
12. Furuse M, Saito K, Kunieda E, et al. Bronchial arteries: CT demonstration with arteriographic correlation. *Radiology* 1987; 162:393–398.
13. Song JW, Im JG, Shim YS, et al. Hypertrophied bronchial artery at thin-section CT in patients with bronchiectasis: correlation with CT angiographic findings. *Radiology* 1998;208:187–191.
14. Murayama S, Haschiguchi N, Murakami J, et al. Helical CT imaging of bronchial arteries with curved reformation technique in comparison with selective bronchial arteriography: preliminary report. *J Comput Assist Tomogr* 1996;20:749–755.
15. Remy-Jardin M, Remy J, Ramon PH, et al. Mediastinal bronchial artery aneurysm: dynamic computed tomography appearance. *Cardiovasc Intervent Radiol* 1991;14:118–120.
16. Jardin M, Remy J. Control of hemoptysis: systemic angiography

and anastomoses of the internal mammary artery. *Radiology* 1988;168:377–383.

17. Casas JD, Prendreu J, Gallart A, et al. Intercostal artery pseudo-aneurysm after a percutaneous biliary procedure: diagnosis with CT and treatment with transarterial embolization. *J Comput Assist Tomogr* 1997;21:729–730.

18. Rumbak M, Kohler G, Eastrige C, et al. Topical treatment of life threatening haemoptysis from aspergillomas. *Thorax* 1996; 51:253–255.

19. Remy J, Lemaitre L, Lafitte JJ, et al. Massive hemoptysis of pulmonary arterial origin: diagnosis and treatment. *AJR* 1984;143: 963–969.

20. Sanyika C, Corr P, Royston D, et al. Pulmonary angiography and embolization for severe hemoptysis due to cavitary pulmonary tuberculosis. *Cardiovasc Intervent Radiol* 1999;22:457–460.

21. Podbielski F, Wiesman IM, Yaghmai B, et al. Pulmonary artery pseudoaneurysm after tube thoracostomy. *Ann Thorac Surg* 1997; 64;1478–1480.

22. Greene RME, Saleh A, Taylor AKM, et al. Noninvasive assessment of bleeding pulmonary artery aneurysms due to Behçet disease. *Eur Radiol* 1998;8:359–363.

23. Urschel JD, Myerowitz PD. Catheter-induced pulmonary artery rupture in the setting of cardiopulmonary bypass. *Ann Thorac Surg* 1993;56:585–589.

24. Ferretti GR, Thony F, Link KM, et al. False aneurysm of the pulmonary artery induced by a Swan-Ganz catheter: clinical presentation and radiologic management. *AJR* 1996;167: 941–945.

25. MacIntosh EL, Parrott JCW, Unruh HW. Fistulas between the aorta and tracheobronchial tree. *Ann Thorac Surg* 1991;51: 515–519.

26. Garniek A, Morag B, Schmahmann S, et al. Aortobronchial fistula as a complication of surgery for correction of congenital aortic anomalies. *Radiology* 1990;175:347–348.

27. Bartter T, Irwin RS, Nash G. Aneurysm of the pulmonary arteries. *Chest* 1988;94:1065–1075.

THORACIC OUTLET DISORDERS

The potential utility of computed tomography (CT) for the examination of the thoracic outlet was suggested more than 10 years ago (1). The increased soft tissue contrast and cross-sectional perspective of CT provide improved visualization of the vascular and bony abnormalities responsible for thoracic outlet pathology. In the majority of patients these abnormalities are undetectable using plain radiographs. However, the slow acquisition time, thick-section collimation, and limited vascular contrast in conventional stop-and-shoot CT gave limited information about the obliquely oriented critical structures of this region including the subclavian and axillary vessels, brachial plexus, and anomalous fibromuscular bands. The introduction of more sophisticated CT imaging (single-slice spiral CT, multislice spiral CT) and visualization tools (multiplanar and curved planar reformatting, surface-shaded display, volume rendering) have greatly improved our understanding of this difficult anatomic region.

AXILLARY AND SUBCLAVIAN VENOUS THROMBOSIS

Prior to the introduction of CT angiography (CTA), the diagnosis of axillary–subclavian vein thrombosis required venography of the upper limbs. However, venography provides limited assessment since the occluded vein is not opacified due to the development of numerous collateral pathways (2). Spiral CT angiography demonstrates the occluded vein and detects the perivascular abnormalities that may be responsible for the venous obstruction. Volumetric thin-slice CT imaging viewed using multiplanar reformatting and three-dimensional reconstructions provides complete assessment of the anatomy surrounding the venous thrombosis and has considerably improved the evaluation of these syndromes (3,4).

Spiral CT Venography Technique

Acquisition Technique

Demonstration of potential compression of the upper thoracic veins requires two CT acquisitions, one obtained in the neutral position (i.e., head straight, both arms alongside the body, retropulsion of the shoulders, deep inspiration), and the second one with 130 degrees of hyperabduction of both arms. Optimal opacification of the upper thoracic systemic veins requires low-concentration contrast agents that provide good venous enhancement without perivenous artifacts. This allows the identification of the vascular lumen, endoluminal clots, and identification of surrounding musculoskeletal abnormalities. We recommend an iodine concentration of 60 mg per mL. This concentration is not commercially available but can be easily obtained by dilution of a 120-mg-per-mL contrast agent with an equivalent volume of sterile water. Using single-slice spiral CT, each acquisition requires a total of 80 mL of contrast media injected at 4 mL per second in each arm.

To optimally visualize the axillary and subclavian vessels at CT venography, the contrast media must be injected via the basilic vein with a tourniquet applied to the upper arm. Injection into the cephalic vein does not provide adequate enhancement of the axillary vein because the contrast media flows directly into the subclavian vein, bypassing the axillary vein. A tourniquet positioned above the venous injection site limits the contrast opacification of the superficial arm veins and ensures adequate contrast enhancement of the deep arm veins. (See Appendix for recommended injection protocols.)

Optimal imaging of the thoracic outlet veins requires the acquisition of thin-collimation transverse sections and analysis of these images using two- and three-dimensional displays targeted to vascular and musculoskeletal structures to improve longitudinal resolution and provide optimal volumetric images. Overlapping reconstructions (1.5-mm spacings) are generated from 3-mm collimation, pitch 1.0 acquisitions (single-slice CT) or contiguous sections generated using 4 × 1-mm collimation (multislice CT). This volumetric data set is then loaded on a workstation and viewed using volumetric display techniques.

Display Technique

Sagittal and curved planar reformations of the volumetric data set are routinely obtained. Since focal lesions may account for the venous thrombosis, continuous sagittal reformations extending from the medial portion of the upper thoracic vertebrae to the head of the humerus are obtained. These are augmented with curved reformations of the axillary, subclavian, and innominate veins which decrease the effect of volume averaging seen in the standard transverse and sagittal images (Figure 9-1). However, caution must be exercised in the interpretation of curved reformations since they are manually prescribed and false stenosis may be generated by the incorrect selection of the reformation plane.

Two types of three-dimensional images are clinically useful in the thoracic outlet region, three-dimensional shaded-surface displays (SSDs) and volume-rendered images. These volumetric display techniques optimally display the venous and bony structures simultaneously. Three-dimensional SSDs can be obtained by means of simple thresholding from unedited images, demonstrating the outer contours of veins and bones as shaded surfaces. The parameter selection for volume-rendered images consists of a standard percentage classification technique. The user has to position and shape two trapezoids relative to the voxel histograms selected. The size and position of the trapezoids relative to the histogram determine the number and attenuation, respectively, of the voxels incorporated into the image. In addition, each anatomic structure is given a degree of opacity (or transparency), enabling the display of opaque veins through transparent bones. In most cases, these volumetric images of the venous and bony structures show the location and cause of the venous obstruction.

Collateral venous pathways that develop around the obstruction may impede the interpretation of the reformatted and volumetric images. Therefore, an awareness of the four common venous collateral pathways (Box 9-1) around this region aids in the accurate interpretation of upper extremity CT venograms. The level of venous obstruction primarily determines which pathway is employed (2). In axillary vein occlusion, 80% of patients demonstrate chest

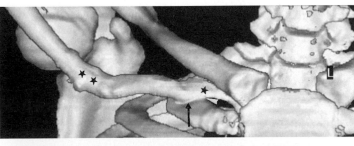

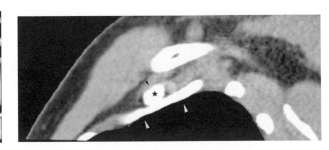

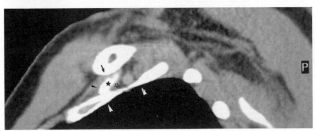

FIGURE 9-1. Spiral CT venography of the right thoracic outlet after postural maneuver illustrating a normal CT venogram. Three-dimensional shaded-surface display of the right outlet (**A**) depicts the axillary (*double stars*) and subclavian (*single star*) veins. Note flattening of the subclavian vein at the level of the costoclavicular space (*arrow*). Saggital reformations obtained at the level of the shaft (**B**, *white arrowheads*) and inner border (**C**, *white arrowheads*) of the first rib. Note the compressive effect of the subclavian muscle (**B** and **C**, *black arrowhead*) on the subclavian vein (**B** and **C**, *dark star*), more pronounced at the level of the inner portion of the costoclavicular space (**C**) where the subclavian vein is located between the clavicle (**C**, *arrow*) and first rib (**C**, *white arrowheads*), behind the subclavius muscle (**C**, *black arrowhead*) and before the medial fibers of the anterior scalene muscle (**C**, *open star*).

wall collaterals (pathway 1). When the occlusion involves the subclavian or brachiocephalic vein, approximately 80% of the collateral pathways occur via the vertebral vein (pathway 3) and/or jugular venous arch (pathway 4). Some of the collateral pathways that develop in the context of systemic venous obstruction can also be seen on a CT scan of the abdomen (5).

Primary Thrombosis of the Axillary–Subclavian Vein (Paget-von Schrötter's Syndrome)

Most cases of axillary–subclavian thrombosis have an identifiable precipitating factor as outlined in Box 9-2. However, 1% to 9% of upper limb deep venous thrombosis have no identifiable inciting event other than arm overuse or minor muscle strain. These cases are referred to as either Paget-von Schrötter's syndrome or primary thrombosis (6). The majority of patients are under 40 years of age and often give a history of vigorous or unusual exercise preceding the onset of symptoms. It is speculated that excessive arm activity in the presence of one or more compressive elements within the thoracic outlet leads to the thrombosis (7).

Spiral CT angiography has become an important diagnostic tool to identify sites of venous compression in primary thrombosis; of particular importance is the analysis of sagittal reformations of the upper thoracic region (3,4). These reformations are helpful in demonstrating the bony, cartilaginous, or soft-tissue abnormalities responsible for the venous obstruction. In addition, they allow analysis of the anatomic relationships between the subclavian vein and the first rib, thus providing the surgeon with precise details on the site and length of first rib resection necessary to relieve the obstruction. These reconstructions are also useful to analyze the functional anatomy of this

region (8) and to recognize the compressive effect of the subclavius muscle on the subclavian vein within, or at the level of the inner portion of the costoclavicular space, during postural maneuvers.

Acute therapy for primary thrombosis is anticoagulation augmented by thrombolytic agents if required. Urgent surgical neurovascular decompression of the thoracic outlet, varying from thrombectomy, angioplasty, surgical bypass, first rib resection, venous stenting, or a combination of several procedures may also be performed (7,9). Because of the controversy regarding the optimal therapeutic approach to this syndrome and the multiplicity of surgical approaches to resect the first rib, an early postoperative spiral CT venogram can be useful to the surgeon. A particularly important postoperative complication is bony or fibrocartilaginous regeneration following incomplete first rib resection. This can compress and inflame the surrounding vascular and nervous structures, leading to recurrence of symptoms. Repeated CT imaging can be useful to identify this postoperative complication. In light of the 10% incidence of pulmonary embolism in patients with primary thrombosis (9), some centers also perform a spiral CT for pulmonary embolism following evaluation of the axillary and subclavian veins.

Venous Thrombosis of Miscellaneous Causes

Among the causes of axillary–subclavian venous obstruction readily identified on clinical and radiologic grounds, particular mention should be made of the SAPHO syndrome because of the marked predominance of radiologic signs over clinical symptoms. The SAPHO syndrome is an increasingly recognized syndrome of synovitis, acne, pustulosis, hyperostosis, and osteitis (10). The osteoarticular manifestations of this syndrome involve the clavicles, first ribs, and sternum as well as the sternoclavicular and manubriosternal joints in the upper anterior chest wall. The most important hallmarks of the SAPHO syndrome are hyperostosis (referring to excessive osteogenesis) and osteitis. This osteogenesis may occur within the medullary canal or subjacent to the cortex from endosteal and periosteal proliferation. Hyperostosis also may be manifested as enthesopathic new bone formation. The sternoclavicular region is the most frequent site of the disease, being affected in 70% to 90% of patients (11). The most serious complication around hyperostotic bones consists of soft-tissue inflammatory involvement leading to a tumorlike mediastinitis with thrombosis of the subclavian vein or superior vena cava (10–12).

Pancoast tumors, because of their location in the apex of the lung, are better imaged in the coronal and sagittal planes than on transverse CT scans. Studies performed in the late 1980s using conventional stop-and-shoot CT scanners concluded that thin-section (5-mm) coronal and sagittal magnetic resonance (MR) images were more accurate than contiguous 10-mm thick CT scans in the evaluation of chest wall, mediastinal, and vascular invasion (13). Since MR imaging of the entire chest and adrenal gland does not result in improved accuracy in staging lung tumors, the authors recommended focused MR imaging of the apices as an adjunct to routine CT scanning of the chest in patients with superior sulcus tumors. The introduction of spiral CT has modified this approach, as it is possible to scan the apices with narrow collimation, improving the CT assessment of chest wall invasion (14). Moreover, high-quality, two-dimensional reformations of this region can also be generated from the same data set, allowing accurate depiction of negative prognostic factors such as involvement of the subclavian vessels, vertebral bodies, or ribs (15).

THORACIC OUTLET SYNDROME

Thoracic outlet syndrome comprises the clinical manifestations in the arm caused by compression of the neurovascular bundle as it leaves the thoracic inlet, the latter being composed of the subclavian and axillary arteries, the subclavian and axillary veins, and the brachial plexus. This clinical syndrome is most often related to compression and/or irritation of the nerves of the brachial plexus, involved in up to 98% of cases, whereas a vascular compression is involved in the remaining 2% of cases. However, the exact mechanism, diagnosis, and treatment of this syndrome are controversial, and cases of this disorder are not easily amenable to appropriate treatment in the absence of an objective diagnostic test.

Owing to the close relationships between the subclavian artery and the nerves of the brachial plexus, compression of the neurovascular bundle can be approached by the evaluation of the arterial component. The difficulty is the lack of an objective and easily reproducible means of demonstrating the presence of arterial stenosis. Angiography, the gold standard for arterial evaluation, is not without risk. Because of this, it is seldom performed in the assessment of these patients. Doppler sonography has gained widespread acceptance but is limited where the bony skeleton overlies the vessels. Moreover, this technique does not allow the operator to provide anatomic details of the structures surrounding the vessels at the level of the several potential sites of neurovascular compression. Spiral CT angiography has recently been shown to be a useful and minimally invasive means of depicting the vascular structures and surrounding musculoskeletal structures of the thoracic outlet (8,16,17). MR imaging of this region is an alternative noninvasive tool, capable of depicting neurovascular vascular structures (18–21), but is less informative than CT in the evaluation of bony abnormalities. Further studies comparing CT and MR imaging are required to determine the role of these imaging modalities in the assessment of patients with thoracic outlet syndrome.

Spiral CT Imaging Protocols

Acquisition

Optimal assessment of patients with thoracic outlet syndrome requires the performance of two spiral CT angiograms at the same session. The examinations are always obtained at full inspiration while the patient is lying in the supine position. The first acquisition is obtained with both arms alongside the body and the head in neutral position. A second acquisition is obtained with the patient's symptomatic arm elevated above the head (130 degrees of hyperabduction with external rotation) and ipsilateral rotation of the head, while the contralateral arm is positioned alongside the body. This positional maneuver combines the characteristics of the Wright and Adson maneuvers.

For each acquisition, the imaged volume extends from the seventh cervical vertebra to the lower extremity of the first rib, selected from a scout view obtained prior to each acquisition. We recommend the use of 3-mm collimation and a pitch of 1 (single-slice spiral CT) or with 4×1 mm and a pitch of 1.7 (multislice CT). The contrast media injection protocol consists of administration of a 30% contrast agent at 4 mL per second, using a scan delay of 17 seconds.

The contrast media should be injected in the asymptomatic arm to obtain an isolated enhancement of the subclavian and axillary arteries. The total amount injected depends on the CT technology used, varying from 70 mL (multislice CT) to 90 mL (single-slice CT) (see Appendix 9).

Display Techniques

A comparison study has been performed to evaluate the relative utility of transverse CT images, sagittal reformations, three-dimensional SSDs, and volume-rendered images for the assessment of arterial stenosis (Figure 9-2). Images were obtained in both the neutral position and after the postural maneuver (9). In this study, volume-rendering was the most valuable technique, demonstrating arterial stenosis with a sensitivity of 95% and a specificity of 100%. Volume-rendering was superior independent of the degree of arterial stenosis. Compared with surface rendering, the main advantage of volume rendering was the variable degree of opacity that can be selected for the anatomic structures retained in the final image. Choosing a high degree of transparency for the clavicle and first rib, it was possible to analyze the arterial

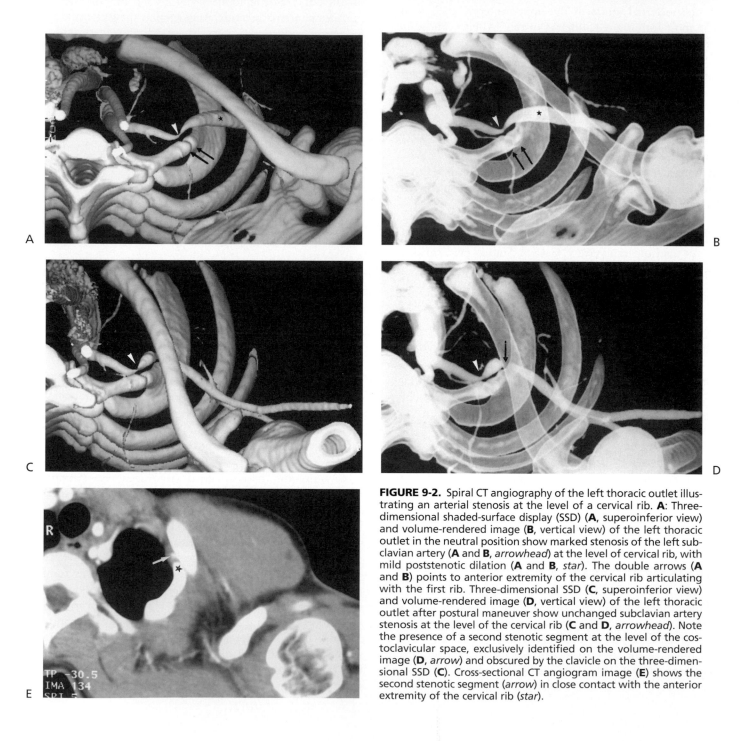

FIGURE 9-2. Spiral CT angiography of the left thoracic outlet illustrating an arterial stenosis at the level of a cervical rib. **A**: Three-dimensional shaded-surface display (SSD) (**A**, superoinferior view) and volume-rendered image (**B**, vertical view) of the left thoracic outlet in the neutral position show marked stenosis of the left subclavian artery (**A** and **B**, *arrowhead*) at the level of cervical rib, with mild poststenotic dilation (**A** and **B**, *star*). The double arrows (**A** and **B**) points to anterior extremity of the cervical rib articulating with the first rib. Three-dimensional SSD (**C**, superoinferior view) and volume-rendered image (**D**, vertical view) of the left thoracic outlet after postural maneuver show unchanged subclavian artery stenosis at the level of the cervical rib (**C** and **D**, *arrowhead*). Note the presence of a second stenotic segment at the level of the costoclavicular space, exclusively identified on the volume-rendered image (**D**, *arrow*) and obscured by the clavicle on the three-dimensional SSD (**C**). Cross-sectional CT angiogram image (**E**) shows the second stenotic segment (*arrow*) in close contact with the anterior extremity of the cervical rib (*star*).

diameters of the subclavian and axillary arteries in every case, especially at the level of the costoclavicular space.

The three-dimensional displays must be interpreted in conjunction with traditional cross-sectional images and multiplanar reformations. This allows the detection of peri-arterial abnormalities and confirms that stenosis seen on the three-dimensional images are not due to image artifact. Sagittal reformations show the relationship between the arteries, surrounding muscles (i.e., the anterior scalene and subclavius muscles), and anomalous fibromuscular bands (also known as Roos fibers), which may be poorly visualized secondary to editing on the three-dimensional images.

Identification of Musculoskeletal Abnormalities

The first *in vivo* CT evaluation of the functional anatomy of the thoracic outlet in a population of symptomatic patients was reported in 2000 (17). Using spiral CT angiographic examinations, the authors analyzed the anatomic characteristics of the three compartments of the thoracic outlet before and after postural maneuver. The most relevant findings concerned the postural changes observed at the level of the costoclavicular space, demonstrating the course of vessels in a narrowed anatomic space after the postural maneuver. A statistically significant difference was found in the distribution of the maximum distances between the clavicle and first rib measured before and after postural maneuver, a finding not observed in a population of asymptomatic volunteers (16, 17). Because the subclavius muscle has also been implicated in restricting the available space at the level of the costoclavicular space, the positional changes in the distance between the inferior border of this muscle and the superior margin of the first rib were also analyzed. A statistically significant difference was found in the distribution of these distances before and after the postural maneuver in the group of male patients. The positional modifications of the first rib were analyzed owing to the well-known influence of the first rib on the orientation of the inferior margin of the interscalene triangle, and thus, on the relationships between the neurovascular structures and the bony boundaries of this narrow space. A statistically significant difference was also found in the distribution of the angle values between the first rib and the horizontal measured before and after the postural maneuver, another finding not observed among a population of asymptomatic volunteers (16,17).

The finding that the anatomic characteristics of the thoracic outlet were smaller in the subgroup of patients with arterial stenosis led the authors to suggest that dynamically induced narrowing of the costoclavicular space could be responsible for neurovascular compression in susceptible patients (17). By the integration of transverse CT scans, multiplanar reformations, and rapid three-dimensional displays of enhanced vascular structures, spiral CT angiography is expected to become an important diagnostic tool of thoracic outlet syndromes which will help elucidate the site of vascular obstruction.

REFERENCES

1. Bilbey JH, Müller NL, Connell DG, et al. Thoracic outlet syndrome: evaluation with CT. *Radiology* 1989;171:381–384.
2. Richard HM, Selby JB, Gay SB, et al. Normal venous anatomy and collateral pathways in upper extremity venous thrombosis. *Radiographics* 1992;12:527–534.
3. Tello R, Scholz E, Finn JP, et al. Subclavian vein thrombosis detected with spiral CT and three-dimensional reconstruction. *AJR* 1993;160:33–34.
4. Remy J, Remy-Jardin M, Artaud D, et al. Multiplanar and three-dimensional reconstruction techniques in CT: impact on chest diseases. *Eur Radiol* 1998;8:335–351.
5. Bashist B, Parisi A, Frager DH, et al. Abdominal CT findings when the superior vena cava, brachiocephalic vein, or subclavian vein is obstructed. *AJR* 1996;167:1457–1463.
6. Grassi CJ, Bettmann MA. Effort thrombosis: role of interventional therapy. *Cardiovasc Intervent Radiol* 1990;13:317–322.
7. Urschel HC, Razzuk MA. Paget-von Schrötter syndrome: what is the best management? *Ann Thorac Surg* 2000;69:1663–1669.
8. Remy-Jardin M, Remy J, Masson P, et al. CT angiography of thoracic outlet syndrome: evaluation of imaging protocols for the detection of arterial stenosis. *J Comput Assist Tomogr* 2000; 24:349–361.
9. Schneider DB, Azakie A, Messina LM, et al. Management of vascular thoracic outlet syndrome. *Chest Surg Clin North Am* 1999;9:781–801.
10. Boutin RD, Resnick D. The SAPHO syndrome: an evolving concept for unifying several idiopathic disorders of bone and skin. *AJR* 1998;170:585–591.
11. Cotten A, Flipo RM, Mentre A, et al. SAPHO syndrome. *Radiographics* 1995;15:1147–1154.
12. Van Holsbeeck M, Martel W, Dequeker J, et al. Soft tissue involvement, mediastinal pseudotumor, and venous thrombosis in pustulotic arthro-osteitis. *Skeletal Radiol* 1989;18:1–8.
13. Heelan RT, Demas BE, Caravelli JF, et al. Superior sulcus tumors: CT and MR imaging. *Radiology* 1989;170:637–641.
14. Uhrmeister P, Allman KH, Wertzel H, et al. Chest wall invasion by lung cancer: value of thin-sectional CT with different reconstruction algorithms. *Eur Radiol* 1999;9:1304–1309.
15. Detterbeck FC. Pancoast (superior sulcus) tumors. *Ann Thorac Surg* 1997;63:1810–1818.
16. Remy-Jardin M, Doyen J, Remy J, et al. Functional anatomy of the thoracic outlet: evaluation with spiral CT. *Radiology* 1997; 205:843–851.
17. Remy-Jardin M, Remy J, Masson P, et al. Helical CT angiography of thoracic outlet syndrome: functional anatomy. *AJR* 2000;174:1667–1674.
18. Dimarkowski S, Bosmans H, Marchal G, et al. Three-dimensional MR angiography in the evaluation of thoracic outlet syndrome. *AJR* 1999;173:1005–1006.
19. Cosottini M, Zampa V, Petruzzi P, et al. Contrast-enhanced three-dimensional MR angiography in the assessment of subclavian artery diseases. *Eur Radiol* 2000;10: 1337–1344.
20. Hagspiel KD, Spinosa DJ, Angle JF, et al. Diagnosis of vascular compression at the thoracic outlet using gadolinium-enhanced high-resolution ultrafast MR angiography in abduction and adduction. *Cardiovasc Intervent Radiol* 2000;23: 152–164.
21. Smedby O, Rostad H, Klaastad O, et al. Functional imaging of the thoracic outlet syndrome in an open MR scanner. *Eur Radiol* 2000;10:597–600.

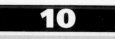

SUPERIOR VENA CAVA SYNDROMES

SPIRAL CT VENOGRAPHY TECHNIQUE

Spiral CT venography (CTV) of the superior vena cava (SVC) employs similar scan acquisition parameters to arterial CT angiography (CTA) studies, but requires a modified contrast-enhancement technique. Since there is no dilution of contrast media in the SVC, a lower iodine concentration should be used. This minimizes the spray artifact that would arise from the use of more concentrated contrast

media (Figures 10-1 and 10-2). Contrast media should be injected at 3 to 4 mL per second into both arms simultaneously via catheters placed in the medial aspect of each antecubital fossa. This injection technique optimally opacifies the axillary, subclavian, and brachiocephalic veins on both sides and outlines the SVC (Figure 10-3). Contrast media may reflux into the azygos vein or unopacified blood from the azygos vein may cause a filling defect in the posterior aspect of the SVC. Scan delays of 5 seconds allow adequate

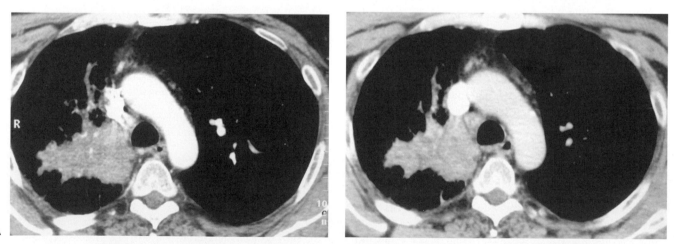

FIGURE 10-1. Comparison between 30% iodine concentration **(A)** and 6% contrast media **(B)** in the same patient. Multiple streak artifacts with the highly concentrated contrast media **(A)** do not allow an optimal analysis of the superior vena cava (SVC) borders and the mediastinal structures. Using diluted contrast media **(B)**, the SVC is optimally opacified while allowing visualization of the posterior wall of the SVC and tumor extension along the anterolateral tracheal wall.

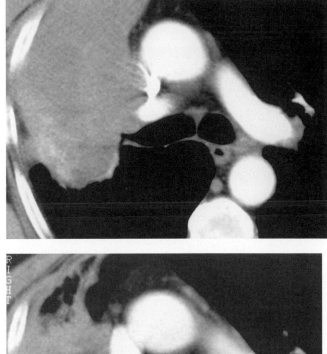

A

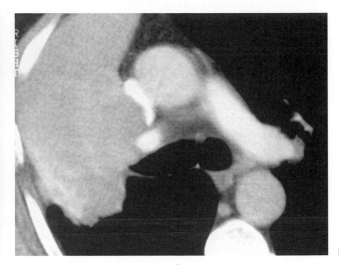

B

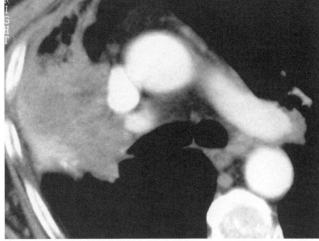

C

FIGURE 10-2. Contrast-enhanced chest CT scans through the superior vena cava (SVC) demonstrate that the use of dilute contrast media can result in a change in the management of a non-small cell carcinoma of the right upper lobe. The first acquisition is performed with a 30% iodine concentration contrast media **(A)**. The walls of the SVC cannot be identified due to the presence of multiple streak artifacts. A second acquisition using 15% iodine concentration contrast media **(B)** eliminates streak artifact and shows the external compression of the posterolateral wall of the SVC. Three months after completion of neoadjuvant chemotherapy **(C)** another acquisition with 15% iodine concentration contrast media shows a normal SVC, which leads to consideration of a right upper lobectomy.

time for the contrast media to opacify the SVC and fill collateral veins if a venous obstruction is present.

Scanner acquisition protocols for SVC venograms are similar to arterial studies (see Appendix 1). On both single-slice and multislice spiral CT scanners, we recommend using a pitch of 1.5 to 2.0 and the narrowest possible collimation or detector aperture with respect to the target volume and duration of the contrast media injection. Images should be reconstructed using the standard algorithm and reviewed using the paging format on a workstation to optimally appreciate occlusions, stenosis, and collateral veins. These images are usually viewed using mediastinal window and level settings (window 350 to 450 HU, level 35 HU). However, wider window settings (window 500 to 700 HU) can help identify filling defects or pacer wires within the contrast column. If a venous abnormality was not suspected at the time of image acquisition and the examination was performed using high-

iodine concentration contrast media (320 mg iodine per mL), viewing the images at wider window settings (window 500 to 700 HU) may permit confident diagnosis and avoid repeating the examination. Sagittal, coronal, and oblique reformations, thick- and thin-slab maximum intensity projection (MIP) reconstructions, surface-shaded displays, and volume rendering can be useful to view the acquired volume data set. These volume-rendering techniques provide sagittal and coronal images with a similar perspective to contrast venograms, which can assist the planning of surgical or endovascular interventions. However, as with arterial studies, these volumetric displays should always be interpreted in conjunction with the source transverse images to minimize the impact of artifact (1). Similar to arterial studies, the quality of the volumetric displays will be enhanced by acquiring the source transverse images using the narrowest possible collimation and performing overlapping reconstructions.

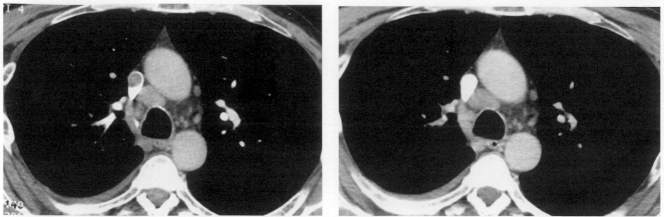

FIGURE 10-3. Contrast-enhanced chest CT through the upper mediastinum in a patient with carcinoma of the right lower lobe. **A:** Preoperative imaging using a unilateral right arm injection of dilute contrast media shows a filling defect within the superior vena cava (SVC), suspicious for thrombus. **B:** A bilateral arm injection with the same diluted contrast media shows a normal SVC. The filling defect in the unilateral arm injection arose from streaming of unopacified blood from the left arm.

CONGENITAL ANOMALIES OF THORACIC VEINS

Left-sided Superior Vena Cava

Abnormalities of the SVC and thoracic veins can be either confined to the chest or be secondary to anomalies of the inferior vena cava (Box 10-1). The most common congenital SVC anomaly is the left-sided SVC, which arises from the confluence of the left subclavian and left jugular veins (Figure 10-4). This anomaly is estimated to occur in 1% to 3% of subjects (2). It courses inferiorly on the left side of the mediastinum, lateral to the aortic arch, and most commonly drains into the coronary sinus. In this configuration, the left-sided SVC represents persistence of the embryologic left anterior and common cardinal veins, which have not normally regressed. Infrequently, the left-sided SVC can cross to the right SVC or right atrium at the level of the right pulmonary artery. A left-sided SVC that drains into the coronary sinus or right atrium has no hemodynamic consequence unless it is associated with congenital heart disease. Rarely, a left-sided SVC can drain into the left atrium (3), in which case it results in a right-to-left shunt. In the majority of cases, the left-sided SVC is an isolated

BOX 10-1. COMMON CONGENITAL ANOMALIES OF THE THORACIC VEINS

- Left-sided superior vena cava (SVC)
  To coronary sinus
  To right-sided SVC
  To right atrium
  To left atrium
- Bilateral SVC
- Azygos continuation of inferior vena cava

asymptomatic variant, but it may be associated with other congenital heart conditions (e.g., atrial septal defect) or systemic venous abnormalities (e.g., anomalies of the inferior vena cava) (2). A left-sided SVC may be seen with a right-sided SVC, with either one being dominant. With bilateral SVC, a small venous connection can often be seen between the two vessels in the superior mediastinum.

Partial anomalous pulmonary venous malformation (PAVM) from the left upper lobe may mimic a left-sided SVC at the level of the aortic arch. In both situations, an aberrant vessel is identified coursing over the left lateral aspect of the aortic arch. These two entities must be distinguished because the majority of left-sided SVC cases have no hemodynamic consequence, whereas PAVM of the left upper lobe results in a left-to-right shunt. In the majority of cases there are no clinical symptoms associated with left upper lobe PAVM, since the shunt is a small fraction of the total pulmonary venous return. However, this small shunt can become clinically significant when the right lung is compromised following lung resection, complete pneumothorax, or during surgical procedures requiring right lung collapse and single left lung ventilation.

Left-sided SVC and left upper lobe PAVM can be distinguished by following the course of the anomalous vessel inferiorly to the level of the left hilum (Table 10-1). In left-sided SVC, at the level of the left main stem bronchus, an additional vessel can be seen anterior to a normal size left upper lobe pulmonary vein (Figure 10-4A). In left upper lobe PAVM, a normal left upper lobe pulmonary vein is not seen at the left hilum, and the only vessel anterior to the left main stem bronchus is a small lingular vein. Most commonly the left-sided SVC drains inferiorly into the coronary sinus, which is usually enlarged. If confident differentiation of left-sided SVC and PAVM from the left upper lobe cannot be

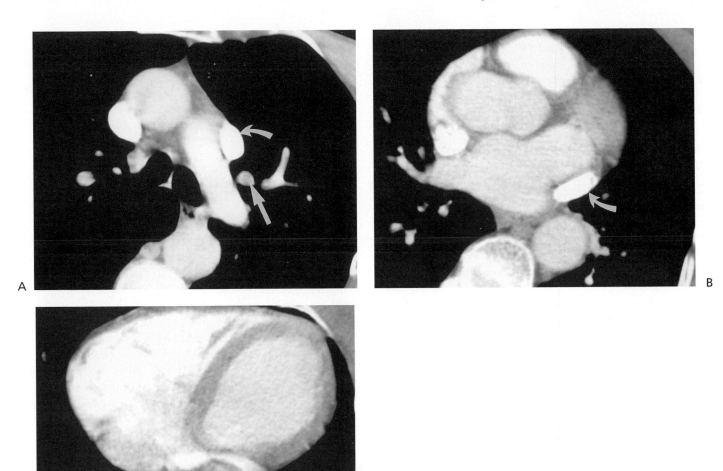

FIGURE 10-4. The diagnosis of left-sided superior vena cava (SVC) can be made with or without contrast media injection. The pathway of this abnormal vein (*curved arrow*) is in front of the left hilum **(A)**, behind the left atrium **(B)**, and in continuity with the coronary sinus **(C)**. At the level of the left hilum, the anomalous left SVC (*curved arrow*) courses anterior to the normal left upper lobe vein (**A**, *straight arrow*).

TABLE 10-1. CT FINDINGS DIFFERENTIATING PARTIAL ANOMALOUS PULMONARY VENOUS DRAINAGE OF THE LEFT UPPER LOBE FROM PERSISTENT LEFT SUPERIOR VENA CAVA DRAINING INTO THE CORONARY SINUS AND PERSISTENT LEFT SUPERIOR VENA CAVA DRAINING INTO THE LEFT ATRIUM

CT Finding	Partial Anomalous Pulmonary Venous Drainage of the Left Upper Lobe	Persistent Left Superior Vena Cava Draining into the Coronary Sinus (i.e., Duplication of the Superior Vena Cava)	Persistent Left Superior Vena Cava Draining into the Left Atrium
Parahilar intraparenchymal pulmonary veins of the left upper lobe	Enters the vertical vein	Enters the left superior pulmonary vein	Enters the left superior pulmonary vein
Blood flow direction in the vertical vein	Caudocranially	Craniocaudally	Craniocaudally
Left superior pulmonary vein	Small-sized or absent	Normal	Normal
Coronary sinus	Normal	Dilated	Normal
Left innominate vein	Normal or dilated	Normal in 20% of cases; absent or small-sized in 80% of cases	Normal, absent, or small-sized

achieved by inspecting the left hilum, a contrast-enhanced CT may be useful. A left-sided SVC enhances promptly following left arm venous injection, while enhancement of PAVM of the left upper lobe will only occur after enhancement of the pulmonary arteries. The spectrum of abnormalities seen in PAVM is discussed in greater detail in Chapter 7.

Azygos Continuation of the Inferior Vena Cava

Thoracic venous abnormalities may also be seen secondary to interruption of the subhepatic inferior vena cava. In this congenital abnormality, all venous blood flow from the lower body, with the exception of the liver, returns to the right atrium via the azygos and hemiazygos veins (4). These veins are prominent up to the level of the azygos arch. Embryologically, this venous anomaly represents a failure of the union of the hepatic veins and the right subhepatic vein. It has been referred to as "absence of the inferior vena cava" (5) but is more correctly termed "infrahepatic interruption of the inferior vena cava with azygos continuation." This venous anomaly may be suspected on the frontal radiograph when a prominent azygos vein is seen. This anomaly can be mistaken for a mediastinal mass (6,7) on chest radiography, with contrast-enhanced CT providing definitive diagnosis. There is no hemodynamic consequence of this venous anomaly when it is an isolated finding. However, when this anomaly is associated with left atrial isomerism syndromes (polysplenia), it can be associated with a wide range of congenital heart defects (8).

ACQUIRED SUPERIOR VENA CAVA OBSTRUCTION

Superior Vena Cava Syndrome

High-grade stenosis or complete obstruction of the SVC results in the SVC syndrome. Clinical findings of SVC syndrome can be highly variable and are primarily determined by the presence and extent of collateral venous pathways. In its most severe form, SVC syndrome can lead to cerebral or laryngeal edema, which may be life-threatening (9). More commonly, patients with inadequate collateral vessels present with facial, neck, and upper extremity swelling. The onset of SVC syndrome can be acute or chronic. The most common collateral venous channels in SVC obstruction are the azygos–hemiazygos, internal mammary, lateral thoracic, and vertebral systems (10,11) (Figure 10-5). Subcutaneous collateral vessels can be visible over the upper chest. Occasionally, systemic-to-pulmonary venous shunting (12) or filling of lymphatic channels can be seen (Figure 10-6).

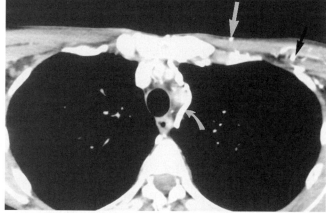

A

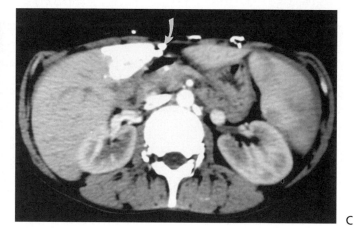

C

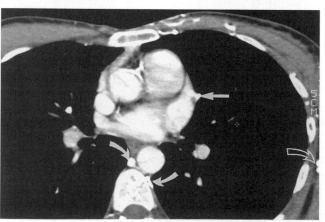

B

FIGURE 10-5. Contrast-enhanced CT scan through the chest and upper abdomen in a patient with obstruction of the left innominate vein following a thymectomy for thymoma. Multiple collateral venous pathways are identified. **A:** Just above the level of the aortic arch, multiple collateral veins are seen over the left anterior chest wall (*straight arrows*). The left upper intercostal vein (*curved arrow*) is also opacified. **B:** The lower superior vena cava fills by collateral channels from the azygos and hemiazygos veins (*curved arrows*), with opacification also noted in the lateral thoracic (*open curved arrow*) and pericardiophrenic vein (*straight arrow*). **C:** At the level of the upper abdomen, there is massive opacification of the left lobe of the liver and filling of paraumbilical veins (*curved arrow*).

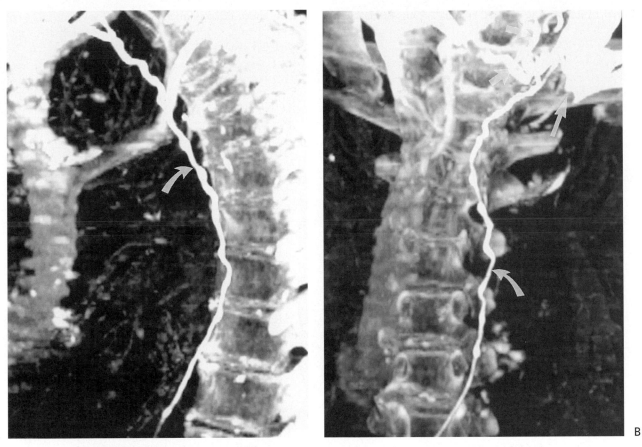

A   B

FIGURE 10-6. A: Sagittal view of a three-dimensional maximum intensity projection of the thorax in a patient with thrombosis of the proximal left innominate vein, showing massive reflux of contrast media into the thoracic duct (*curved arrow*). **B:** Coronal view of the same reconstruction shows obstruction of the left innominate vein (*straight arrow*), filling of multiple collaterals at the base of the neck (*short arrows*), and reflux of contrast down the moderately dilated thoracic duct (*curved arrow*).

Identification of enlarged collateral channels on routine chest or abdominal CT studies should raise the possibility of SVC stenosis or obstruction.

The SVC is easily narrowed or obstructed by neoplastic invasion (Figure 10-7) or compression (Figure 10-8), wall fibrosis or intraluminal thrombus (Figure 10-9) (Box 10-2). Extrinsic masses in the mediastinum can compress the SVC due to its low intraluminal pressure. The low flow velocity in the SVC makes it susceptible to thrombosis in the presence of a hypercoagulable state, which may be isolated or be secondary to a malignancy. Additionally, the SVC is a favored site for the placement of large diameter indwelling chemotherapy or dialysis catheter and pacemaker wires. These devices can incite a fibrotic reaction that can lead to stenosis and obstruction. These devices can also mechanically obstruct flow, which can precipitate thrombosis. In many cases more than one of the above factors may contribute to the SVC obstruction.

In the past the most common etiology for SVC syndrome has been malignancy, with lung cancer and lym-phoma accounting for the vast majority of cases (13). However, recent series have noted an increase in the number of SVC obstructions associated with placement of central venous lines in oncology and dialysis patients (10). Fibrosing mediastinitis can also cause SVC syndrome (10,14,15).

Although venography has previously been the examination of choice for the diagnosis of SVC abnormalities, vessel overlap and failure to visualize slowly flowing collateral veins limit this technique. Additionally, venography only provides information about the patent intraluminal portions of the SVC. In comparison, spiral CT can show the cause of SVC syndrome, the extent of the abnormality and the site and degree of venous obstruction (1,10,11). The size and extent of collateral vessels can also be determined. The addition of volume-rendering techniques to stacks of transverse CT slices provide the same perspective as conventional venography. These volume-rendered images can assist in planning surgical or radiologic endovascular procedures (16).

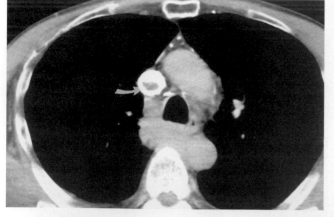

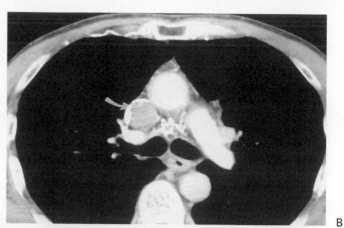

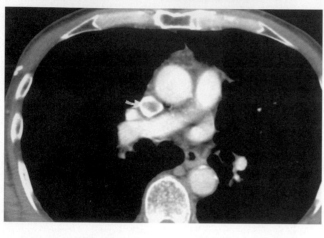

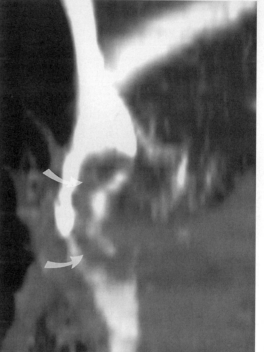

FIGURE 10-7. Contrast-enhanced CT scan through the superior mediastinum showing intracaval extension of a squamous cell carcinoma of the right upper lobe. Tumor thrombus (*curved arrow*), proven by intracaval sampling, is seen within the superior vena cava (SVC) at the level of the aortic arch **(A)**, level of the left pulmonary artery **(B)**, and at the level of the right pulmonary artery **(C)**. A coronal reformat **(D)** shows the ovoid shape of the intraluminal thrombus (*curved arrows*) within the SVC.

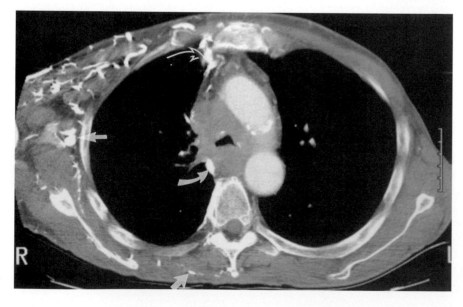

FIGURE 10-8. Contrast-enhanced chest CT scan at the level of the aortic arch showing complete occlusion of the superior vena cava secondary to extensive mediastinal lymphadenopathy in a patient with lung cancer. Extensive collateral vessels are seen in the azygos (*curved arrow*), lateral thoracic (*straight arrow*), internal mammary (*open arrow*), and vertebral regions (*short arrow*).

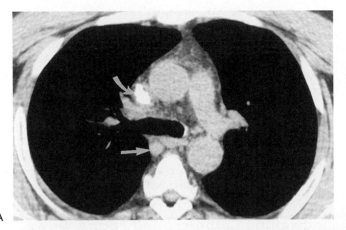
A

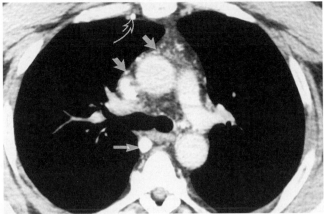
B

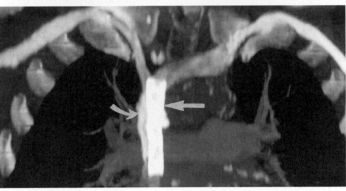
C

FIGURE 10-9. An initial noncontrast chest CT **(A)** through the upper mediastinum in a patient with superior vena cava (SVC) syndrome demonstrates a calcified thrombus within the SVC (*curved arrow*) and associated dilation of the azygos vein (*straight arrow*). **B:** Following contrast injection, the calcified thrombus in the SVC is unchanged, but multiple collateral channels are now outlined including small mediastinal veins (*short arrows*), right internal mammary vein (*open curved arrow*), and azygos vein (*straight arrow*). **C:** A coronal reformat of a contrast-enhanced CT obtained following intracaval stent placement (*straight arrow*) shows the calcified thrombus (*curved arrow*) pushed against the right wall of the SVC.

Neoplastic Superior Vena Cava Obstruction

Most cases (more than 85%) of SVC syndrome are caused by an underlying malignancy, either a primary lung cancer, lymphoma, or metastatic tumor. Either tumor invasion (Figure 10-7) or extrinsic compression (Figure 10-8) of the SVC (17) causes the obstruction. Within the lung cancer category, small cell carcinoma is the most common histologic type (18). Typically, lung cancer obstructs the SVC through compression by enlarged right paratracheal lymph nodes or by direct medi-

astinal invasion of the tumor. In most cases, the SVC is compressed, although frank tumor invasion of the SVC wall can also occur. A narrowed SVC may progress to complete obstruction secondary to intraluminal thrombosis. Spiral CT assists in patient management by demonstrating the location and extent of narrowing or obstruction, the presence of collateral venous channels, and the location of surrounding masses. The two common therapies used in malignant SVC obstruction, radiation therapy (19) and endovascular stenting (1,20), rely on spiral CT diagnostic images for planning. CT-guided fine needle or core biopsy is often performed to establish the histologic diagnosis prior to therapy.

Recent series have indicated that endovascular stent therapy provides more rapid palliation of SVC syndrome symptoms with fewer side effects than the previous standard approach of radiation therapy (1,20). For this reason, many centers now use endovascular therapy as the first-line treatment for malignant SVC syndrome.

BOX 10-2. CAUSES OF ACQUIRED SUPERIOR VENA CAVA OBSTRUCTION

- Extrinsic compression
  Lung cancer
  Lymphoma
  Metastatic disease
  Fibrosing mediastinitis
- Wall scarring
  Indwelling catheter
  Pacing wire
- Thrombosis
  Hypercoagulable state:
    Malignancy-associated
    Nonmalignant

Fibrosing Mediastinitis

Fibrosing mediastinitis is a rare condition characterized by the proliferation of fibrous tissue within the mediastinum (15) (Box 10-3). It is believed to represent a delayed hypersensitivity reaction to fungal, mycobacterial, or other unknown antigens and occurs most commonly as a com-

BOX 10-3. FIBROSING MEDIASTINITIS—ETIOLOGY

- Localized calcified masses
  - Histoplasmosis
  - Tuberculosis
- Diffuse
  - Retroperitoneal fibrosis
  - Orbital pseudotumors
  - Riedel's sclerosing thyroiditis
  - Methysergide therapy
  - Histoplasmosis

plication of histoplasmosis (21) or tuberculosis (22). Usually no active granulomas or infectious agents are found in biopsied tissues. An idiopathic form has been described that may be associated with other conditions including retroperitoneal fibrosis (23), orbital pseudotumors (24), Riedel's sclerosing thyroiditis (24), and methysergide therapy (25). This form may represent an autoimmune process.

Fibrosing mediastinitis occurs in two distinct forms, a localized mass that is often calcified and a diffuse infiltration of the mediastinum. It is has been observed that the localized form is most commonly associated with granulomatous infection, while the diffuse form is more commonly idiopathic. Response to medical therapy with steroids is more likely with the diffuse form than with the focal form (15).

The clinical manifestations of fibrosing mediastinitis can include stenosis of the trachea, main stem bronchi, right pulmonary artery, esophagus, or SVC. A recent series of localized and diffuse fibrosing mediastinitis found that 39% of patients presented with SVC syndrome (15). In all cases, CT

(Figure 10-10) or MRI studies showed SVC narrowing or obstruction, with collateral vessels identified in the majority of cases. In the appropriate clinical context, the presence of a localized mediastinal soft tissue mass with calcification is virtually diagnostic of fibrosing mediastinitis and a biopsy is not required (26). However, if the mass is not calcified or if there is clinical or radiologic evidence of disease progression, biopsy may be required to exclude a neoplasm. If SVC obstruction is unresponsive to steroid therapy and symptoms warrant aggressive management, surgical reconstruction of the SVC using a spiral vein graft technique (27) or intervascular stent therapy (1) should be considered.

Indwelling Catheters and Pacing Wires

SVC stenosis or obstruction can occur secondary to placement of central catheters or pacing wires (Figure 10-11) (1,28,29). The incidence of this complication appears to be increasing (10). This is likely secondary to the greater use of central line placement in oncologic and dialysis patients. It is speculated that these indwelling devices injure the intima and incite a fibrotic reaction. If the devices remain *in situ* for sufficient time, irreversible stenosis or complete obstruction can occur leading to SVC syndrome. Once the fibrotic reaction is established, removal of the device may not restore the vessel caliber. Pacing wires can become incorporated into the fibrotic reaction and may not be removable. Management of these iatrogenic injuries initially consists of removal of the device, if possible. Once removed, surgical reconstruction or endovascular stent placement can be attempted if the symptoms warrant aggressive management.

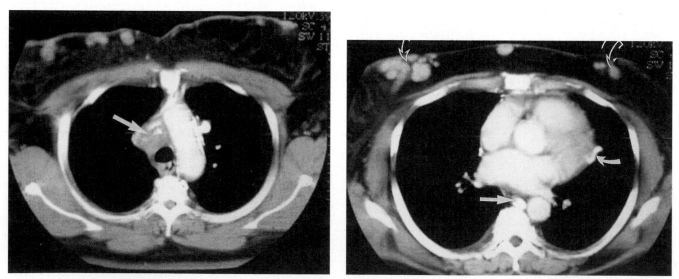

A   B

FIGURE 10-10. A: A contrast-enhanced CT in a patient with histoplasmosis-associated fibrosing mediastinitis shows a complete obstruction of the superior vena cava by a calcified fibrotic mass (*straight arrow*). An enlarged left superior intercostal vein is identified to the left of the aortic arch. **B:** CT scan at a more caudal level shows extensive collateral circulation through the left pericardiophrenic vein (*curved arrow*), azygos vein (*straight arrow*), and chest wall veins (*open curved arrows*). (Case courtesy of Dr. Robert Tarver, Indiana University Medical Center, Indianapolis, IN.)

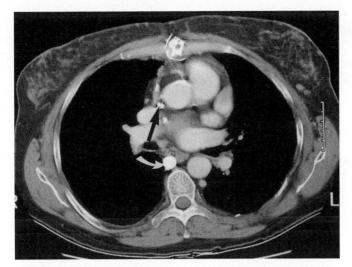

FIGURE 10-11. A 53-year-old woman with a complete obstruction of the superior vena cava secondary to fibrosis around pacemaker wires. A contrast-enhanced CT scan demonstrates two pacing wires within a completely occluded SVC (*straight arrow*). Collateral flow is seen in a dilated azygos vein (*curved arrow*).

However, as collateral venous pathways may develop in time, careful timing of interventions in benign SVC obstruction is essential (1). It is noted that either surgical or endovascular therapy may aggravate the situation by irreversibly damaging collateral venous pathways. Further research into the long-term efficacy of either surgical or endovascular treatment of these benign lesions is required.

REFERENCES

1. Vedantham S. Endovascular strategies for superior vena cava obstruction. *Tech Vasc Intervent Radiol* 2000;3(1):29–39.
2. Luzsa G. Thoracic veins (veins of the greater circulation): system of the superior vena cava and the azygos vein. In: Luzsa G, ed. *X-ray anatomy of the vascular system*. Philadelphia: JB Lippincott Co, 1974:44.
3. Friedrich A, Bing RJ, Blount SG Jr. Physiological studies in congenital heart disease. IX. Circulatory dynamics in the anomalies of venous return to the heart including pulmonary arteriovenous fistula. *Bull Johns Hopkins Hosp* 1950;86:20.
4. Mayo JR, Gray R, St. Louis E, et al. Anomalies of the inferior vena cava. *AJR* 1983;140:339–345.
5. Milledge RD. Absence of the inferior vena cava. *Radiology* 1965; 85:860–865.
6. Castellino RA, Blank N, Adams DF. Dilated azygos and hemiazygos veins presenting as paravertebral intrathoracic masses. *N Engl J Med* 1968;278:1087–1091.
7. Magbitang NH, Hayford FC, Blake JM. Dilated azygos vein simulating mediastinal tumour. Report of a case. *N Engl J Med* 1960;263:598–600.
8. Freedom RM, Yoo S-J, Mawson JB, et al. Azygous continuation of the inferior vena cava: absence of the hepatic segment of the inferior vena cava. In: *Congenital heart disease: textbook of angiocardiography*. Armonk, NY: Futura Publishing Co, 1997: 305.
9. McFadden PM, Jammplis RW. Superior vena cava syndrome. In: Shield TW, ed. *General thoracic surgery*. Philadelphia: Williams & Wilkins, 1994:1716–1723.
10. Cihangiroglu M, Lin BHJ, Dachman AH. Collateral pathways in superior vena caval obstruction as seen on CT. *J Comput Assist Tomogr* 2001;25(1):1–8.
11. Kim H-J, Kim HS, Chung SH. CT diagnosis of superior vena cava syndrome: importance of collateral vessels. *AJR* 1993;161: 539–542.
12. Grayet D, Benoit G, Szapiro D, et al. Systemic-to-pulmonary venous shunt in superior vena cava obstruction revealed on dynamic helical CT. *AJR* 2001;176:211–213.
13. Lochridge SK, Knibbe WP, Doty DB. Obstruction of the superior vena cava. *Surgery* 1979;85:14.
14. Rodríguez E, Soler R, Pombo F, et al. Fibrosing mediastinitis: CT and MR findings. *Clin Radiol* 1998;53:907–910.
15. Sherrick AD, Brown LR, Harms GF, et al. The radiographic findings of fibrosing mediastinitis. *Chest* 1994;106:484–489.
16. Hennequin LM, Fade O, Fays JG, et al. Superior vena cava stent placement: results with the Wallstent endoprosthesis. *Radiology* 1995;196:353–361.
17. Escalante CP. Causes and management of superior vena cava syndrome. *Oncology* 1993;7:61–68.
18. Chan RH, Dar AR, Yu E, et al. Superior vena cava obstruction in small-cell lung cancer. *Int J Radiat Oncol* 1997;38:513.
19. Armstrong B, Perez C, Simpson J, et al. Role of irradiation in the management of superior vena cava syndrome. *Intern J Radiat Oncol Biol Physics* 1987;13:531–539.
20. Nicholson AA, Ettles DF, Arnold A, et al. Treatment of malignant superior vena cava obstruction: metal stents or radiation therapy. *J Vasc Intervent Radiol* 1997;8:781–788.
21. Rubin SA, Winer-Muram H. Thoracic histoplasmosis. *J Thorac Imag* 1992;7:39.
22. Mole TM, Glover J, Sheppard MN. Sclerosing mediastinitis: a report of 18 cases. *Thorax* 1995;50:280–283.
23. Kittredge RD, Nash AD. The many facets of sclerosing fibrosis. *AJR* 1974;122:288–298.
24. Comings DE, Skubi KB, Van Eyes J, Motulsky AG. Familial multifocal fibrosclerosis findings suggesting that retroperitoneal fibrosis, mediastinal fibrosis, sclerosing cholangitis, Riedel's thyroiditis, and pseudotumor of the orbit may be different manifestations of a single disease. *Ann Intern Med* 1967;66:884–892.
25. Graham JR. Fibrotic disorders associated with methysergide therapy for headache. *N Engl J Med* 1966;274:359–368.
26. Weinstein JB, Aronberg DJ, Sagel SS. CT of fibrosing mediastinitis: findings and their utility. *AJR* 1983;141:247–251.
27. Doty JR, Flores JH, Doty DB. Superior vena cava obstruction: bypass using spiral vein graft. *Ann Thorac Surg* 1999;67: 1111–1116.
28. Rosenthal E, Qureshi SA, Tynan M, et al. Percutaneous pacemaker lead extraction and stent implantation for superior vena cava occlusion due to pacemaker leads. *Am J Cardiol* 1996;77: 670–672.
29. Francis CM, Starkey IR, Errington ML, et al. Venous stenting as treatment for pacemaker-induced superior vena cava syndrome. *Am Heart J* 1995;129:836–837.

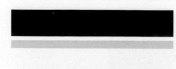

APPENDIX

PROTOCOLS FOR CT ANGIOGRAPHY

APPENDIX 3: THORACIC AORTA

1. **Recommended protocol for routine assessment of thoracic aorta**
   - Patient position:
     - head midline
     - deep inspiration
   - Acquisition parameters:
     - region of interest: sternal notch to diaphragm
     - collimation 7 mm, pitch 1.5 on SSCT
     - collimation 5 mm, pitch 1.5 on MSCT
     - acquisition direction: craniocaudal
     - scan delay 20 seconds or, preferably, timed bolus
   - Reconstruction parameters:
     - contiguous transverse sections
     - MPRs and three-dimensional reconstructions
2. **Recommended protocol for assessment of aortic trauma**
   - Patient position:
     - head midline
     - deep inspiration
   - Acquisition parameters:
     - sternal notch to tracheal carina:
       - 3-mm collimation, pitch 1.5, overlapping reconstructions at 1.5-mm intervals on SSCT
       - 1.25- to 2-mm collimation, pitch 1.5 on MSCT
     - carina to diaphragm
       - 7-mm collimation on SSCT
       - 5-mm collimation on MSCT
     - acquisition direction: craniocaudal
     - scan delay 20 seconds or, preferably, timed bolus
   - Reconstruction parameters:
     - contiguous transverse sections
     - MPRs and three-dimensional reconstructions

APPENDIX 4: ACUTE PULMONARY EMBOLISM

1. **Recommended protocol for detection of acute pulmonary embolism using single-slice CT**
   - Patient position:
     - head medially located
       - deep inspiration
   - Acquisition parameters:
     - collimation: 2 mm (alternative: 3 mm)
     - pitch: 1.7 to 2.0
     - x-ray tube:
       - 120 kV
       - 100 mAs per slice
     - acquisition direction: craniocaudal (alternative: caudocranial)
     - region-of-interest:
       - 10 to 12 cm
       - from the level of the aortic arch to 2 cm below the inferior pulmonary veins
   - Injection parameters:
     a. according to the injection site:
       - via an antecubital vein
         - contrast concentration: 240 mg iodine per mL
         - contrast volume: 120 to 140 mL
         - contrast flow rate: 4 mL per second
       - via a peripheral venous access:
         - contrast concentration: 300 mg iodine per mL
         - contrast volume: 120 to 140 mL
         - contrast flow rate: 2 to 3 mL per second
     b. choice of the start delay:
       - patient with a normal hemodynamic status: 12 to 15 seconds
       - patient with patent or suspected pulmonary hypertension and/or right heart failure:
         - 18 to 20 seconds
         - alternative: automatic triggering of data acquisition
   - Reconstruction parameters:
     - contiguous transverse CT scans
     - optional:
       - overlapping CT scans (to exclude pseudo-filling defects due to partial volume effects)
       - two-dimensional reformations (to differentiate hilar lymph nodes from mural defects)
2. **Recommended protocol for detection of acute pulmonary embolism using multislice CT**
   - Patient position: similar
   - Scanning protocols:

a. Apnea possible:
- survey of the entire thorax with simultaneous administration of contrast material with:
  - collimation: 4 × 1 mm; pitch: 2.0 (maximum breath-hold: 20 seconds)
  - x-ray tube:
    - 120 kV
    - 100 mAs per slice
  - acquisition direction: craniocaudal (or caudocranial)
- same injection protocols as with single-slice CT, except:
  - a reduced volume of contrast material administered: 80 to 100 mL
  - the start delay: 18 seconds

b. Apnea impossible:
- noncontrast spiral CT examination of the entire thorax with:
  - collimation: 4 × 2.5 mm; pitch: 2.0 (data acquisition: around 8 seconds)
  - x-ray tube:
    - 120 kV
    - 80 mAs per slice
  - acquisition direction: craniocaudal (or caudocranial)
- CT angiography of the pulmonary vasculature:
  - region-of-interest:
    - 10 to 12 cm
    - from the level of the aortic arch to 2 cm below the inferior pulmonary veins
  - collimation: 4 × 1 mm; pitch: 2.0 (data acquisition: 10 seconds maximum)
  - x-ray tube:
    - 120 kV
    - 100 mAs per slice
  - acquisition direction: craniocaudal (or caudocranial)
  - same injection protocols as with single-slice CT, except a reduced volume of contrast material administered: 80 to 100 mL
- Reconstruction parameters:
  - contiguous transverse CT scans (1-mm thick reconstructed scans)

APPENDIX 5: PULMONARY HYPERTENSION

Summary of the reconstruction protocols useful for spiral CT imaging of chronic thromboembolism
- Transverse CT scans:
  - systematically generated
  - contiguous thin-collimated scans
  - recommended collimation: 1 mm
- Multiplanar reformations:
  - recommended for an adequate evaluation of the arterial lumen without volume averaging

- obtained along the long axis of questionable arterial branches
- objectives:
  - depiction of vascular signs of chronic pulmonary embolism
    - residual mural thrombi
    - mild arterial stenosis
    - mild poststenotic dilation
  - surgical accessibility of chronic thrombi
    - removal if proximal location extends to the main, lobar, and segmental arteries
    - determination of thrombi extension on angiogramlike views
- Maximum intensity projections (MIPs):
  - recommended for an adequate depiction of calcifications on proximal pulmonary arteries on enhanced CT scans
  - alternative: viewing of transverse CT scans with large window settings
- Sliding thin slab-MIP:
  - recommended for an adequate depiction of calcified thrombi within peripheral pulmonary arteries (beyond fifth-order branches)
  - MIP algorithm applied on 3-mm to 5-mm thick slabs

APPENDIX 7: VASCULAR ANOMALIES OF THE LUNG

Pretherapeutic Evaluation of Pulmonary Arteriovenous Malformations (PAVMs)
1. Screening examination
- Patient position:
  - head medially located
  - deep inspiration
- Acquisition parameters:
  - collimation: 4 × 2.5 mm (MSCT); 5 mm (SSCT)
  - pitch: 2.0 (MSCT; SSCT)
  - x-ray tube:
    - 120 kV
    - low milliamperage (10 to 20 mAs per slice)
  - recommended use of automatic dose reduction device (if available)
  - acquisition direction: craniocaudal (caudocranial)
  - region-of-interest: entire thorax
- Noncontrast CT examination
- Reconstruction parameters:
  - transverse CT scans: contiguous 5-mm thick scans
2. Suspicion of small-sized PAVMs
- Patient position:
  - head medially located
  - deep inspiration
- Acquisition parameters:
  - collimation: 4 × 1 mm (MSCT); 2 mm (SSCT)

- pitch: 2.0 (MSCT; SSCT)
- x-ray tube:
  - 120 kV
  - low milliamperage (10 to 20 mAs per slice)
  - recommended use of automatic dose reduction device (if available)
- acquisition direction: craniocaudal (caudocranial)
- focal region-of-interest; must include the vessels connected to the aneurysmal sac
- Noncontrast CT examination:
- Reconstruction parameters:
  - transverse CT scans:
    - contiguous 1-mm thick scans (MSCT)
    - contiguous 2-mm thick scans (SSCT)
  - slabs of 3 to 5 mm on which is applied the maximum intensity projection (MIP) algorithm (sliding thin slab-MIP technique)
3. Determination of PAVM angioarchitecture
- Patient position:
  - head medially located
  - deep inspiration
- Acquisition parameters:
  - collimation: 4 × 1 mm (MSCT); 2 mm (SSCT)
  - pitch: 2.0 (MSCT; SSCT)
  - x-ray tube:
    - 120 kV
    - 100 mAs per slice
    - recommended use of automatic dose reduction device (if available)
  - acquisition direction: craniocaudal
  - focal region-of-interest
- Injection parameters:
  - injection site: antecubital vein
  - contrast concentration: 240 mg iodine per mL
  - contrast volume: 120 mL
  - contrast flow rate: 4 mL per second
  - scan delay: 15 seconds
- Reconstruction parameters:
  - contiguous transverse CT scans
  - three-dimensional (3D) reconstructions:
    - three-dimensional shaded-surface display (SSD): 3DSSD:
    - VRT

APPENDIX 8: HEMOPTYSIS

1. Detection of bronchial arteries
- Patient position:
  - head medially located
  - deep inspiration
- Acquisition parameters:
  - collimation: 4 × 1 mm (MSCT); 2 mm (SSCT)
  - pitch: 2.0 (MSCT; SSCT)

- x-ray tube:
  - 120 kV
  - 100 mAs per slice
- acquisition direction: caudocranial
- region-of-interest
  - must cover the sites of origin of bronchial arteries (from proximal descending aorta to great vessels)
  - must detect the anterior spinal artery (including the cervical region)
- Injection parameters:
  - injection site: antecubital vein
  - contrast concentration: 300 mg iodine per mL
  - contrast volume: 140 mL
  - contrast flow rate: 4 mL per second
  - scan delay: 18 seconds
- Reconstruction parameters:
  - contiguous transverse CT scans
  - curved reformations
  - three-dimensional reconstructions (three-dimensional shaded-surface display, VRT, and/or maximum intensity projection)
2. Detection of pulmonary artery pseudoaneurysms
a. depiction of large-sized lesions: compare with evaluation of acute pulmonary embolism
b. depiction of small-sized lesions:
- Patient position:
  - head medially located
  - deep inspiration
- Acquisition parameters:
  - collimation: 4 × 1 mm (MSCT); 2 mm (SSCT)
  - pitch: 2.0 (MSCT; SSCT)
  - x-ray tube:
    - 120 kV
    - 100 mAs per slice
  - acquisition direction: caudocranial
  - region-of-interest: area of destructive process of the lung parenchyma
- Injection parameters:
  - injection site: antecubital vein
  - contrast concentration: 300 mg iodine per mL
  - contrast volume: 100 mL (MSCT); 120 mL (SSCT)
  - contrast flow rate: 4 mL per second
  - scan delay: 15 seconds
- Reconstruction parameters:
  - contiguous transverse CT scans
  - curved reformations (depends on the location of the pseudoaneurysm)

APPENDIX 9: THORACIC OUTLET DISORDERS

1. **CT venography (thoracic outlet venous disorders)**
- Patient position:
  - neutral position:

- both arms alongside the body
- head medially located
- retropulsion of the shoulders
- deep inspiration
- postural maneuver:
  - 130 degrees of hyperabduction of both arms
  - same other positional characteristics as those described for the neutral position
- Acquisition parameters:
  - similar for the acquisitions in the neutral position and after postural maneuver
  - collimation: 4 × 1 mm (MSCT); 3 mm (SSCT)
  - pitch: 2.0 (MSCT); 1.0 (SSCT)
  - x-ray tube:
    - 140 kV;140 mAs per slice
    - recommended use of automatic dose reduction device (if available)
  - acquisition direction: craniocaudal
  - region-of-interest: C7, inner extremity of the first rib
- Injection parameters:
  - injection site:
    - basilic vein
    - use of a tourniquet during data acquisition
  - contrast concentration: 60 mg iodine per mL
  - contrast volume: 80 mL
  - contrast flow rate: 4 mL per second
  - scan delay: 10 to 12 sesonds
- Reconstruction parameters:
  - transverse CT scans:
    - contiguous with MSCT
    - overlapped images with SSCT
  - two-dimensional images:
    - contiguous sagittal reformations on both sides
    - curved reformations along the main axis of the axillary, subclavian, and innominate veins on both sides
  - three-dimensional reconstructions
    - three-dimensional surface-shaded display (3DSSD): simple thresholding classification (150 HU)
    - VR images:
      - trapezoid for the display of bony structures:
        - width: 1,250 to 1,400 HU
        - center: 555 to 615 HU
        - opacity: 10%
      - trapezoid for the display of venous structures:
        - width: 555 to 615 HU
        - center: 125 to 135 HU
        - opacity:9 0%

2. CT angiography of thoracic outlet arteries (thoracic outlet arterial disorders)
- Patient position:
  - neutral position:
    - both arms alongside the body
    - head medially located

- retropulsion of the shoulders
- deep inspiration
- postural maneuver:
  - 130 degrees of hyperabduction of the symptomatic arm; contralateral arm alongside the body
  - retropulsion of the shoulders
  - deep inspiration
  - ipsilateral rotation of the head
- Acquisition parameters:
  - similar for the acquisitions in the neutral position and after postural maneuver
  - collimation: 4 × 1 mm (MSCT); 3 mm (SSCT)
  - pitch: 2.0 (MSCT; SSCT)
  - x-ray tube:
    - 140 kV;140 mAs per slice
    - recommended use of automatic dose reduction device (if available)
  - acquisition direction: craniocaudal
  - region-of-interest: C7, inner extremity of the first rib
- Injection parameters:
  - injection site:
    - antecubital vein
    - contralateral to the side to be analyzed
  - contrast concentration: 300 mg iodine per mL
  - contrast volume: 70 mL (MSCT); 90 mL (SSCT)
  - contrast flow rate: 4 mL per second
  - scan delay: 17 second
- Reconstruction parameters:
  - transverse CT scans:
    - contiguous with MSCT
    - overlapped images with SSCT
  - two-dimensional images:
    - contiguous sagittal reformations of the symptomatic arm
    - curved reformation along the main axis of the axillary and subclavian artery of the symptomatic arm
  - three-dimensional reconstructions:
    - three-dimensional surface-shaded displays: simple thresholding classification (150 HU)
    - VR images:
      - trapezoid for the display of bony structures:
        - width: 1,250 to 1,400 HU
        - center: 555 to 615 HU
        - opacity: 10%
      - trapezoid for the display of arterial structures:
        - width: 555 to 615 HU
        - center: 125 to 135 HU
        - opacity: 90%

APPENDIX 10: SUPERIOR VENA CAVA SYNDROMES

- Patient position:
  - both arms alongside the body

- head medially located
- deep inspiration
- Acquisition parameters:
  - collimation: 4 × 2.5 mm (MSCT); 2 to 3 mm (SSCT)
  - pitch: 2.0 (MSCT); 1.7 to 2.0 (SSCT)
  - x-ray tube: 140 kV and 80 mAs (MSCT); 140 kV and 140 mAs per slice (SSCT)
  - acquisition direction: craniocaudal
  - region-of-interest: subclavicular region—right atrium
- Injection parameters:
  - injection site: antecubital vein
  - contrast concentration: 60 mg iodine per mL
  - contrast volume: 90 mL
  - contrast flow rate: 4 mL per second
  - scan delay: 10 seconds (15 seconds if SVC obstruction is clinically patent)
- Reconstruction parameters:
  - transverse CT scans: overlapped images with MSCT and SSCT

- two-dimensional (2D) images:
  - contiguous sagittal reformations on both sides
  - optional: curved reformations along the main axis of the subclavian and innominate veins on both sides and/or along the main axis of the SVC
- three-dimensional reconstructions
  - three-dimensional surface-shaded display (3DSSD): simple thresholding classification (150 HU)
  - optional:
    - maximum intensity projection
    - VR images:
      - trapezoid for the display of bony structures:
        - width: 1,250 to 1,400 HU
        - center: 550 to 610 HU
        - opacity: 10%
      - trapezoid for the display of venous structures:
        - width: 550 to 610 HU
        - center: 125 to 135 HU
        - opacity: 90%

SUBJECT INDEX

Note: page numbers with *b* indicate a box, with *f,* a figure, and with *t,* a table.